THE COMPLETE FAMILY GUIDE
TO HEALTHY LIVING

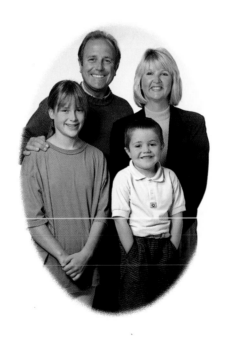

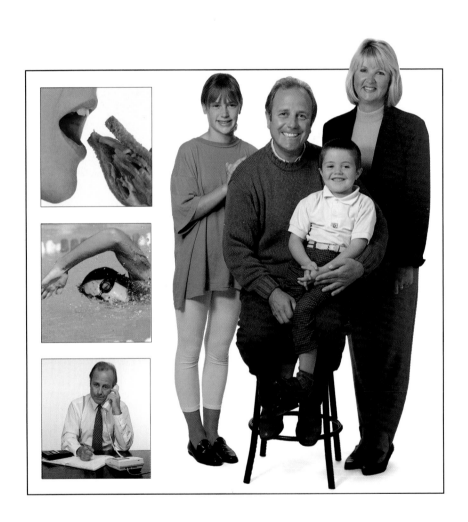

THE COMPLETE FAMILY GUIDE TO HEALTHY LIVING

Dr. Stephen Carroll

Dr. Tony Smith MEDICAL EDITOR

DK PUBLISHING, INC

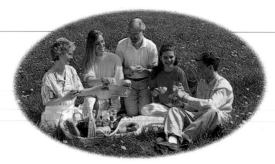

The Complete Family Guide to Healthy Living
has been conceived, edited, and designed by
DK Direct Limited

A DK PUBLISHING INC BOOK

First American Edition, 1995
4 6 8 10 9 7 5

Published in the United States
by Dorling Kindersley Publishing Inc.,
95 Madison Avenue, New York, NY 10016

Visit us on the World Wide Web at
http://www.dk.com

MEDICAL EDITOR Dr. Tony Smith
MEDICAL CONSULTANT Dr. Patricia Last

PROJECT EDITORS Ellen Dupont, Sarah Miller
U.S. EDITORS Julee Binder, Mary Sutherland
SENIOR ART EDITOR Simon Webb
ART EDITOR Andrew Walker
DESIGNER Tuong Nguyen
PICTURE RESEARCHER Julia Tacey
PRODUCTION MANAGER Ian Paton

PUBLISHER Jonathan Reed
DESIGN DIRECTOR Ed Day

CIP data is available
ISBN 0-7894-0114-2

Color reproduction by Colourscan, Singapore
Printed and bound by R.R. Donnelley & Sons Company, United States

FOREWORD

PEOPLE ARE LIVING LONGER than ever before. Many, however, are not in perfect health – they are overweight, smoke tobacco, drink too much alcohol, and do not exercise sufficiently. In addition to these self-inflicted health risks, living in a modern congested and competitive society can cause high levels of stress and expose people to all sorts of other hazards, from road accidents to industrial smog, from infectious diseases to food poisoning.

In recent years doctors have greatly increased their understanding of how the human body is actually affected by these various factors and have devised screening tests that can reveal early warning signs of illness. With the benefit of this knowledge, doctors can do far more than just treat the sick – they can explain how harmful smoking or being overweight can be and advise people on how they can change their way of life to improve their long-term health and increase their life expectancy.

Using the most up-to-date medical information, this book will provide the whole family with all the facts they need to adopt a lifestyle that will not only make them healthier, but will also help them to look and feel better.

DR. TONY SMITH   DR. PATRICIA LAST

CONTENTS

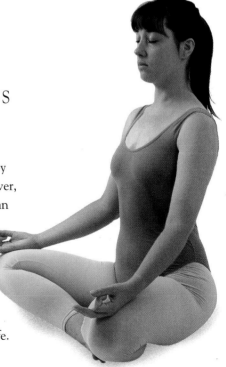

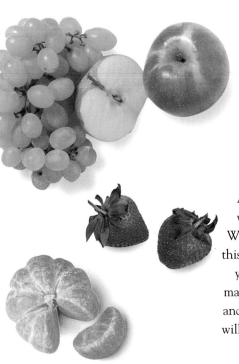

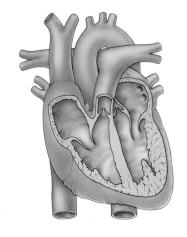

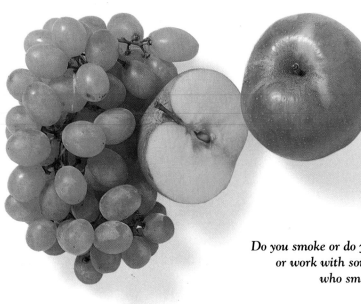

Is the food you eat helping or harming your health?

Do you smoke or do you live or work with someone who smokes?

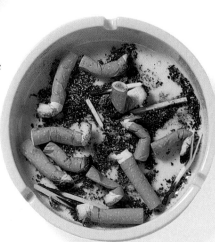

Do you make time every day to sit down and relax?

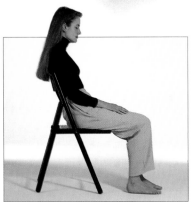

Do you weigh the right amount for your sex, age, and height?

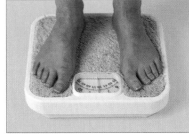

When you exercise, do you wear the recommended clothing and use the proper safety equipment?

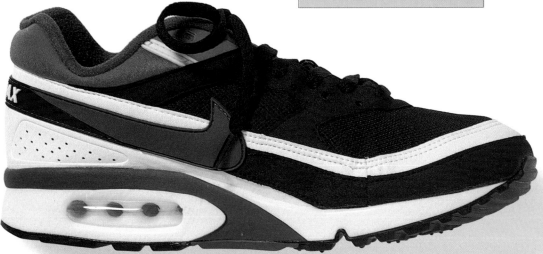

CHAPTER ONE

Have all your family been given all the recommended vaccinations?

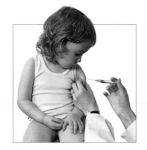

HOW HEALTHY ARE YOU?

If you experience some unusual symptoms, such as feeling dizzy and tired, do you always go to ask your doctor's advice?

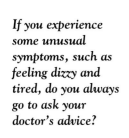

MOST PEOPLE DO NOT really know if they are healthy or not. By answering the questions in this chapter, you will be able to assess whether the foods you eat, the exercise you get, the stresses you are under, how you relate to those around you, and the way you use the health-care system are keeping you in good health or paving the way for problems in the future.

Maintaining health is not only about eating well and staying fit. It also means getting the right medical care. You need to know when to visit your doctor, what symptoms to report, and what questions to ask. You should also be well-informed about self-examination and how it can help you recognize the early warning signs of disease. Do you know what screening tests you should have and how often you should have them? By taking a few sensible precautions now, you may be able to avoid many future illnesses. Immunization, accident prevention, safe sex, drinking alcohol only in moderation, and not smoking are all part of maintaining good health. Taking the steps outlined in this chapter will help you gain control of your life and make the right choices for your physical health and emotional wellbeing.

GOOD HEALTH: CHOICE OR CHANCE?

MANY DIFFERENT FACTORS determine how healthy you will be. Some, such as the genes you inherit from your parents, are a matter of chance. But there are many choices you can make that will help determine whether you enjoy good health or bad.

The two main choices you can make are to adopt a healthy lifestyle and to learn how to recognize the possible early warning symptoms of illness. If you do, you will reduce your chances of dying at an early age from heart disease and improve the quality of your life in later years by staying healthier longer.

The decisions you make about how much exercise you get, what foods you eat, which habits such as smoking and drinking you acquire, what risks you take in your sex life, and how much effort you put into avoiding accidents at work, at home, on the road, or during your leisure time, can all directly benefit or harm your health and wellbeing.

To help determine whether you are making the right choices and to enable you to identify those areas of your lifestyle which may be endangering your health, try answering the following questions.

CHOICE

1 *Do you eat mostly fresh or mostly convenience foods?*

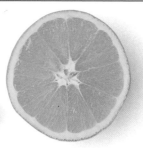

A varied diet of fresh foods, including plenty of fruit and vegetables, is better for your health. A diet consisting predominantly of convenience foods is likely to be low in fiber and high in fats and added sugars.

2 *How often do you exercise strenuously?*

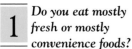

Getting any form of vigorous exercise for at least 20 minutes, three times a week, improves your overall fitness. It also decreases stress and reduces your risk of becoming ill.

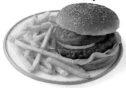

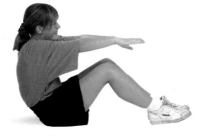

3 *Do you smoke?*

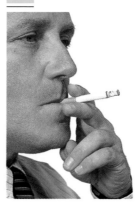

Smoking is a major risk factor for bronchitis and lung cancer as well as for other diseases including coronary heart disease, peptic ulcers, and premature aging of the skin. If you smoke, you should stop for the sake of your health.

4 *Do you keep your alcohol intake within the recommended limits?*

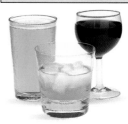

In the long term, drinking too much can harm your health and your emotional wellbeing. Because alcohol effects your judgment, it is a major cause of accidents.

5 *Do you weigh far too much?*

Being obese greatly increases your risk of developing heart disease, stroke, arthritis, diabetes, and other diseases.

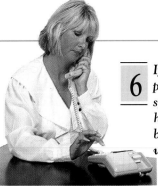

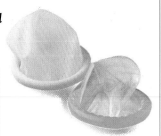

6 *If you developed any persistent distressing symptoms, such as headaches or breathlessness, would you make an appointment to see your doctor?*

Persistent or recurrent symptoms could signify a disease for which prompt treatment may be more effective. See your doctor now.

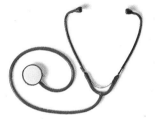

7 *Have you had all the health checks and screening tests you should have?*

Early detection of disease improves your chances of achieving a successful cure.

8 *Are you protected against high-risk sexual activities?*

Practice safe sex by using condoms during sexual intercourse if you are not involved in a mutually monogamous relationship.

9 *Have you received all the recommended immunizations?*

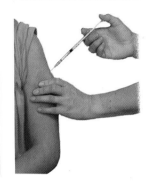

Without immunization you are at risk of a variety of serious, and potentially fatal, infectious diseases. Ask your doctor if you need to be vaccinated.

CHANCE

1 *Did your parents and grandparents live to a very old age?*

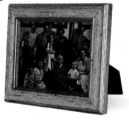

Life expectancy is largely determined by genetic inheritance but an unhealthy lifestyle can work against this genetic advantage by introducing behavior-related diseases.

2 *Are you between 15 and 24?*

Accident rates are highest among people in this age group, but everyone should learn to prevent accidents.

3 *Do you live in a polluted environment?*

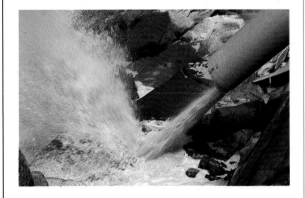

Although you can improve your local environment by recycling or switching to lead-free petrol, global pollution of the air, water, or food supply represent potential causes of ill-health beyond your control.

HOW HEALTHY IS YOUR LIFESTYLE?

CHANGING TO A HEALTHIER lifestyle will improve your chances of living longer and enhance your quality of life. To find out exactly how healthy your current lifestyle is, answer the following questions. They relate to key lifestyle choices about diet, exercise, alcohol, smoking, and stress.

Identify those aspects of your life that you want to change, then set yourself realistic targets to help boost your future health and wellbeing. To help you achieve your personal targets, turn to the pages listed where more detailed information and advice on that particular issue is provided.

ARE YOU EATING A HEALTHY DIET?

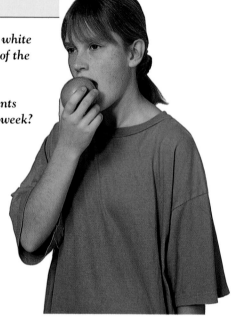

- *Do you eat a lot of processed, convenience foods?*

- *Do you treat yourself to sweet snacks such as chocolate or cookies?*

- *Do you skip meals?*

- *Do you eat late-night snacks ?*

- *Do you go on diets, then gain the weight back in a few weeks?*

- *Do you usually choose white bread and pasta instead of the whole wheat varieties?*

- *Do you eat in restaurants more than three times a week?*

- *Do you need to take nutrient supplements?*

- *Do you often eat on the run?*

If you answered YES to most of these questions, you are eating badly and need to learn more about nutrition so that you can change your diet to a healthier, and probably tastier one (see p22-83).

DO YOU EXERCISE ENOUGH?

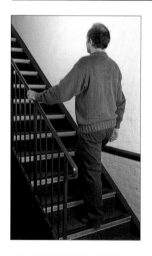

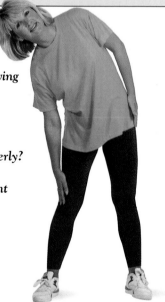

- **Can you climb three flights of stairs without becoming breathless and exhausted?**

- **Do you sometimes walk or cycle instead of driving or taking the bus or train?**

- **Do you exercise three times a week?**

- **When exercising do you always warm up properly?**

- **Do you wear all the necessary safety equipment when exercising or playing a sport?**

If you answered NO to the first three questions, you are out of shape. To keep fit, you should exercise vigorously for 20 minutes, three times a week. It is easy to start (see p146-155). Answering NO to the last two questions means you are not exercising safely and could injure yourself. Learn to exercise safely (see p156-163).

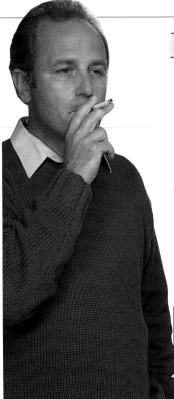

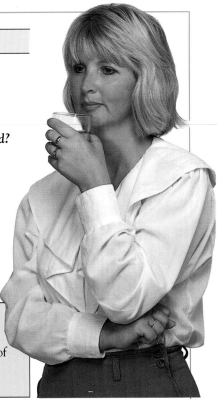

ARE YOU ABUSING YOUR BODY?

- *Do you smoke cigarettes?*

- *Do you smoke cigars or a pipe?*

- *Have you tried to stop smoking and failed?*

- *Do you regularly drink more than the recommended limits for alcohol intake?*

- *Do you drink when you are alone?*

- *Do you have trouble remembering what happened the night before when you have been out drinking?*

If you answered YES to the first two questions you should stop smoking (see p106-107). If you answered YES to any of the last three questions, you need to cut down on your drinking (see p100-103).

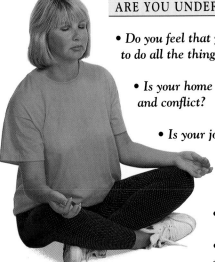

ARE YOU UNDER STRESS?

- *Do you feel that you never have enough time to do all the things you have to do?*

- *Is your home life a source of stress and conflict?*

- *Is your job highly stressful?*

- *Do you worry all the time?*

- *Do you find it hard to relax?*

- *Do you have trouble falling asleep at night?*

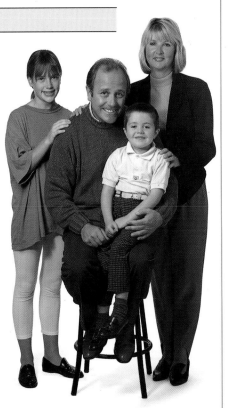

If you answered YES to any of these questions, you may not be dealing with stress very well. Find out how to cope with stress better (see p180-195), see if you have any of the early signs of too much stress (see p176-177), discover how stress can make you ill (see p178-179), and learn what to do if stress is making you anxious or depressed (see p196-201).

IS YOUR HEART AT RISK?

No ONE IS ABLE to foretell who will develop heart disease in later life. What is known, however, is that heart disease is more likely to strike when certain factors are present than when they are not.

Some coronary risk factors – such as your age, sex, and family history – cannot be changed. Death from heart disease is much more common in men than women before the age of 60. After menopause, the risk to women goes up rapidly as the protective effect of estrogen is lost. But although the risk for women is not as great until later in life, even young women should protect their hearts.

To see which of the areas under your control may be putting your heart at risk, answer the questions below. Then you can start taking action to reduce your risk of heart disease.

DOES YOUR MEDICAL HISTORY PUT YOU AT RISK OF HEART DISEASE?

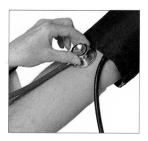

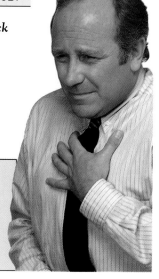

- *Have any of your close relatives had a heart attack or stroke before the age of 50?*

- *Do you have diabetes?*

- *Do you have a history of high blood pressure?*

- *Were your parents overweight?*

If you answered YES to any of these questions, you may have a greater risk of developing coronary heart disease. Having a family history of heart disease means it is even more important to have regular checks on your cholesterol level and blood pressure, and to keep your weight and alcohol intake under control. If you have diabetes or a raised blood pressure, you can reduce your risk of heart disease by following the treatment recommended by your doctor.

DOES YOUR PERSONALITY PUT YOU AT RISK OF HEART DISEASE?

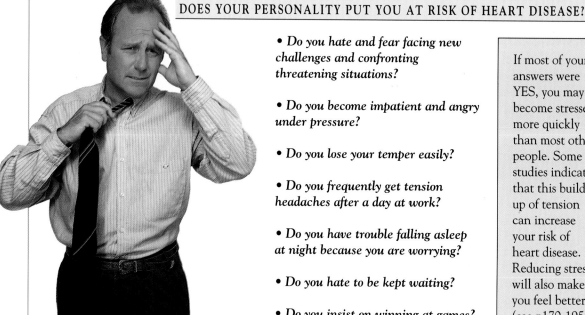

- *Do you hate and fear facing new challenges and confronting threatening situations?*

- *Do you become impatient and angry under pressure?*

- *Do you lose your temper easily?*

- *Do you frequently get tension headaches after a day at work?*

- *Do you have trouble falling asleep at night because you are worrying?*

- *Do you hate to be kept waiting?*

- *Do you insist on winning at games?*

If most of your answers were YES, you may become stressed more quickly than most other people. Some studies indicate that this build-up of tension can increase your risk of heart disease. Reducing stress will also make you feel better (see p170-195).

ARE YOU MAKING THE RIGHT CHOICES FOR YOUR HEART?

• *Is exercise an important part of the way you spend your leisure time?*

• *Do you get vigorous aerobic exercise three times a week for at least twenty minutes?*

• *Do you smoke more than ten cigarettes a day?*

• *Have you smoked in the last five years?*

• *Do you sometimes eat fish rather than red meat?*

• *Do you steer clear of fatty foods?*

• *Does your diet include plenty of fiber-rich foods such as fruit and whole grains?*

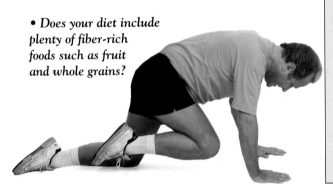

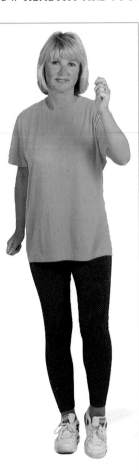

If you answered NO to the exercise questions, you are putting your heart at risk. Exercise prevents the build-up of cholesterol in the bloodstream, so reducing the risk of heart disease. Make exercise a part of your life (see p146-155).

If you smoke, try to give up smoking for good (see p106).

If you answered NO to the last three questions, learn how to change to a healthier diet (see p42-53).

ARE YOU MONITORING YOUR HEART'S HEALTH?

• *Do you know your resting blood pressure?*

• *Is your blood pressure within normal limits (140/90 or lower)?*

• *If you have high blood pressure, is it being treated?*

• *Have you had your blood cholesterol level measured?*

• *Is your blood cholesterol level within normal limits?*

• *If you are over 50, have you talked to your doctor about whether or not you are at risk of heart disease?*

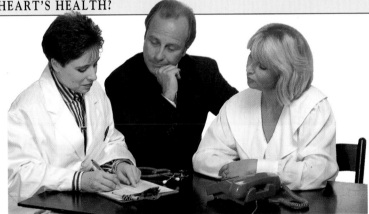

If you answered NO to any of these questions, you may not be taking the best care of your heart. Learn more about all the tests that are available and whether or not you need them (see p262-265). Talking to your doctor about the steps you can take to prevent heart disease is an important part of a routine physical.

YOUR PHYSICAL WELLBEING

PHYSICAL WELLBEING IS not just a matter of leading a healthy lifestyle by eating well and exercising enough. You must also be sure to get the right medical care. Are you well-informed about health care screening and self-examination? Do you know how to take medications sensibly and how to get the most from your doctor?

To find out more about these essential components of your health care, try answering the following questions. Once you have identified those areas that might benefit from extra care and attention, turn to the pages listed. There you will learn more about the subject and find useful information that will enhance your medical knowledge.

DO YOU PROTECT YOUR BODY?

- *Do you brush and floss your teeth daily?*

- *Do you visit the dentist at least once a year?*

- *Do you use sunscreen when you are out in the sun?*

- *Do you replace your exercise shoes when they get worn?*

- *Do you wear proper safety equipment when exercising?*

Answering NO may mean that you are not taking good care of your body. Learn how to prevent tooth decay (see p260), protect your skin (see p288), and avoid injuries (see p160-163).

DO YOU EXAMINE YOURSELF REGULARLY?

- *Do you know how to examine your skin for the early warning signs of skin cancer?*

- *Do you know the early signs of mouth cancer?*

- *For women: do you examine your breasts carefully once a month?*

- *For men: do you examine your testicles once a month?*

If you do not know how to examine yourself, learn how: testicles (see p226), skin (see p270), mouth (see p272), and breasts (see p274).

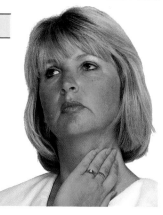

ARE YOU GETTING THE BEST FROM HEALTH SCREENING?

- *Do you know if you should have your blood cholesterol level checked?*

- *Have you had your vision tested recently?*

- *For women under 65: have you had a cervical smear in the past three years?*

- *Do you know what a mammogram is and when and how often you should have one?*

Answering NO to these questions means that you may not be taking care of your health. Ask your doctor for a routine physical (see p250).

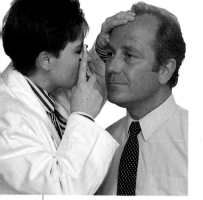

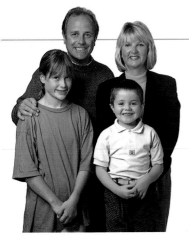

DO YOU KNOW YOUR FAMILY MEDICAL HISTORY?

• *Do you have a close relative with any of the following conditions?*

Heart attack or angina before the age of 50, high blood pressure needing treatment, raised blood cholesterol, diabetes, breast cancer, bowel cancer, or glaucoma.

• *Have any relatives in your or your partner's family suffered or died from a genetic disorder?*

Knowing your family's medical history lets you find out if there is a risk of you passing on a disorder to your children (see p280).

ARE YOUR IMMUNIZATIONS UP TO DATE?

• *Are all your children up to date with their immunization programs?*

• *If you are planning to become pregnant, have you been tested to confirm that you are immune to rubella?*

• *Do you check to see if you need an immunization before traveling to a foreign country?*

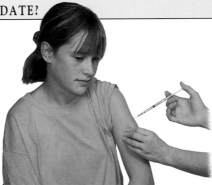

If you answered NO to any of these questions, learn about travel vaccines (see p288) and other immunizations (see p308).

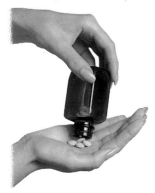

ARE YOU WELL-INFORMED ABOUT YOUR MEDICATIONS?

• *Do you know that you should not take drugs that belong to someone else?*

• *Do you know how to store drugs properly?*

• *Do you know how to safely dispose of old medicines?*

If you do not know why you have been prescribed a particular medication, do not realize how important it is to take the drug exactly as prescribed, and do not know how to store the medicine (see p295), you are less likely to gain the maximum benefit from your treatment.

MAKING THE MOST OF YOUR DOCTOR

• Try to visit your usual doctor, especially if you are already being seen for an illness.
• Be prepared to explain in detail what you mean by a symptom.
• Do not try to exaggerate or interpret your symptoms yourself.
• Write a summary of what you want to say and any questions you want to ask before you go in.

• Ask how long your problem will last and if you should visit your doctor again.
• Take notes of what the doctor says.
• Do not expect your doctor to have all the answers – he or she may need to wait for test results.
• If you want a second opinion, ask to be referred to another doctor.
• Do not always expect a prescription.

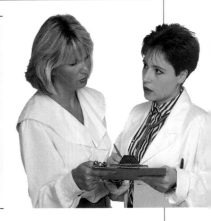

YOUR EMOTIONAL WELLBEING

HOWEVER PHYSICALLY FIT and healthy you are, you will not feel your best unless you take good care of yourself emotionally too. To find out more about your current mental state, try answering the questions under each of the different categories of anxiety, depression, loving relationships, coping with stress, and how you feel about yourself.

Having identified those areas of your emotional outlook and self-image that might benefit from extra care and attention, turn to the pages that cover these issues in greater detail. There you will find advice on how to resolve any difficulties you might be experiencing at home, at work, in your personal relationships, or deep within yourself.

HOW DO YOU FEEL ABOUT YOURSELF?

• *Do you need a lot of reassurance?*

• *Do you only feel at ease with people you consider inferior?*

• *Do you tend not to believe compliments?*

• *Do you often question your value as a person?*

• *Do you get upset if someone criticizes you?*

• *Do you regularly wish you were someone else?*

If you answered YES to most of these questions, you have low self-esteem. Having a poor opinion of yourself can be extremely damaging to your emotional wellbeing. Find out how to develop a more positive outlook on yourself and on life (see p198).

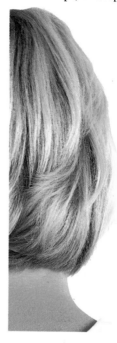
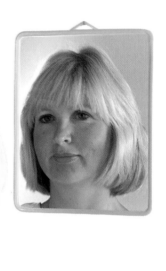

DO YOU HAVE HAPPY, LOVING RELATIONSHIPS?

• *Do you find it difficult to talk about personal matters to your partner?*

• *Do you often lose your temper with a loved one, then regret it?*

• *Do you think your relationship is emotionally one-sided?*

• *Do you often feel jealous?*

• *Do you avoid physical contact with your partner?*

• *Do you dread going home?*

• *Are you unable to hold down lasting relationships?*

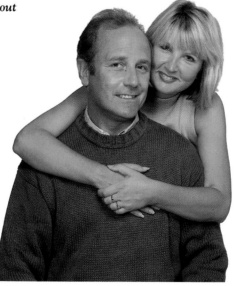

Most relationship difficulties are due to a failure either to communicate, or to see things from the other person's point of view. If you answered YES to these questions, you should learn how to ease tension at home and relate better to your partner (see p188).

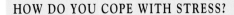

HOW DO YOU COPE WITH STRESS?

- *Do you feel irritable and uptight?*

- *Do you harbor regrets and resentments?*

- *Do you dislike meeting new people?*

- *Do you feel your life is out of control?*

- *Is it hard for you to make decisions?*

- *Do you go out of your way to avoid awkward situations?*

- *Do you regularly feel tired or lacking in enthusiasm?*

If you answered YES to most of these questions, you are under too much stress. Learn how to cushion the harmful effects of stress through relaxation, exercise, yoga, meditation, and massage (see p180-187).

ARE YOU OVER-ANXIOUS?

- *Do you find it difficult to relax?*

- *Do you worry about trivial things?*

- *Do you get upset when plans fall through?*

- *Do you lie awake worrying about your troubles?*

- *Do you have too many problems to overcome?*

- *Do you often get restless and fidgety?*

- *Do you sweat and shake in social situations?*

If you answered YES to most of these questions, you may be plagued by tension or deep-rooted fears. Find out how to cope with your anxiety (see p196).

ARE YOU DEPRESSED?

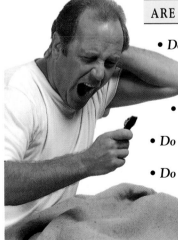
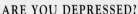

- *Do you feel lonely, even when you are not alone?*

- *Do you wake up early every morning?*

- *Does your future appear gloomy?*

- *Do you think you are getting a raw deal in life?*

- *Do things often seem hopeless to you?*

- *Do you wish you were dead?*

- *Do you often feel like an outsider?*

If you answered YES to any of these questions, you may be feeling sad and despairing. Find out what can cause this and the steps you can take to overcome your depression (see p200).

PLOTTING YOUR ENERGY CHART

ARE YOU REALIZING your full potential in life and responding positively to all its challenges, or do you constantly feel drained and under too much pressure? You can discover how well your personality is able to cope with the trials of life by working out how much energy you devote to each of the six areas (shown below) that make up your personality profile.

If you put too much or too little energy into one area, your approach to life may not be well-balanced.

Answer the following questions to assess the amount of energy you put into each area of your life. Score one point for YES, and zero for NO. Add up your score for each type of energy and then plot these figures on the star chart opposite.

INTELLECTUAL ENERGY | YES | NO

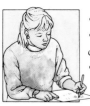

- Do you enjoy a debate?
- Do you regularly do quizzes or crossword puzzles?
- Does your job involve problem solving?
- Do you read every day?
- Do you visit museums or art galleries?
- Do you play card or board games that do not rely purely on chance?
- Do you find it easy to concentrate?

PHYSICAL ENERGY

- Do you exercise for 20 minutes three times a week?
- Do you walk or cycle part of the way to work?
- Do you still feel energetic at the end of the day?
- Would you climb three flights of stairs?
- Do you enjoy active vacations?
- Do you soon get bored when you sit still?
- Does your job involve any manual work?

EMOTIONAL ENERGY

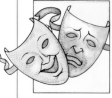

- Do you fall in love easily or are you in love with someone at the moment?
- Do you find it easy to laugh out loud?
- Do you burst into tears when you see or hear something sad?
- Would you say that you are romantic?
- Are you close to your family?
- Have you made any new friends during the last year?
- Do you have difficulty controlling your feelings and emotions?

SEXUAL ENERGY | YES | NO

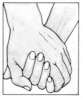

- Do you have sex more than twice a week?
- Do you hug or kiss people to show affection?
- Do you have sex outside the bedroom?
- Do you often think about sex?
- Do you talk about sex to other people?
- Do you like to be touched all over?
- Do you experience orgasm during sex?

NEUROTIC ENERGY

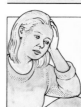

- Do you dwell on the past?
- Do you suffer from insomnia?
- Do you check things over and over again?
- Do you get moody or irritable for no good reason?
- Do you quickly become impatient?
- Do you have any nervous mannerisms?
- Do you find it hard to relax and unwind?

COMMUNICATION ENERGY

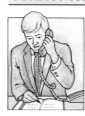

- Do you find it easy to make friends?
- Would you rather ask someone a question than look up the answer in a reference book?
- Do you look forward to meeting new people?
- Are you relaxed about using the telephone?
- Given the choice, would you prefer to spend the evening with a group of people rather than on your own?
- Do you interrupt to voice your opinions?
- Would you enjoy being interviewed?

PLOT YOUR ENERGY STAR CHART

Mark your score for each area of your personality on the chart shown below. For instance, if your score is 5 in the physical energy section, put a cross on the number 5 of the physical energy line. Next draw a straight line from this cross to the two nearest black dots in the center of the chart. Repeat this for all six sections and you will find that you have drawn a star – this is your own personal energy star chart. The length of each arm of the star reflects the amount of that particular energy you have in your personality.

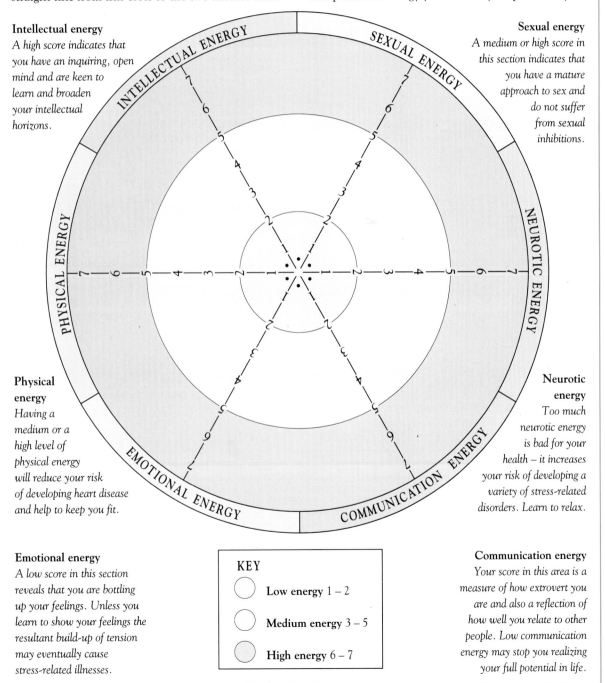

Intellectual energy
A high score indicates that you have an inquiring, open mind and are keen to learn and broaden your intellectual horizons.

Sexual energy
A medium or high score in this section indicates that you have a mature approach to sex and do not suffer from sexual inhibitions.

Physical energy
Having a medium or a high level of physical energy will reduce your risk of developing heart disease and help to keep you fit.

Neurotic energy
Too much neurotic energy is bad for your health – it increases your risk of developing a variety of stress-related disorders. Learn to relax.

Emotional energy
A low score in this section reveals that you are bottling up your feelings. Unless you learn to show your feelings the resultant build-up of tension may eventually cause stress-related illnesses.

KEY
◯ **Low energy** 1 – 2
◯ **Medium energy** 3 – 5
◯ **High energy** 6 – 7

Communication energy
Your score in this area is a measure of how extrovert you are and also a reflection of how well you relate to other people. Low communication energy may stop you realizing your full potential in life.

21

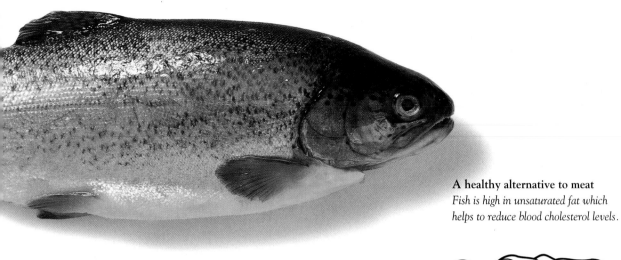

A healthy alternative to meat
Fish is high in unsaturated fat which helps to reduce blood cholesterol levels.

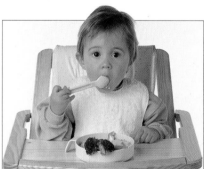

A pattern for life
If children are brought up to enjoy eating fruit, vegetables, and lean meats they are likely to continue this healthy habit throughout the rest of their lives.

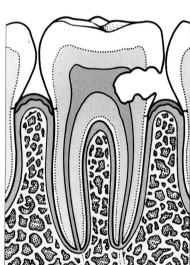

Vitamin-rich
Like many other vegetables, carrots and spinach are excellent fiber-rich, low-calorie, sources of vitamins.

Preventing tooth decay
Eating a varied, balanced diet will help to keep your teeth strong and healthy. However, sugary foods increase your risk of suffering from tooth decay.

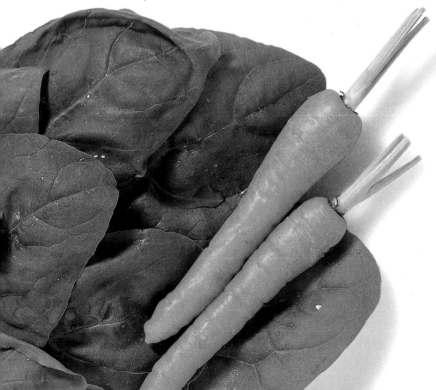

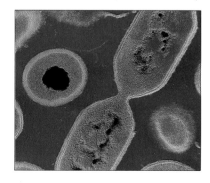

Food hygiene
Listeria can cause food poisoning when lots of the bacteria are consumed, for example in prepared salads.

CHAPTER TWO

EATING FOR HEALTH

DEBATE ABOUT THE influence of diet on your health has never been greater. Newspapers and magazines are full of conflicting advice on what makes up a healthy diet, which can be confusing.

But the principles of healthy eating are very simple. Eating a wide variety of foods in the right balance is the key. In this chapter you will find information about how to choose wisely from the foods that provide you with the essential nutrients for the growth, maintenance, and repair of blood, tissues, and vital organs.

Good nutrition is important for good health. Eating the right foods can help protect you from heart disease and some cancers. But too many people in the West eat the wrong foods. Today's dietary problems come from eating too much saturated fat and refined carbohydrates, too many calories, and not enough fiber. Many people are overweight or put their hearts at risk by clogging their arteries with fats and cholesterol. Dieting is not the solution. Rigid eating programs do not work since no one can stay on them forever. It is better to make a few small but important changes to your eating habits that will stay with you for a lifetime. These will improve your nutritional balance, your health, and solve any weight problems you may have.

Food for energy
Apples and grapes, like most fruit, contain starch, sugar, and fiber. They are digested by the body slowly and therefore provide a steady flow of energy.

ARE YOU EATING FOR GOOD HEALTH?

Examining your eating habits is the first step to a healthy diet.

THE FOODS YOU EAT influence your health, so making the right decisions about your eating behavior and about what and how much you eat, are in your best interests. Answering the following questions will enable you to assess just how healthy your diet really is and discover which areas could be altered to improve your health.

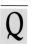

Q *How many proper meals a day do you eat on average?*

A
- Two or three.
- More than three.
- One.

It is better to eat two or three moderate-size meals during the day, rather than one large feast. Your body's metabolism works more efficiently with a regular supply of nutrients. If you eat too many large meals, or one big meal a day, you are more likely to become obese, and to suffer from indigestion and peptic ulcers.

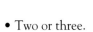

Q *How many snacks do you eat during the day between meals?*

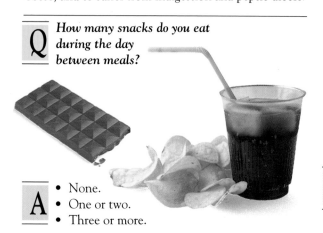

A
- None.
- One or two.
- Three or more.

Although snacking is a bad habit that you should try to avoid, what you eat between meals is more important than whether or not you snack. Sweets, cookies, potato chips, chocolates, and cakes are high in calories, refined sugar, and fats. So, if you do snack, choose a piece of fresh fruit or a raw vegetable which will provide you with vitamins, minerals, and fiber.

Q *Are you overweight?*

A
- Not at all.
- Just a little.
- Seriously.

If you are overweight you should reduce your weight by eating less fat and more fiber and exercising more. People who are overweight tend to die earlier than those who are of average weight. They are also more prone to coronary heart disease, stroke, hernias, some cancers, diabetes, arthritis, and high blood pressure.

Q *How often do you eat red or fatty meats, such as beef, lamb, and pork?*

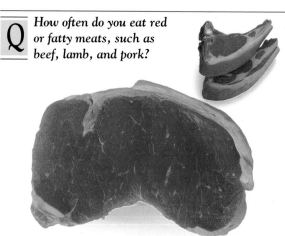

A
- Twice a week, or less.
- Three to four times a week.
- Almost every day.

Red and fatty meats (including processed meats such as sausages and hamburgers) contain large amounts of saturated fat, so you should not eat them more than twice a week. Introduce as many alternative sources of protein as possible into your diet, for example from fish and poultry. Also, aim to have at least one completely meat-free day a week, by preparing nutritious dishes containing a mixture of grains.

Q *How often do you eat fresh fruit and vegetables?*

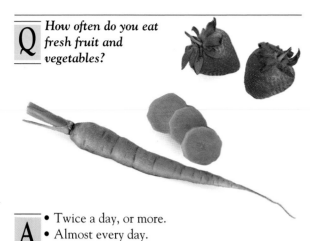

A
• Twice a day, or more.
• Almost every day.
• Less than four times a week.

Eating vegetables at least twice a day is good for you. They provide minerals and essential vitamins, particularly if eaten raw or lightly cooked. They also boost your fiber intake, without adding many calories. Of course, to balance your diet, you will also need to eat foods that are sources of energy, protein, and fat.

Q *How often do you eat unrefined starchy products such as brown rice, whole grain cereals, bread, and pasta?*

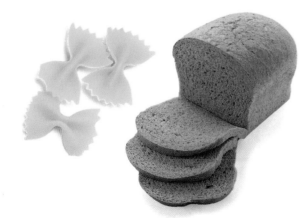

A
• At least once a day.
• Between three and six times a week.
• Less than three times a week.

Try to eat unrefined foods, rather than more refined alternatives, every day. Avoid polished white rice, processed cereals with added sugar, and white bread. Eating unrefined foods will improve your diet because the refining processes remove a lot of the fiber, vitamin, and mineral content, leaving a product high in calories but lacking in nutrients.

Q *How many times a week do you eat fried food?*

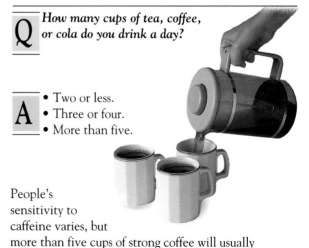

A
• Once a week, or less.
• Around three times a week.
• Almost every day.

To reduce your intake of fat do not eat fried foods more than once a week. It is better to grill or bake food rather than fry it. When you do fry, use olive oil or polyunsaturated vegetable oil, rather than butter.

Q *How often do you eat butter, cream, or whole milk?*

A
• Twice a week, or less.
• Most days.
• More than once a day.

Only eat whole milk products occasionally. They are very high in saturated fats. These can increase your risk of heart disease. They are high in calories too, which can cause weight problems. It is better to replace butter with polyunsaturated margarine, cream with low-fat yogurt, and whole milk with skimmed.

Q *How many cups of tea, coffee, or cola do you drink a day?*

A
• Two or less.
• Three or four.
• More than five.

People's sensitivity to caffeine varies, but more than five cups of strong coffee will usually cause some unpleasant side effects, such as irritability, sleeping difficulties, and tremors. Reduce your caffeine intake by drinking water, diluted fruit juices, or decaffeinated products.

FOOD FOR ENERGY AND GROWTH

FOOD COMES IN many forms, but it all has the same basic chemical functions – to supply body cells with a source of energy, and also to act as the raw material for growth, repair, and maintenance of vital organs and tissues. The substances in food that fulfill these functions are called nutrients. As carbohydrates and fats are the main sources of energy in the diet, the value of any particular type of food for energy and growth depends mainly on its content of these two nutrients.

The sensations of hunger and of having overeaten are designed to ensure that you take in the correct amount of food to fulfill your own particular energy requirements.

Additional energy also comes from the body's stores of glycogen (starch) and fat. Glycogen is made from the glucose molecules that were absorbed from carbohydrates and were not required for the immediate production of energy. Any surplus that cannot be stored as glycogen is stored as body fat.

Food provides the body with the energy needed to sustain life.

SIX VITAL COMPONENTS OF FOOD

Vitamins
Used in numerous cell activities; vitamins aid the release of energy from glucose, and assist growth and repair mechanisms.

Minerals
Sixteen different minerals facilitate growth and repair mechanisms, the release of energy from nutrients, and help form new tissues.

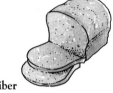

Fiber
Fiber regulates cell metabolism by influencing the digestion and absorption of other energy-producing nutrients.

Carbohydrates
Sugars and starches are broken down to provide energy. Rapid absorption means that they are ideal foods to eat before exercise.

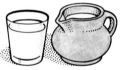

Fats
Fats supply concentrated energy. They also help form chemical messengers, such as hormones and prostaglandins.

Proteins
Amino acids, released from the digestion of proteins, are used as building blocks in the formation of new cells.

ENERGY PRODUCTION FROM FOOD

Every activity requires energy. Your body needs to be able to convert your food into stores of energy that will be available at all times. This complex chain of events begins when your food is broken down by digestive processes in your stomach and intestines to release nutrients, such as glucose, fatty acids, and amino acids.

1 Nutrients from food are absorbed directly into the bloodstream and distributed to cells throughout the body.

2 The cells then use glucose and fatty acids as fuel for a complex sequence of chemical reactions that leads to the release of energy. This energy is stored as ATP (adenosine triphosphate) molecules.

3 When cells undertake a particular activity, such as the contraction of a muscle, ATP is broken down to ADP (adenosine diphosphate), freeing the stored energy.

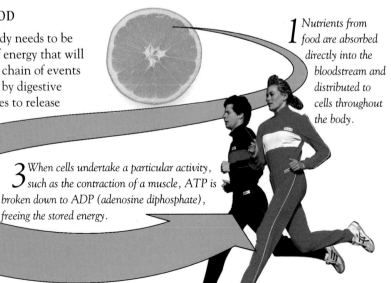

ENERGY FOR LIFE

Energy requirements depend partly on the physical activity you undertake, but the average person in a sedentary job burns up 70 percent of his or her daily energy expenditure just keeping the heart and other organs working and maintaining body temperature.

Activity burns up energy

Regular exercise increases the demand for energy even while you are at rest, thus helping to reduce body fat.

Growth is a continuous process in your body tissues, throughout your life. Cells are continually replaced as part of a routine maintenance program in most tissues and organs. Tissue damage also increases this regeneration.

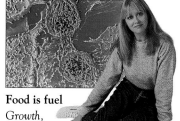

Food is fuel

Growth, repair, and maintenance of cells, such as this one, constantly uses up small amounts of your energy stores.

WHAT IS A CALORIE?

Food energy is traditionally measured in calories, where one calorie is the amount of energy needed to raise the temperature of one gram of water by one degree Centigrade. As the calorie is an extremely small unit, when referring to measurements of the energy value of food, the kilocalorie – equivalent to 1,000 calories – is often used instead. Kilocalories are sometimes called Calories, with a capital C. The number of calories needed each day depends on your level of activity and your basal energy expenditure. The resting energy required by an adult woman averages about 1,300 Calories and for a man about 1,600. All exercise needs extra energy and therefore increases your total calorie requirements.

THE PERFECT FOOD?

Most foods contain a variety of nutrients, but no single food can supply all the nutrients you need for energy and growth. Milk, for example, is an excellent source of protein, and also contains a good amount of carbohydrate. Whole milk is rich in saturated fats, while skim and low-fat milk contain only a little fat. All varieties provide a high percentage of the recommended daily allowance of calcium, vitamin B12, and riboflavin, in just one glass. Milk is also fortified with vitamins A and D. But, even a nutritious food like milk is deficient in iron and vitamin C.

Protein *8 g*

Fat *8 g*

Carbohydrate *11 g*

Calories *150*

Protein *9 g*

Fat *1 g*

Carbohydrate *13 g*

Calories *90*

1 glass (8 oz) of whole milk	1 glass (8 oz) of skim milk

CARBOHYDRATES

Carbohydrates are the body's main source of energy.

CARBOHYDRATES ARE a group of chemicals formed from single molecules known as saccharides. These are linked together to form the two main types of carbohydrates – sugars and starches.

Sugars are simple carbohydrates made of either one or two linked saccharide molecules, called monosaccharides or disaccharides. They taste sweet. Two of the most common sugars are sucrose, or cane sugar, and lactose, or milk sugar.

Starches are complex carbohydrates made up from at least 10 saccharide molecules that must be broken down before they can be absorbed by the body. They are found in many plant foods. Good sources include fruit; vegetables, like potatoes; and grain-based foods like bread, pasta, and cereals.

Metabolizing carbohydrates

The body can only use glucose which is found in plant juices and some fruit. All other carbohydrates must be broken down into single units and converted into glucose in the liver before they can be used.

Complex carbohydrates (starches)

Starches are formed by a long chain of saccharide molecules and can be found in pasta, potatoes, and most fruit.

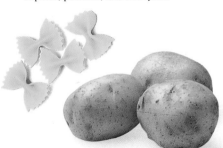

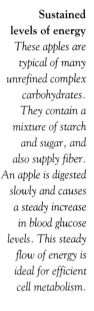

Sustained levels of energy
These apples are typical of many unrefined complex carbohydrates. They contain a mixture of starch and sugar, and also supply fiber. An apple is digested slowly and causes a steady increase in blood glucose levels. This steady flow of energy is ideal for efficient cell metabolism.

CARBOHYDRATES AND ENERGY PRODUCTION

The speed at which saccharides are absorbed, and so able to provide the body with energy, depends on the type of carbohydrate that has been eaten. Only single saccharides can be absorbed through the wall of the intestine into the bloodstream. It takes time for the

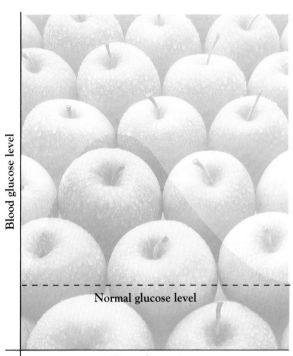

Blood glucose level

- - - - - Normal glucose level

Time after eating

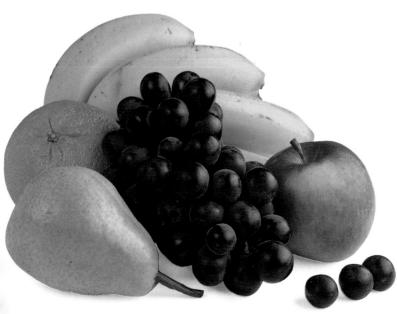

digestive enzymes to break down starch into single saccharide molecules, whereas sugars are absorbed much more rapidly. The high-fiber content of most starchy foods also slows down the absorption and energy production from complex carbohydrates.

The body responds to the increase in blood glucose, which occurs when you eat carbohydrates, by releasing insulin from the pancreas. This hormone stimulates the up-take of glucose into the cells. Most of the glucose that is not needed for the immediate production of energy is changed into body fat.

Refined or unrefined – which is healthier?

Unrefined carbohydrates such as whole wheat bread and brown pasta have a higher nutrient value than refined carbohydrates.

To produce a refined carbohydrate, for example white sugar or white rice, the manufacturer uses a process which actually removes a large percentage of the food's fiber content, and also causes a loss of other nutrients such as vitamins and minerals.

You should therefore always choose to eat unrefined carbohydrates and cut down on all refined foods, especially those that have added sugar.

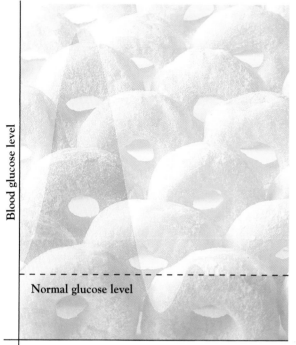

Bursts of energy
After eating a food which is high in sugar, such as a doughnut, there is a rapid surge in the blood glucose levels within the body, followed by an almost equally rapid drop. Hypoglycemia, an abnormally low level of glucose in the blood, may result, causing symptoms such as hunger, weakness, and dizziness.

Blood glucose level

Normal glucose level

Time after eating

VITAL FOR HEALTH

Experts believe that carbohydrates should make up approximately 55 percent of a healthy diet. Starch is the optimum source for energy and should always be eaten in preference to sugars. Even when dieting starch should play a major role in your diet.

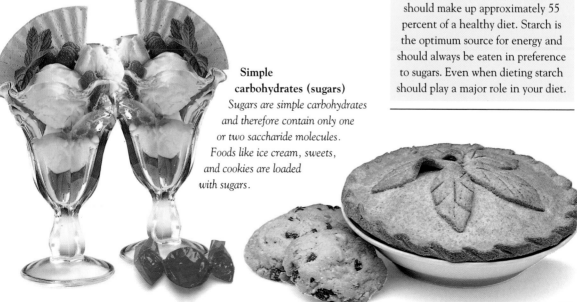

Simple carbohydrates (sugars)
Sugars are simple carbohydrates and therefore contain only one or two saccharide molecules. Foods like ice cream, sweets, and cookies are loaded with sugars.

FATS

Fats are a highly concentrated energy source and are used to power the body's chemical reactions.

THERE ARE TWO types of fats, saturated and unsaturated. They vary in their chemical composition and in the way they effect your body. Saturated fats are found in animal and dairy products. They increase the amount of cholesterol in the blood which in turn increases the risk of developing coronary heart disease. Most vegetable fats provide larger amounts of the healthier unsaturated fat.

A fatty diet

Most people in the West eat far too much of both types. A healthy diet should provide no more than 30 percent of the total calorie intake as fat. Unsaturated fats should be chosen instead of saturated fats whenever possible in order to reduce the risk of heart disease.

An important nutrient

Although too much fat is bad for you, some fat is necessary for the healthy functioning of the body. Small amounts of fatty acids released from digested fats are used as a structural component of cells, and are therefore important in cell growth and repair. Some dietary fats are also valuable sources of vitamins A, D, E, and K.

How your body breaks down dietary fat

The fats that you eat pass through the stomach into the intestine, where they are dissolved by the action of bile salts released from the liver. Enzymes that are secreted by the pancreas then break the fat down into fatty acids and glycerol which can enter the wall of the intestine. There they recombine in the ratio of three molecules of fatty acid to one glycerol molecule, to form triglycerides, which can be used by the body to provide energy.

These triglycerides are absorbed by the lymphatic system and passed

SATURATED FATS

Butter, lard, pork, beef, lamb, eggs, and whole milk are high in saturated fats, as are some vegetable oils, including coconut, palm, and palm kernel. These fats are solid at room temperature. A high intake of saturated fats tends to raise your blood cholesterol, which in turn increases your risk of developing coronary heart disease.

Sirloin steak

Pork

Butter

Eggs

into the bloodstream, which carries them, bound to protein and cholesterol, to cells throughout the body.

A source of energy

Cells use the fatty acids and the glycerol as a source of energy. Any excess fat is stored under the skin causing weight gain and obesity. Some triglycerides are also carried to the liver where they are used to manufacture cholesterol.

FAT FACT

Fats are packed with calories. They provide you with roughly 9 Calories per gram compared with only 4 Calories for each gram of carbohydrate you eat. So you can eat twice as much carbohydrate-rich food as fat-rich food, and still save calories.

THE HIDDEN FATS

Because fats make food more palatable and also more filling, they are added to a variety of processed foods, including pot pies, sausages, hamburgers, cakes, and cookies. If you read the labels carefully, you should be able to find out the amount of saturated fat and also the total fat content in all these types of food.

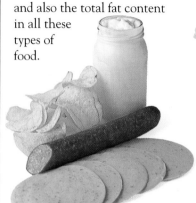

Do you know what you are really eating?
Most people know that foods such as ice cream are loaded with fat, but few people realize just how much fat is added to foods like luncheon meat, chips, salami, and mayonnaise.

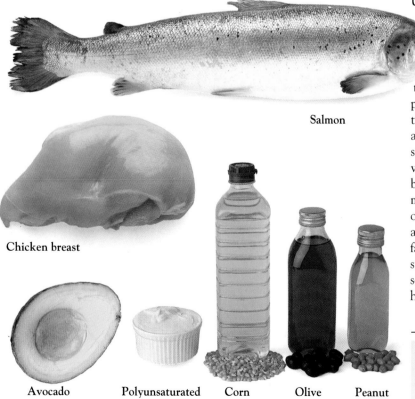

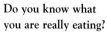

Salmon

Chicken breast

Avocado

Polyunsaturated margarine

Corn oil

Olive oil

Peanut oil

UNSATURATED FATS

Many types of food contain high levels of unsaturated fats. These fats are liquid at room temperature. The fat in fish and poultry is largely unsaturated and the levels in soft margarines are also usually high. But the major source of unsaturated fats is vegetable oil. These oils can be divided into two categories: monounsaturated fats, found in olive oil, peanut oil, canola oil, and avocados, and polyunsaturated fats, which come from corn oil, sunflower oil, safflower oil, and soy bean oil. Both types are healthy for your heart.

TOO MUCH!

The average American consumes 30 precent of total calories from fat.

CHOLESTEROL

The link between cholesterol and heart disease is well known, but did you know that most blood cholesterol is made in the liver from saturated fats?

CHOLESTEROL-PRODUCING FOODS

Foods that are naturally rich in cholesterol include eggs, liver, kidneys, and some shellfish. However, the main sources of cholesterol are actually those foods that are high in saturated fats, for example, cream, butter, hard cheese, and fatty meats like pork, lamb, and beef. The body turns these into cholesterol in the liver.

CELLS THROUGHOUT the body use cholesterol to produce a number of important hormones that are needed for growth and reproduction. During the formation of new cells within different parts of the body, cholesterol is used as a vital component of the cell wall. Cholesterol is also an essential ingredient of bile salts produced in the liver, which are later passed into the intestines to help with the digestion of fats.

A surplus of cholesterol

Nearly all the cholesterol that reaches the bloodstream is actually made in the liver from the metabolism of a wide variety of foods, especially saturated fats. Since the daily requirement of cholesterol for cell function is more than adequately supplied by the cholesterol

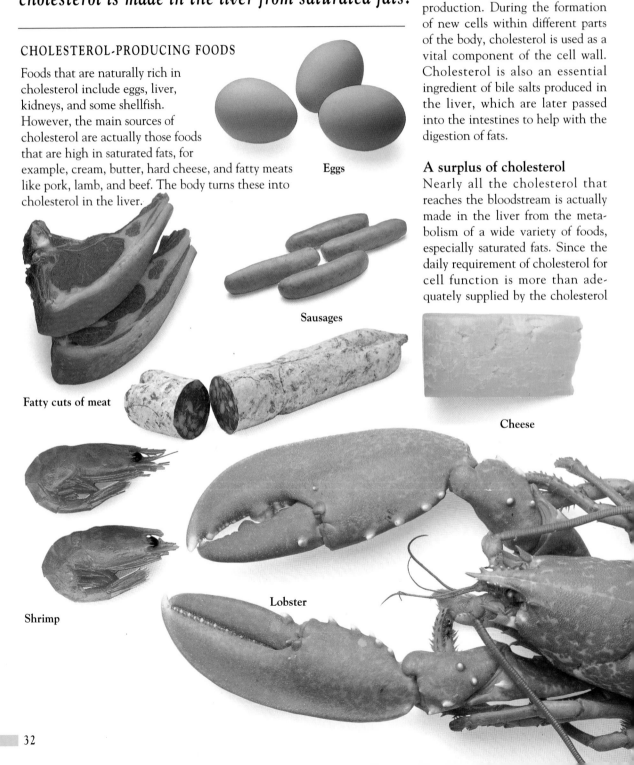

Eggs

Sausages

Cheese

Fatty cuts of meat

Shrimp

Lobster

WHERE DOES CHOLESTEROL COME FROM?

The cholesterol levels in your blood increase according to the amount of saturated fats you eat. Your body goes on making cholesterol from fat regardless of how much cholesterol is actually being eaten. There are many foods which contain no cholesterol, but which are rich in saturated fats and therefore raise the level of cholesterol in your blood. The liver produces almost all the body's cholesterol from the metabolism of digested fats. To prevent a build up of cholesterol in the blood, you must cut down on both cholesterol-containing foods and saturated fats in your diet.

Food enters the stomach
The digestion of foods containing fats and cholesterol begins inside the stomach and continues in the intestines.

From the intestines to the liver
Fatty acids and glycerol, released from fatty foods, and dietary cholesterol are absorbed through the wall of the intestine directly into lymphatic vessels, and then into the bloodstream. They are eventually carried to the liver.

The liver produces cholesterol
Fatty acids and glycerol are metabolized within the liver and used as building blocks to produce cholesterol.

Cholesterol in the blood
The cholesterol that the liver has produced is then added to the cholesterol that is already in the bloodstream, some of which comes directly from cholesterol-rich food. Other factors that influence levels include your genetic characteristics and fitness.

manufactured in the liver, the body does not need dietary cholesterol. Only a small proportion is absorbed directly from cholesterol-rich foods such as eggs and shellfish.

Critical levels

Cholesterol is transported around the body in the bloodstream and all body cells are able to take the cholesterol they need directly from this source. Cholesterol that is sur-plus to requirements remains in the circulation and may soon build up to abnormally high levels.

There is clear evidence that people with high blood cholesterol levels have a much greater risk of suffering from heart attacks, angina, stroke, or circulation disorders. The excess cholesterol clings to the artery walls as fatty deposits and then obstructs the flow of blood to organs, such as the heart and brain.

Most people can quite easily lower their blood cholesterol levels by changing their diet. It is not simply a matter of eating fewer choles-terol-rich foods, because these have only a minimal effect on the actual level in the blood. To lower your blood cholesterol level you must eat fewer fatty foods, particularly those containing a lot of saturated fats since your liver uses these to produce cholesterol.

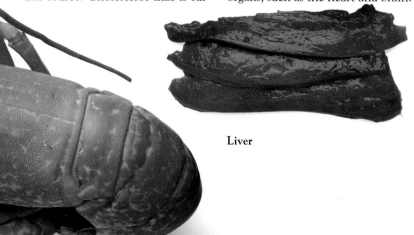

Liver

FATS AT FAULT

Only three percent of the cholesterol in your blood comes directly from the cholesterol in your foods – the majority is manufactured in your own liver from foods rich in saturated fats.

PROTEINS

Proteins are the basic material from which our bodies' cells and tissues are made.

PROTEINS ARE LARGE molecules that consist of hundreds or thousands of chemical units, called amino acids, that are linked together in long, folded chains. Each type of protein has a specific sequence of amino acids.

How your body uses protein

A regular intake of protein in the diet provides your body cells with an adequate supply of amino acids. Cells then use these chemical units as building blocks to form new proteins. Proteins also assist in the growth, repair, and replacement of different body tissues, such as bones, muscles, connective tissues, and the walls of hollow organs. Each cell makes its own specific range of proteins, with the code that determines the sequence of amino acids held on genetic material inside the cell nucleus. Some of these proteins are enzymes which trigger the chemical reactions that produce energy for muscle contraction and other cell activities.

The effects of starvation

In people who are well nourished, the amino acids released from the protein in food, and that stored in muscles, are not required for energy production. Carbohydrates and fats are a more efficient fuel.

In cases of starvation, where fat and glycogen (starch) stores are depleted, amino acids will act as an energy source, at the cost of tissue maintenance, growth, and repair.

Crayfish

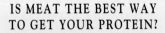

Milk

Poultry

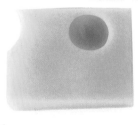

Animal sources of protein
The proteins supplied by foods of animal origin are called complete proteins because they contain all the so-called essential amino acids which the body cannot make for itself. Meat, poultry, fish, eggs, and dairy products all provide substantial quantities of complete protein.

Cheese

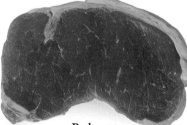

Red meat

IS MEAT THE BEST WAY TO GET YOUR PROTEIN?

Meat provides all the essential amino acids in approximately the same proportions as needed by the body, and also supplies many vitamins and minerals. But meat also contains saturated fats which increase the risk of heart disease. For a healthy diet, the recommended intake of meat is 4-6 oz (100-150 g) a day at most. Choose lean meats and have at least one meat-free day a week.

Fish

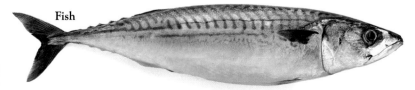

Protein-rich foods

Protein is supplied by both animal and plant foods. The recommended amount of protein in the diet is determined primarily by your age and your weight (see RDA chart p307). Most people in the Western world eat at least twice the recommended allowance because of the greater availability of fresh, inexpensive food, particularly meat.

Eating to excess

Consuming too much protein on a regular basis may cause various problems for people with liver and kidney disorders, as these organs are involved in the removal of waste products from protein metabolism. Animal foods, particularly red meat and dairy products, that are rich in protein also tend to be high in saturated fats which provide excessive amounts of calories and elevate blood cholesterol levels, thereby increasing the risk of suffering from heart disease.

COMBINING PLANT PROTEINS

Foods from plant sources such as nuts and beans all contain protein but none of them have the complete protein that is found in meat. A complete protein is one that contains all the essential amino acids in about the same proportions needed by the body. Proteins from plant sources are known as partially complete proteins because they are deficient in one or more essential amino acids. But the amino acids missing in one plant food are often present in another. In order to obtain a complete protein from these foods, they must be eaten in combination with one another, as shown.

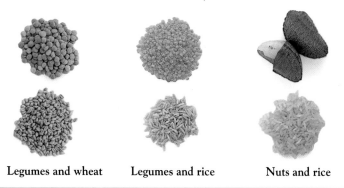

Legumes and wheat   **Legumes and rice**   **Nuts and rice**

Crisp bread

Plant sources of protein
Proteins from plant sources, such as peas, beans, nuts, and the grain in cereals and bread, are known as partially complete proteins, because they are lacking in one or more of the essential amino acids. However even those who do not eat meat, fish, or dairy products (vegans) can avoid becoming deficient in any one amino acid, simply by consuming a diet containing a wide variety of plant proteins.

Bread   **Tofu (Soy bean curd)**

Almonds

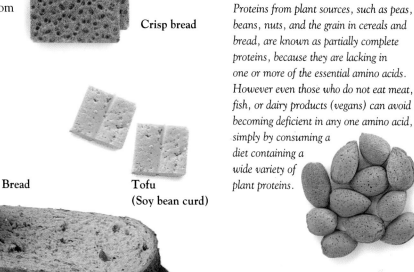

Potatoes   **Pasta**   **Rice**   **Dried beans**   **Whole grain cereals**

VITAMINS

Without the vitamins obtained from the food you eat, your body would not function normally.

VITAMINS ARE VITAL. Your health will suffer if you do not take in your Recommended Daily Amount (RDA) of every single vitamin. Most of these vitamins must be obtained from your diet.

A balanced, mixed diet will naturally contain all the vitamins needed by the body and therefore supplements are needed only by those people who are in poor health, suffer from a chronic illness, or do not eat well. In general, vitamins ensure that the body's cells work properly by controlling the growth and repair of tissues and by stimulating energy production.

VITAMIN A

Various animal foods, including liver, fish-liver oils, egg yolk, and fortified milk products contain this vitamin. Retinol, an active form of vitamin A, is made in the body from the beta-carotene found in green leafy vegetables and yellow-orange colored fruit and vegetables.

Functions

- *forms bones and teeth.*
- *keeps skin and hair healthy.*
- *protects lining of respiratory, digestive, and urinary tracts against infection.*
- *maintains night vision.*

Functions

- *helps stimulate release of energy from nutrients.*
- *promotes the production of hormones by the adrenal glands.*
- *maintains a healthy mouth, tongue, and skin.*

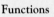

VITAMIN B2 (RIBOFLAVIN)

Also known as riboflavin, vitamin B2 is found in many animal and plant foods. Sources of this vitamin include milk, liver, cheese, eggs, green vegetables, brewer's yeast, whole grains, enriched cereals, and wheatgerm.

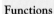

VITAMIN B1 (THIAMINE)

Vitamin B1, also known as thiamine, is found in both animal and plant foods. Good sources include whole wheat bread, brown rice, pasta, whole grain cereals, bran, liver, kidney, pork, fish, peas, nuts, beans, and eggs.

Functions

- *controls the enzymes involved in stimulating the chemical reactions which convert glucose (sugar) into energy.*
- *promotes the production of energy, needed for functioning of the nerves, muscles, and heart.*

NIACIN

Niacin, occasionally referred to as vitamin B3, has two forms – nicotinamide, and nicotinic acid. The major sources of niacin in the diet are liver, lean meats, poultry, fish, nuts, and dried beans. The body can also manufacture small amounts of niacin from tryptophan, which is an amino acid released during the digestion of proteins.

Functions

- *aids energy production from fats and carbohydrates.*
- *assists the functioning of the nervous and digestive systems.*
- *promotes the production of the sex hormones.*
- *helps maintain a healthy skin.*

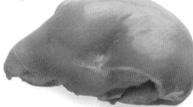
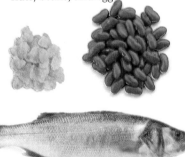
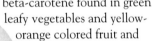

VITAMIN B6 (PYRIDOXINE)

Functions

- *helps produce energy from nutrients.*
- *helps form red blood cells and antibodies.*
- *aids digestive and nervous systems.*
- *maintains healthy skin.*

Vitamin B6, pyridoxine, is found in liver, poultry, pork, fish, bananas, potatoes, dried beans, whole grain products, and most other fruit and vegetables.

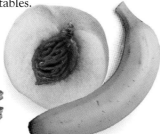

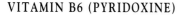

VITAMIN C

Vitamin C is found in fruit and vegetables, especially citrus fruit, strawberries, blackcurrants, green peppers, green leafy vegetables, and potatoes. The processing and cooking of these foods loses much of the vitamin C; they are best eaten raw.

Functions

- *maintains gums, teeth, bones, and blood vessels.*
- *improves iron absorption.*
- *aids the immune system.*
- *enhances wound healing.*

VITAMIN B12

Vitamin B12 is only found in products of animal origin, such as liver, pork, fish, yeast, eggs, and dairy products. Vegetarians who do not eat any animal produce (vegans) must take a supplement of this vitamin.

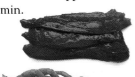

Functions

- *aids production of genetic matter inside cells – essential for the formation of new cells, like red and white blood cells, cells in the hair follicles and intestine.*
- *helps keep the nervous system healthy.*

Functions

- *aids calcium absorption from food.*
- *forms strong teeth and bones.*
- *maintains healthy blood clotting, muscles, and nerves by controlling blood levels of calcium.*

VITAMIN D

Food sources of vitamin D include oily fish, such as salmon, milk, liver, eggs, cod-liver oil, and some cereals. It is also added to margarine. However, the major supply of vitamin D comes from sunlight, through its action on a chemical in the skin.

FOLIC ACID

Functions

- *aids production of genetic material inside cells – needed for the growth and repair of cells, and for the formation of new red blood cells in bone marrow.*
- *helps maintain a healthy nervous system.*

One of the B-complex vitamins, the main sources of folic acid are green leafy vegetables, mushrooms, liver, nuts, dried beans, peas, and whole wheat bread.

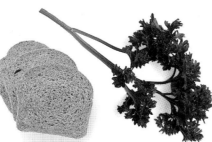

VITAMIN E

Margarine, whole grain cereals, dried beans, green leafy vegetables, nuts, fish, and meat are among the many sources of this vitamin; deficiency is virtually unknown.

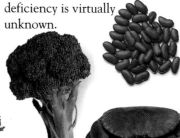

Functions

- *assists in the formation of new red blood cells and protects them from being destroyed in the bloodstream.*
- *protects cell linings in the lungs and other tissues.*
- *may slow down cell aging.*

MINERALS

Minerals are just as important as vitamins, making an essential contribution to your body's health.

AT LEAST 20 different minerals are known to play a role in controlling the metabolism or maintaining the function of specific body tissues. Some minerals, like magnesium, potassium, calcium, and sodium, are needed in fairly large amounts. Others, like iron, zinc, copper, selenium, fluoride, and iodine are only needed in tiny quantities, but are still required for numerous chemical processes in the body. A balanced diet usually supplies all the necessary minerals, but deficiencies of iron, calcium, and iodine are not uncommon and supplements are often included in staple foods like bread and flour.

SODIUM

Almost all foods contain sodium. Apart from table salt, which is added for flavor, the main dietary sources are processed foods, smoked or cured meats and fish, snack foods, pickles, bread, cereals, cheese, and water treated with a water-softener.

Functions
- *controls body's water balance.*
- *maintains normal heart rhythm.*
- *helps in the generation of nerve impulses, and muscle contraction.*

Functions
- *forms and maintains teeth and bones.*
- *controls transmission of nerve impulses.*
- *aids efficiency of muscle contraction.*
- *assists blood clotting.*

CALCIUM

Sources of calcium in the diet include milk, both whole and non-fat, dairy products, green leafy vegetables, dried peas, beans, nuts, citrus fruit, fish with edible bones such as sardines and tinned salmon, and hard water.

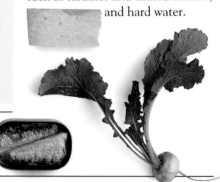

POTASSIUM

The main sources of potassium in the diet are bread and whole grain cereals, green leafy vegetables, legumes and beans, meat, milk, and fruit, particularly bananas and oranges.

Functions
- *controls body's water balance.*
- *maintains normal heart rhythm.*
- *helps in the generation of nerve impulses and muscle contraction.*

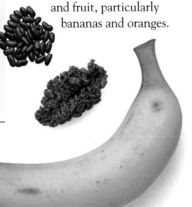

MAGNESIUM

Magnesium-rich foods include nuts, soy beans, milk, fish, green vegetables, whole grain cereals, bread, and hard water.

Functions
- *forms and maintains healthy teeth and bones.*
- *controls transmission of nerve impulses and contraction of muscles.*
- *activates energy-producing chemical reactions inside cells.*

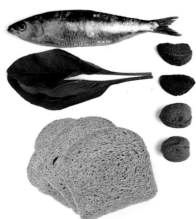

IRON

Iron is found in meat, fish, liver, egg yolks, bread, some green leafy vegetables, cereals, nuts, and beans. Deficiency may occur in children on a poor diet and some women.

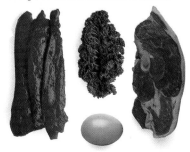

FLUORIDE

Fish provides a rich source of fluoride. This mineral is also found in tea, coffee, and soy beans. Also, drinking water may contain a naturally high level of fluoride, or it may have been added artificially.

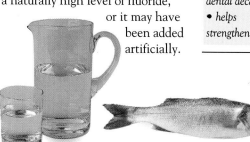

ZINC

Tiny amounts of zinc are found in many different foods. The main dietary sources are lean meats, fish, and other sea foods such as oysters. It is also found in beans, whole grain cereals, eggs, nuts, and whole wheat bread.

Functions

• *assists wound healing.*

• *maintains skin and hair.*

• *enables growth and sexual development to occur normally.*

• *helps to control the activities of many different enzymes.*

Functions

• *protects cells against damage from oxidizing substances found in the blood.*

• *may reduce the risk of developing some cancers.*

• *may help to preserve the elasticity of body tissues.*

SELENIUM

The main sources of this mineral are meat, fish, shellfish, whole grain cereals, and dairy products. The amount of selenium provided by any particular vegetable varies according to the selenium content of the soil it was grown in.

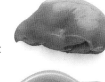

COPPER

The minute quantities of copper required by the body are found in liver, shellfish, peas, nuts, dried beans, mushrooms, grapes, whole grain cereals, and bread.

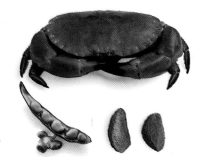

IODINE

The best sources of iodine are salt-water fish and shellfish. Levels in other foods depend entirely on the iodine in the soil or in animal feeds. Iodine may be added to salt and bread in areas where the soil is deficient.

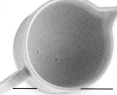

THE IMPORTANCE OF FIBER

Fiber consists of the indigestible parts of plant foods and helps prevent coronary heart disease and cancer of the bowel.

THE FIBER WE EAT, also called roughage, comes from grain husks, the skins and flesh of fruit, and the tough, fibrous material in vegetables. It cannot be broken down by digestive enzymes and is therefore not absorbed by the body as it passes through the stomach and intestine.

Although it has no nutritional or energy value, it is a vital part of your diet. High-fiber foods are filling, but low in calories, so they aid weight loss.

Fiber has a key role to play in maintaining a healthy body. By increasing the bulk of the feces, it encourages the efficient passage of waste products through the intestine. It also draws in water from the surrounding blood vessels, which softens the stools.

The absorption of nutrients from the intestine into the bloodstream is also modified by fiber. By reducing the absorption of digested fats it slightly lowers blood cholesterol levels, thereby reducing the risk of coronary heart disease.

Every adult should eat about 25 grams of fiber a day. However, the typical Western diet, which is high in animal fats and refined carbohydrates, is often lacking in fiber.

FIBER-RICH FOODS

This chart lists the approximate amount of fibre, measured in grams, that can be found in 100 gram portions of various high-fiber foods.

FOOD	FIBER CONTENT
(grams of fiber per 100 grams of food)	
Bran, unprocessed	**44 g**
Apricots, dried and pitted	**24 g**
Prunes	**14 g**
Almonds	**14 g**
Raisins	**7 g**
Whole grain bread	**7 g**
Baked beans, canned	**7 g**
Spinach, boiled	**7 g**
Peas	**7 g**
Peanut butter	**7 g**
Sweet corn	**6 g**
Celery	**5 g**
Leeks or broccoli	**3.5 g**
Lentils, boiled	**3.5 g**
Apples, bananas, and strawberries	**2 g**

Fiber's structure
Like all other types of fiber, cellulose consists of parallel, interlinked chains of sugar molecules. Because these links are resistant to attack from digestive enzymes, they cannot be broken down and absorbed into the bloodstream by humans.

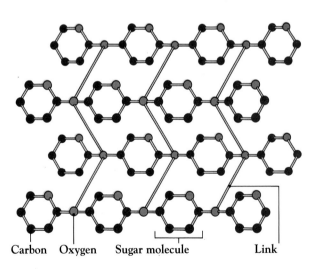

Carbon   Oxygen   Sugar molecule   Link

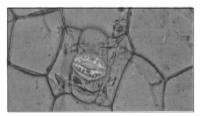

Cellulose under the microscope
Electron microscope pictures of cellulose reveal parallel chains of sugar molecules.

HOW TO MEET YOUR FIBER REQUIREMENTS

To ensure you are eating the recommended daily intake of around 25 grams of fiber, there are a number of simple ways you can improve your diet.

- Eat plenty of fresh fruit and vegetables.

- Rather than drink a glass of fruit juice, eat a whole fruit.

- Do not overcook vegetables; eat some raw.

- Eat the skins of fruit and vegetables, such as apples and baked potatoes – but wash them first.

- Choose whole grain cereals, whole wheat bread, and brown rice, rather than highly refined alternatives.

- Remember that the outer leaves of a lettuce, and the strings running through a stick of celery, contain more fiber than the other parts.

WARNING

Introduce fiber-rich foods gradually or your digestive system will not have time to adapt and you are likely to suffer from abdominal cramps and flatulence. Concentrated sources of fiber, such as unprocessed bran or fiber supplements should only be taken if advised by your doctor.

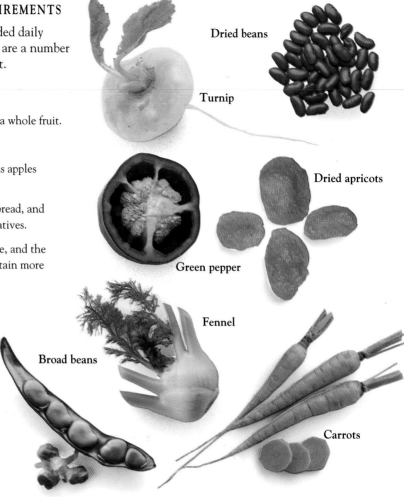

Dried beans

Turnip

Dried apricots

Green pepper

Fennel

Broad beans

Carrots

YOUR FIBER FOR THE DAY

This selection of everyday foods will provide an adult's recommended daily fiber intake of 25 grams.

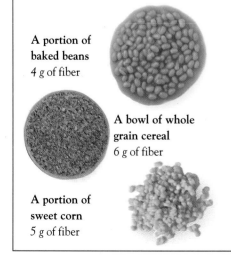

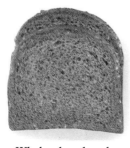

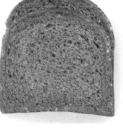

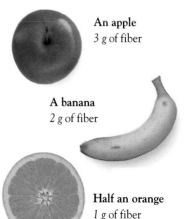

A portion of baked beans
4 g of fiber

A bowl of whole grain cereal
6 g of fiber

A portion of sweet corn
5 g of fiber

Whole wheat bread
(two slices)
4 g of fiber

TOTAL DIETARY FIBER
25 g

An apple
3 g of fiber

A banana
2 g of fiber

Half an orange
1 g of fiber

YOUR HEALTHY EATING PLAN

THE KEY TO HEALTHY eating is a varied and balanced diet, which provides the right mixture of carbohydrates, fats, and proteins; and the recommended amount of all the vitamins and minerals. This ideal diet has enough calories to fulfill your energy requirements, but not an excess that would cause you to put on weight. It also supplies the right quantity of fiber, sometimes called roughage, and water to keep your digestive system working efficiently.

A healthy balance
By eating a wide variety of foods, from each of the major food groups, you should satisfy all your nutritional requirements. Simply eat a range of foods every day from the five separate categories – bread, cereals and other grain products; fruit; vegetables; meat, poultry, fish, eggs, and plant protein sources such as dried beans, peas, nuts, and seeds; and dairy produce.

Healthy eating habits play a vital role in allowing you and your family to lead life to the full.

Carbohydrates should provide about 50 to 55 percent of your energy needs, proteins about 15 percent, and fats 30 percent or less. However, many people in the West consume far too much fat and eat most of their carbohydrate in the form of refined sugar, which lacks vitamins, minerals, and fiber.

Reducing fats
Cutting down on fats reduces the risk of heart disease. Try to choose unsaturated instead of saturated fats wherever possible. Saturated fats are found in red meat, milk, cheese, coconut oil, palm oil, and butter, and are also added to processed foods. They increase your blood cholesterol level, which increases the risk of fatty deposits clogging up your arteries. Unsaturated

fats, contained in oily fish, chicken, nuts, and most types of vegetable oil do not raise your blood cholesterol, and may even have a protective effect on your heart and circulation.

Increasing fibre
Healthy eating need not always mean eating less. High-fiber foods such as whole wheat bread, brown rice, fresh fruit, and vegetables fill you up without adding empty calories to your diet. They are also a good source of vitamins and minerals. A high intake of dietary fiber prevents constipation and also helps regulate the absorption of glucose and fatty acids from your digestive system.

If possible, carbohydrates should come from low-calorie, high-fiber foods. Cut down on cookies and

A week's food intake
An average woman aged between 18 and 54 years would eat the foods shown here in the course of just one week. Different people have different nutritional requirements which vary according to sex, age, size, activity level, and with any special needs such as pregnancy. For instance, a sedentary adult woman needs to consume about 12,000 Calories a week, as compared to 25,000 Calories for a man doing a physically demanding job.

sweets since they contain calories without the benefit of other nutrients. They also increase your risk of obesity and tooth decay.

All in a day

Another key to healthy eating is to have three meals a day, rather than a lot of snacks and one big meal. Do not be tempted to skip breakfast since your body's metabolism works more efficiently on a steady supply of foods. People who do not usually eat three regular meals a day are more likely to put on weight.

Planning a healthy diet

Careful shopping and cooking can ensure that you eat a healthier diet. Simply reducing the amount of red meat in your diet will mean you eat less fat, as all red meats are high in saturated fats as well as protein. Try to eat meat only once a day, or to have a completely meat-free day once a week. To cut down on cholesterol eat no more than four eggs a week.

Low calorie foods

Because fish and salad are low in fat and therefore calories, you can eat far more of them than of foods like butter or red meat.

The smart shopper

When shopping, buy fresh rather than processed foods because they have a higher nutritional value and are free of added sugar and salt. Check the labels on canned foods, selecting those that do not have salt or sugar added. Choose fish that is packed in water rather than oil. Select low-fat dairy products like skimmed milk and low-fat yogurts, spreads, and cheeses. When buying meat, choose lean cuts. Fish and poultry, which contain less fat than red meat, pork, sausages, and processed meats, are a nutritionally sound choice.

The health-conscious cook

In the kitchen, trim all visible fat from meat and remove chicken skin. Bake, boil, grill, stir-fry, or steam food rather than frying it. If you choose to fry, use olive oil or a polyunsaturated vegetable oil rather than butter or lard. Two generous portions of foods that are high in fiber, such as whole wheat bread and cereal, fresh fruit, raw or lightly cooked vegetables, whole wheat pasta, brown rice, and dried beans, should be eaten every day. Salads supply vitamins, minerals, and even fiber; they are healthiest when served with lemon juice or a low-fat dressing.

Sugary foods and alcohol are both high in calories and should be consumed in moderation. Although small amounts of alcohol are good for your heart and circulation, you should limit your intake to two measures of wine, beer, or spirits each day.

A healthy diet

The Mediterranean diet is far healthier than the high-fat diet of most other people in the West. This pasta with a seafood sauce is low in fat but high in nutrients.

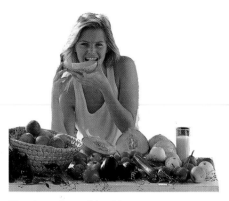

Keeping trim and healthy

Eat plenty of vegetables and salads, and finish your meals with fruit rather than rich desserts that are high in calories.

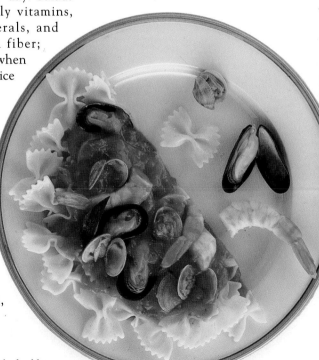

A BALANCED DIET FOR LIFE

A HEALTHY BREAKFAST

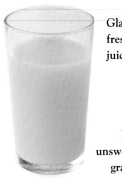

Glass of
fresh orange
juice

Half an
unsweetened
grapefruit

Eating breakfast will provide you
and your family with energy for the
day ahead. Cereal, toast, and grapefruit is an
excellent nutrient-rich choice, and just as filling as a
fried breakfast. The muesli is loaded with vitamins and
fiber, and the whole wheat toast is high in protein, fiber,
and carbohydrate. If you use skimmed milk, a low-fat
spread, and only a little marmalade your meal will
not be high in refined sugars, fats, or calories either.

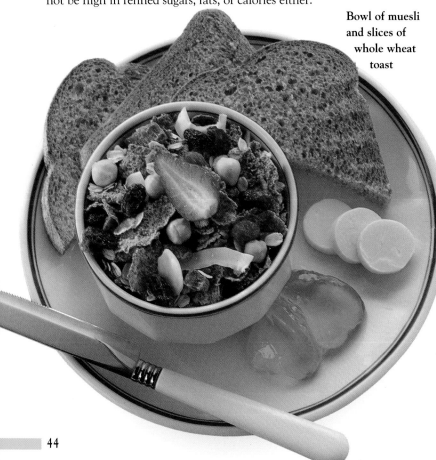

Bowl of muesli
and slices of
whole wheat
toast

Eating the right foods in the right amounts will help ensure good health.

HEALTHY EATING means having a low-fat, high-fiber diet that also has the right balance of foods to provide all the essential nutrients and energy needed by your body. Maintaining a nutritionally balanced diet is an important part of leading a healthy lifestyle, and a major step toward keeping you and your family fit and well. To achieve this balanced diet, you should eat as wide a variety of foods as possible, from all the five major food groups – grain products; fruit; vegetables; meat, eggs, and plant protein sources such as nuts or beans; and finally dairy produce. You must also make an effort to cut down on sugar and salt.

COOKING FOR GOOD HEALTH

• Grill, steam, boil, or bake food to minimize its fat content.
• Use polyunsaturated vegetable oil when you do fry food.
• Cook stews and soups slowly, skimming off the fat regularly.
• Drain off as much fat as you can from the pan before making gravy.
• Make your own salt-free stock; processed stock cubes usually contain added salt.
• Only add a small amount of salt, if any, to your cooking.
• To help preserve vitamins, cook fruit and vegetables in their skins, and try not to overcook them.
• Instead of cooking with cream, use plain yogurt.

A HEALTHY LUNCH

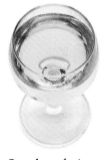

Glass of low-fat milk

Always make time to eat a filling lunch. A snack simply is not sufficient. An easy to prepare yet nutritious lunch is provided, for example, by a vegetable soup, which is low in fat but high in protein, followed by chicken sandwiches and a glass of milk. The whole wheat bread is an unrefined carbohydrate and rich in protein and vitamins. The lean, skinless meat also provides protein and the salad supplies additional vitamins, minerals, and fiber.

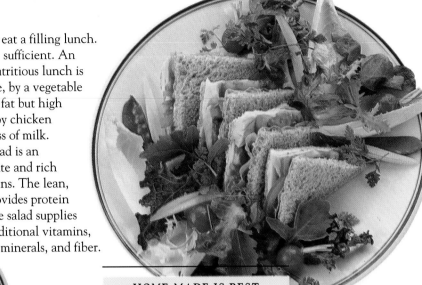

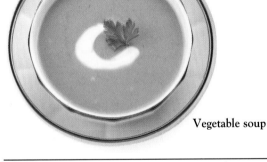

Vegetable soup

HOME-MADE IS BEST

Beware of processed soups from cans or packets; they often contain large amounts of added fat and salt. Choose a brand that is low in fat and salt-free; or better still, make your own soup using fresh ingredients.

Green salad, with a low-calorie dressing, and a round of chicken sandwiches

A HEALTHY DINNER

Fresh fruit salad served with yogurt

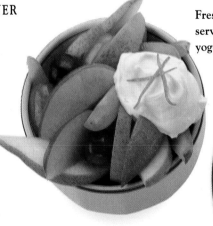

One glass of wine

Grilled sole followed by a fruit salad will complement and complete your healthy balanced menu for the day. Fish is high in protein, vitamins, and minerals; the rice is a rich source of carbohydrate and fiber; and the broccoli has been steamed to preserve its nutrient content. A fresh fruit salad is not only vitamin-rich and tasty, but low in calories. The occasional glass of wine or beer may even reduce the risk of heart disease.

Sole dressed with thyme, parsley, and lemon juice

45

SNACKS AND DRINKS

Avoiding high-calorie snacks and drinks by always choosing nutritious alternatives will keep you trim and healthy.

THE WRONG CHOICE

Many mass-produced foods contain large amounts of sugar and saturated fats, and are therefore high in calories. Cutting down on processed food helps reduce your risk of obesity and heart disease. Reducing the amount of sugar in your diet may help prevent the development of tooth decay and diabetes. Read the labels on processed food, checking the amount of sugar and fat.

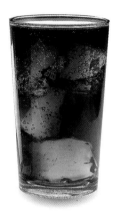

Cola

Chocolate

Added sugar
Sweet-tasting foods have sugar added, but so do many savory foods such as relishes, burgers, and baked beans.

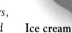

Ice cream

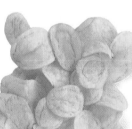

Crisps

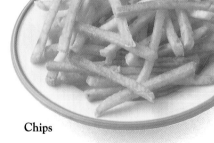

Chips

Hot dog

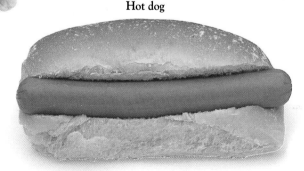

Added fats
Chips, sausages, hamburgers, and fries are low in nutrients and also contain a great deal of fat, sugar, and salt.

FOR MANY PEOPLE, convenience has become the most important consideration when choosing which food products to buy. Unfortunately many convenience foods are high in calories, with a lot of saturated fats, added sugar, and salt, but low in fiber, and short of essential nutrients. Eaten on a regular basis they increase your risk of obesity, heart disease, and deficiencies of some vitamins and minerals.

Be sure to read the labels on all the food you eat between meals. If you are worried about your weight you should also remember to check the ingredients of your drinks. Many soft drinks have added sugars and they should not be part of a healthy diet.

Healthy alternatives

Store nutritious convenience foods in your freezer. When you do have time to prepare a meal from scratch, with all sorts of fresh ingredients, cook more than you need and freeze the leftovers. Then when you are hungry and pressed for time, rather than snacking on fast foods, there will be a ready-made nutritious meal waiting.

IMPROVING YOUR HEALTH
How healthy is your diet?

Take the time to think about your snacking habits. This will help you make a healthy choice.
- Do you eat high-fiber alternatives to chips like baked potatoes, brown rice, or pasta?
- Do you make burgers from lean ground beef or buy ready-made ones with added salt, fat, and sugar?
- Do you grill burgers or fry them?
- Do you snack on vegetables or fruit, rather than chips or cookies?

CAFFEINE – ARE YOU DRINKING TOO MUCH EACH DAY?

Caffeine is a stimulant that reduces fatigue and improves concentration. However, just three or four cups of tea a day may be enough to produce adverse effects, including tremors, irritability, restlessness, sleeping difficulties, anxiety, and diarrhea in some people. Reducing your caffeine intake gradually will help minimize withdrawal symptoms.

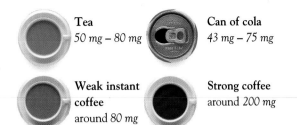

Tea
50 mg – 80 mg

Can of cola
43 mg – 75 mg

Weak instant coffee
around 80 mg

Strong coffee
around 200 mg

Caffeine levels in milligrams *(mg)* **per cup**

THE RIGHT CHOICE

Snacks can be healthy and nutritious, as well as tasty and easy to prepare. The quickest, and perhaps healthiest of all, is fruit. Plain, lightly-salted air-popped popcorn is another favorite. Sandwiches make more substantial snacks. Choose lean sandwich fillings such as tuna, low-fat cottage cheese, and chicken (without its skin). For something different, try some shredded vegetables with a low-fat salad dressing that adds taste not excess calories.

Raw vegetables
Carrots, celery sticks, cherry tomatoes, pepper rings, and cucumber slices may be eaten in a side salad, or as a low calorie snack between meals.

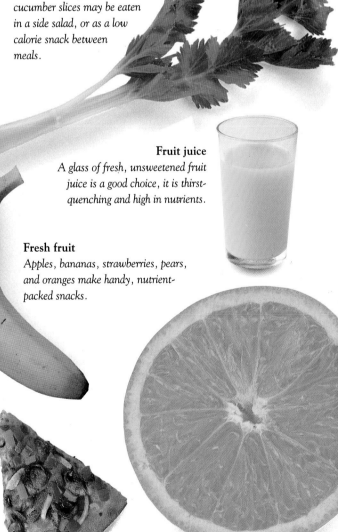

Fruit juice
A glass of fresh, unsweetened fruit juice is a good choice, it is thirst-quenching and high in nutrients.

Fresh fruit
Apples, bananas, strawberries, pears, and oranges make handy, nutrient-packed snacks.

Yogurt
A low-fat yogurt is a healthy dessert either on its own or with fruit.

Filling snacks
Pairing whole grain bread with salad makes a well-balanced snack. Whole wheat pizza is also a healthy choice.

MAKING THE RIGHT CHOICE

Eating out is very popular, but how healthy is the food other people prepare for us?

THE FOOD IN a restaurant may look and taste delicious, but much of it is high in calories and saturated fats, and low in fiber. For those who only eat out once in a while, overindulging on one meal can easily be corrected later; but if your social or business life involves dining out often your health could suffer if you do not choose carefully from the menu.

Many restaurants are aware of the growing public interest in diet and nutrition and have now adjusted their cooking by offering more low-fat meals. Some even offer a daily special for health-conscious diners. If you eat in restaurants several times a week, be sure to read the menu carefully so that you can choose the most nutritious dishes.

The healthy choice

Choosing healthy options from the menu does not have to spoil your enjoyment of eating out. There is certainly no need to cut out your favorite foods or to eat a monotonous diet of salads.

High-fat foods, not starches, are the real bane of a healthy diet. Butter, cream, cheese, and fatty meats are all rich in saturated fats and should be avoided for the sake of your heart and health. Starches such as whole grain bread, pasta, potatoes, and legumes provide nutrients and fiber and should make up the bulk of your diet.

For a main dish that is not too high in fat and calories, look for foods that have been poached, steamed, grilled, or stir-fried, and avoid those with rich, creamy sauces. Also, try not to eat unnecessary fat; remove the skin from poultry and do not choose fatty cuts of meat. Ask for vegetables that are not buttered or fried; opt for baked potatoes, these are lower in calories and high in starch. If you do choose a high-fat dish, cut down your fat intake the next day to balance out your diet.

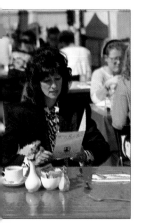

Time to think
Before you order, study the menu. Take into account both the ingredients and the preparation of each dish. Try to select a range of courses that are part of a balanced diet, and not too high in calories, fats, or sugar.

READING THE MENU

Here is a typical menu, with codes to indicate those dishes which are high in fats, sugar, and salt. The other foods on the menu are lower in these ingredients, and generally provide fewer calories. By studying this menu, you can learn to identify which dishes are high in fats, salt, or sugar, and thereby ensure that you always make the right choice for a healthy diet.

KEY
 High in fats   High in sugar   High in salt

menu

APPETIZERS

Fresh melon

Fried wonton
Served with sweet and sour sauce
 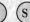

Chicken liver pâté
Served with melba toast
 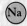

Gazpacho
A crunchy soup of blended tomatoes, cucumbers, garlic, green peppers, and onion, served chilled

Shrimp cocktail
Served with a spicy cocktail sauce on the side

◊

ENTRÉES

Baked chicken breast
Boneless breast of chicken baked in a delicate lemon basil sauce

Southern-style chicken
Fried to a crispy, golden brown
 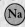

Beef en brochette
Skewered cubes of beef with fresh mushroom caps

Barbecued ribs
A hefty rack of broiled pork ribs smothered with hickory-smoked barbecue sauce

Fish and chips

Fresh filet of sole dipped in a special beer batter and deep-fried, served with french-fried potatoes

◊

VEGETABLES

French-fried potatoes

Herbed new potatoes

Creamy coleslaw

Garden fresh peas

Served with pearl onions

◊

DESSERTS

Fresh fruit sorbet

Assorted flavors

Poached pears

Served with raspberry glaze

Assorted fresh pastries

Rich, flaky pastries with assorted fillings

Apple dumpling

Whole apple baked in a flaky cinnamon pastry, topped with whipped cream and chopped pecans

Ice cream sundae

A rich French vanilla, topped with fudge sauce and whipped cream

Beware of calorie-rich cream

When you select a dessert, choose fresh or poached fruit. These are healthy alternatives as long as you do not smother them in calorie-laden toppings such as cream or ice cream. Fruit sorbets or yogurts are another light, tasty ending to a meal. Cream-filled cakes and rich flaky pastries should be reserved for treats or special occasions. Finally, do not forget that alcohol is high in calories, so only allow yourself to have one or two glasses of wine with your meal, at the most.

Restrict salt intake

Some people need to restrict their salt intake, because of high blood pressure or heart disease. As well as not adding salt to their food, they should only use small amounts of soy sauce, and other condiments, which are often high in sodium.

TIPS FOR EATING OUT

• To cut down on the amount you eat, ask whether it is possible to have only a half-portion.

• Choose one of the appetizers as a main course, or share a main dish with one of your companions.

• Choose clear soups rather than creamy ones that are high in fat.

• Make sure your vegetables are not going to be prepared with butter.

• To reduce your fat intake, always choose grilled, steamed, poached, or stir-fried foods.

• Ask for any rich or creamy sauce or dressing to be served on the side, so you can eat less.

• Ask for a low-fat salad dressing.

• If all the desserts on the menu are high in fat and sugar, ask for plain yogurt or a piece of fruit.

FOOD LABELS AND SHOPPING

While you are shopping, it is certainly worthwhile checking all food and drink labels carefully. Many processed and convenience foods contain large amounts of added fats, sugar, and salt. Just a few moments thought will enable you to choose the healthy products. You will generally discover that there are far healthier alternatives available nearby – that will not cost you any more.

• Always look for canned foods that do not have "added salt or sugar."

• If you do buy canned fruit, choose one that is prepared in "water or natural juices."

• Pick "low-calorie" soft drinks.

• Make sure your whole grain or bran cereal does not contain added sugar.

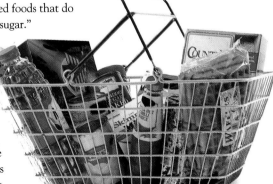

THE VEGETARIAN OPTION

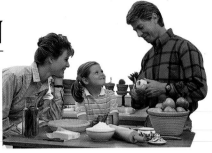

You do not need to eat meat to stay healthy; plants can provide all the nutrients you need and give extra protection against some diseases.

VEGETARIANS DO NOT eat meat or fish. Most vegetarians will eat some foods from animals, such as eggs and dairy produce, while excluding all types of meat and fish from their diet. If special care is taken to eat a wide variety of plant products, including cereals, nuts, and grains, vegetarians should get all the amino acids, vitamins, and minerals they need.

Are vegetarians healthier?
People who do not eat any meat are often healthier than those who do. They may have lower cholesterol levels and blood pressure readings, and so be less prone to heart disease.

The vegetarian diet is healthier because it is normally low in fat since it does not contain fatty cuts of meat. It is also richer in fiber from beans, legumes, and grains, which not only aids bowel function, but also reduces the absorption of fat and cholesterol from foods. A vegetarian diet usually has less sodium and more potassium, which may help to lower blood pressure.

But their diet may not be the only reason vegetarians are healthier. They may also tend to be more health conscious than meat eaters which will reduce their risk of high blood pressure and heart disease. They may extend their interest in health from the foods they eat to

Vegetarian children
A vegetarian diet may not provide enough calories for normal growth, so more dairy produce should be eaten to provide the extra energy needed.

other areas in their lives – exercising more, drinking less alcohol, and not smoking at all.

The vegan diet
Vegans are people who avoid all animal products including milk and eggs. They must be sure to eat a wide range of plant foods to avoid becoming deficient in basic nutrients. Even so, some may need extra vitamins and minerals.

DO VEGETARIANS NEED SUPPLEMENTS?

• Vegetarians who eat dairy products rarely need supplements.
• Vegans may need vitamin B12 supplements.
• Women who are pregnant or breast-feeding and eat a vegan diet will normally be advised to take a calcium supplement.

COOKING FOR A VEGETARIAN

A vegetarian in the family need not totally disrupt your cooking routine, or force you to prepare two different meals each evening.

• Prepare the same meat-free sauce for everyone; then divide it up, cooking one portion with meat, the other with lentils or beans.
• Serve baked potatoes with a choice of meat or vegetarian toppings.
• Keep healthy snacks, such as vegetarian burgers, in the freezer.
• Add vegetables to one part of a risotto and cooked meat or fish to the rest.
• Have at least one meat-free day each week, cooking more than you need, and freezing the left-overs in individual portions.

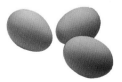
Eggs
Do not eat more than an egg a day. They are very high in cholesterol.

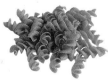
Brown pasta
Eat with beans for a complete protein.

Cottage cheese
Provides a low-fat protein source.

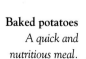
Baked potatoes
A quick and nutritious meal.

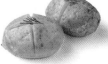

Tofu (bean curd)
High in protein but very low in fat.

Dried beans
High in protein, fiber, and iron.

MEATLESS MENUS

Having one meat-free day a week adds variety to your diet. Vegetarian foods are not only easy to prepare but are also healthy and nutritious. They tend to be lower in calories and fats, and higher in fiber.

The choice is wide. For lunch you could have a vegetable or bean soup, a meat-free sandwich with a cheese, cottage cheese, egg, tomato and lettuce, or cucumber filling; and fruit or yogurt to follow. For dinner, walnuts and mushrooms in a casserole make a combination that will please even meat eaters. It can be served with rice and vegetables.

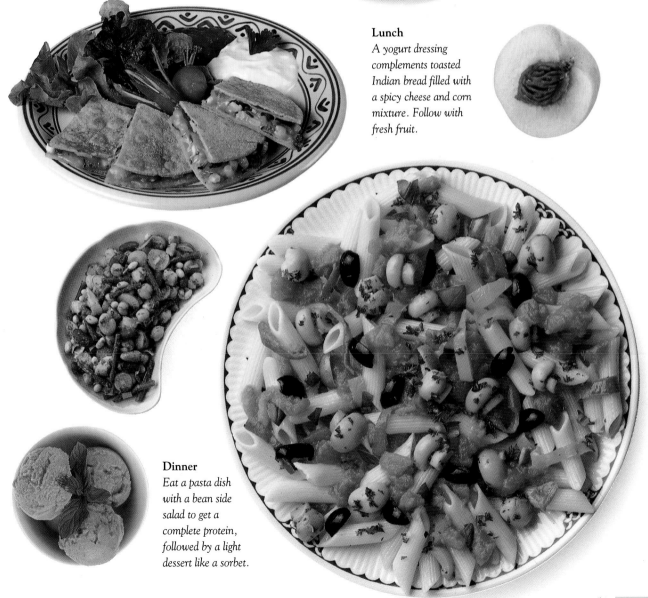

Breakfast
Choose bran flakes, skimmed milk, grapefruit, and coffee.

Lunch
A yogurt dressing complements toasted Indian bread filled with a spicy cheese and corn mixture. Follow with fresh fruit.

Dinner
Eat a pasta dish with a bean side salad to get a complete protein, followed by a light dessert like a sorbet.

FOOD SUPPLEMENTS

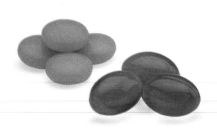

Most of us do not need supplements; a varied and balanced diet, containing plenty of fresh foods, gives us all the nutrients we need.

SOME PEOPLE WORRY that their diet is inadequate and take one of the many supplements on the market. These preparations contain one or more nutrients (vitamins, minerals, and carbohydrates) and are taken in addition to food. They are unlikely to improve your health, unless for some reason you have become deficient in a particular nutrient.

Who needs supplements?

Although doctors do not encourage the routine use of vitamin and mineral supplements, they might recommend them under certain circumstances, like pregnancy. Chronic illness or disease may also cause deficiencies. Only take supplements on medical advice, which may be based on blood tests that show a deficiency.

Poverty remains a cause of nutritional deficiencies. Sometimes, however, people do not eat well for other reasons, such as alcoholism, drug abuse, or mental illness.

Illness and supplements

Some stomach, intestinal, pancreatic, and liver disorders may lead to the impairment of the digestion or absorption of a particular nutrient. Persistent diarrhea can produce a deficiency in potassium and magnesium. Kidney diseases may also cause deficiencies. With any of these conditions, even if the underlying disorder cannot be treated, supplements can help supply all the nutrients that are needed.

Certain drugs may also interfere with the absorption or metabolism of a nutrient. The combined contraceptive pill increases the need for several B vitamins, vitamin C, and vitamin E, but these extra needs are easily met from a healthy diet. Some anticonvulsant drugs increase the need for vitamin D and folic acid. If you are on any long term medication, ask your doctor if you need a supplement.

Refined and processed foods

Eating a lot of processed or refined foods may cause a slight deficiency in a variety of nutrients, such as vitamins B6 and E, chromium, zinc, copper, and selenium. These deficiencies only show up in blood tests and rarely cause symptoms

The modern life-style with its stressful pace and emphasis on fast food means that many people rely on refined and processed foods

High-energy drinks

A sugary high energy drink may help keep your muscles supplied with glucose during prolonged exercise, such as running a marathon. However, for short exercise sessions, it is better to drink water to replace body fluids lost through perspiration.

The benefits of a balanced diet

Vitamin pills and other food supplements are no substitute for a well-balanced diet rich in fresh, unrefined foods. Even if supplements provide essential nutrients, they do not contain fiber which protects you from heart disease and some forms of cancer. If you are lacking nutrients, you should improve your diet rather than take supplements.

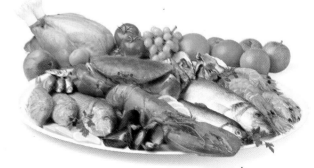

from which most of the nutrients have been lost. These lost nutrients may not be fully replaced even in foods that are later enriched with vitamins and minerals. The answer, however, is to eat a healthier diet, not to take supplements.

Time for a supplement?

Some healthy people may require supplements at specific times. Women who have heavy periods may lack iron. Changes in the digestive systems of the elderly due to aging may interfere with the absorption of certain nutrients.

Losing weight by going on crash diets may mean you are not getting enough nutrients. Even those on a long-term balanced low-calorie diet may need supplements. Food fads that involve a very low intake of food, or that restrict the types of food being eaten can also deprive the body of essential nutrients.

PROTEIN SUPPLEMENTS

Some athletes and body builders believe that extra amino acids, which are found in protein, will develop their muscle bulk and eat extra protein or take protein supplements. These efforts are likely to be futile as there is a limit to how much protein the body can use. Most supplements that contain specific amino acids have not been shown to increase muscle growth and development. Two amino acids, arginine and ornithine, do stimulate growth hormone production, and hence muscle growth, but only in dangerously high doses.

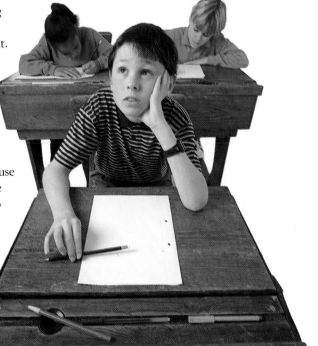

Building muscle

Most people, even body builders and athletes, eat more protein than their bodies can use. Excess protein is broken down in the liver and passed out of the body in the urine. Some is stored as fat.

CHILDREN AND VITAMINS

Healthy children eating a varied diet, containing fresh fruit and vegetables, bread, cereals, and dairy products, do not need a vitamin supplement. However, children who live on processed foods such as fries, chips, burgers, sweets, and canned drinks can become vitamin-deficient. Evidence is now being debated by scientists that a lack of vitamins in the diet can cause bad behavior and poor performance at school. The answer to this should lie in improving your children's diet, but if they refuse to eat more healthy food, the next best move is to give them a daily vitamin supplement.

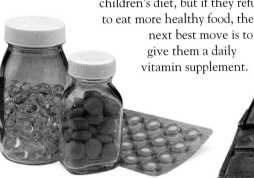

CURING NUTRIENT DEFICIENCIES

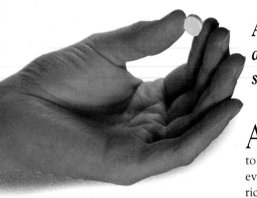

Although most people in the Western world have access to a good diet, nutrient deficiencies can still sometimes occur.

How to choose a supplement
Multi-vitamin and mineral preparations with a variety of nutrients in different doses and combinations are available. Some contain many times the recommended daily dose, so see a doctor before starting yourself, or your children, on a course of supplements. Supplements of only one vitamin or mineral may cause problems by increasing the demand for other nutrients.

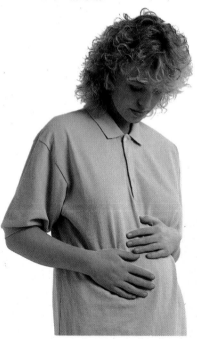

Supplements during pregnancy
The requirements for iron, folic acid, calcium, and other nutrients are higher in women who are pregnant or breast-feeding, which is why supplements are frequently recommended at this time.

A BALANCED DIET supplies all the nutrients that the body needs to function properly. However, not everyone eats a healthy diet that is rich in a wide variety of fresh, unprocessed foods. Some people suffer from illnesses which interfere with the absorption of nutrients, and this also leads to deficiencies.

Remember that it is always best to avoid supplements. They can cause vitamins to build up to toxic levels in the body, while some may even cause a deficiency by increasing the demand for other nutrients.

The traditional nutrient deficiency diseases such as scurvy (caused by a lack of vitamin C), rickets (due to a lack of vitamin D), and iodine-deficiency goitre, are now very rare in the West.

VITAMIN OVERDOSE

Taking too much of a vitamin or mineral can be dangerous. Vitamins that the body is able to store can build up to a toxic level. Vitamin A in excess may cause bone deformities in children and skin irritation with hair loss in adults. Very high doses have caused liver failure and death. Too much vitamin D can lead to an abnormal build up of calcium in the blood, causing nausea, vomiting, and muscle spasms. Excess vitamin B6 (pyridoxine) may damage nerves, resulting in numbness and weakness. Large doses of some minerals may cause side effects. Iron often causes diarrhea or constipation.

Not enough iron in the diet

Iron-deficiency anemia is the most common deficiency in the developed world. About one woman in every 10 has a mild form of this condition, while another three out of 10 are close to developing it. Men rarely lack this mineral.

Iron is used to make the oxygen-carrying pigment hemoglobin during the formation of red blood cells, so reserves may be rapidly used up through the need to replace a loss of blood. Women who have heavy periods can therefore drain their stores of iron within a few months. A lack of iron-containing foods in the diet is often a major contributory factor.

As a result of iron deficiency, the body's resistance to the effects of illness or injury are weakened, and in severe cases symptoms such as chest pain or breathlessness are caused. Generally, fatigue is the first noticeable sign of anemia.

Illness and anaemia

Anemia may also develop in response to a deficiency of either folic acid or vitamin B12. A lack of folic acid is normally the result of a poor diet or a prolonged illness. Vitamin B12 is found in many animal products; a deficiency is usually caused by a disorder of the stomach or intestine, which prevents the nutrient from being absorbed properly. Because the liver contains large stores of vitamin B12, it can take as long as three years for symptoms of anemia to appear.

SYMPTOMS OF THE MOST COMMON NUTRIENT DEFICIENCIES

Some doctors believe that many vague symptoms and minor skin problems are due to marginal deficiencies in one, or several nutrients, caused by eating a lot of processed foods or a highly restricted diet. Such deficiencies should be confirmed by your doctor before treatment is started. Other deficiencies may occur when the body is put under additional strain during pregnancy or breast-feeding. Older people too may risk incurring deficiencies from a poor diet or through changes in their digestive systems due to aging.

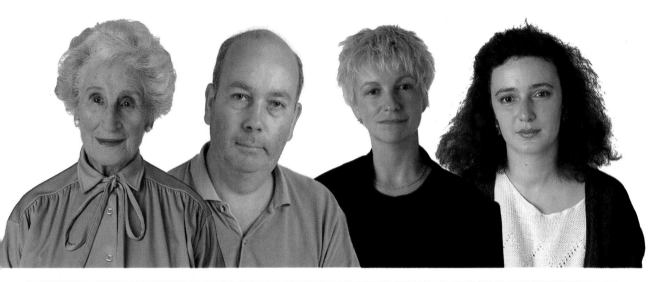

NUTRIENT	MAIN SOURCES	SYMPTOMS	PEOPLE AT RISK
Iron	Meat, eggs, whole grain cereals, and bread.	Tiredness, pale skin, sore mouth, and nail changes.	Those who eat a poor diet, women with heavy periods, and the elderly.
Calcium	Milk, dairy products, green vegetables, and fish with edible bones.	Increased risk of fractures in later life due to osteoporosis.	Needed during growth spurts, pregnancy, and breast-feeding.
Potassium	Bananas, oranges, vegetables, milk, and meat.	Weakness and palpitations.	Individuals with chronic diarrhea or taking some types of diuretic.
Zinc	Seafood, meat, nuts, and eggs.	Loss of appetite and delayed wound healing.	Those who eat a poor diet or a lot of processed foods.
Vitamin B2 (riboflavin)	Milk, liver, cheese, eggs, and whole grains.	Chapped lips and sore tongue.	Those who eat a poor diet or a lot of overcooked foods.
Folic acid	Peas, green leafy vegetables, nuts, mushrooms, and liver.	Reduced resistance to infection and fatigue.	Pregnant women or anyone with a prolonged illness.

FOOD ADDITIVES

A food additive is any substance put into food either to improve its color, texture, flavor, or to help keep it fresh longer – but are they safe to eat?

ALTHOUGH SOME PEOPLE are wary of food additives, without them many of our favorite foods could not be eaten. In the modern world it is just not possible for everyone to eat all their foods fresh from a garden or farm. Without the use of additives, certain foods would begin to spoil after just a day or two of storage, due to contamination from bacteria, yeasts, or molds. Some additives, therefore, protect us from food poisoning.

Many additives are in fact naturally occurring substances; salt, saffron, turmeric, vitamin C, and lecithin are common examples. Others are synthetic copies of a natural substance that are produced in a pure, highly concentrated form, such as riboflavin and ascorbic acid. However, the majority of additives are now produced artificially in the laboratory. These include tartrazine and artificial sweeteners such as saccharin and aspartame. All these

SECRET INGREDIENTS OF PROCESSED FOODS

This commercially-prepared cheesecake mix is a good example of how food additives may be used in the preparation of a processed food. The ingredients list includes at least one of each different type of additive.

Preservatives
Without adding a preservative, many foods would begin to spoil within a day or two of storage. Citric acid has been included in this mix to help the cheesecake stay fresh. The most common preservatives added to processed foods are nitrates and sulphites.

Flavorings
The cheesecake mix contains both natural and artificial flavorings. Manufacturers tend to prefer artificial flavorings, because of their reduced moisture content and greater stability at high temperatures.

Antioxidants
To stop the fat in the cheesecake turning rancid, a common synthetic antioxidant, butylated hydroxyanisole, has been added to the mix.

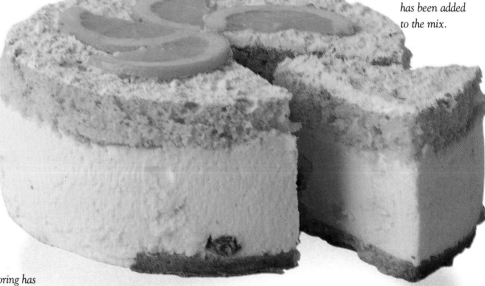

Colorings
An artificial yellow coloring has been added to the mix to help make the cheesecake look more attractive. Colorings are also used in foods to put back color lost during processing. Many food colorings are natural pigments, for example beetroot red, saffron, turmeric, and cochineal.

Emulsifiers
Prepared from soy beans, hydroxylated lecithin is just one of several different emulsifiers used in this cheesecake. Like all emulsifiers its purpose is to stop the fat and water within the food from separating, and thus ruining the dish.

Thickeners
Thickeners are added to food to improve its texture. In this cheesecake, sodium phosphates have been used as thickeners. The most popular types are produced from plant material, for example pectin, methylcellulose, and guar gum.

substances have their own code numbers and these must be clearly printed in the list of ingredients on the food label.

Are additives harmful?

All additives undergo rigorous testing. Any additive that produces harmful side-effects is prohibited. For every substance, a safety level is established which must never be exceeded by the manufacturer. This safety level is set well below the amount known to be safe in humans assuming they eat reasonable quantities of the food it is in.

Additives and cancer

Research into the relationship between diet and specific diseases has suggested that as many as 35 percent of all cancers may in fact be associated with diet. But the foods suspected of being harmful are "natural," such as smoked meats and alcohol. Food additives are not thought to contribute significantly to the incidence of cancer.

Preservatives that inhibit the formation of molds may actually help prevent cancer, since mold has been associated with an increased risk of developing cancer of the stomach and the esophagus. Antioxidants may help prevent certain other types of cancer.

Additives and hyperactivity

Common food additives, such as the yellow coloring tartrazine, are sometimes blamed for causing hyperactivity in children. A small number of children do seem to develop allergic reactions to certain additives, that in some cases may dramatically alter their behavior. However, for the majority of hyperactive children, there is not yet any scientifically proven link between the additives within their diet and their condition.

IRRADIATION OF FOOD

Food irradiation is a new processing technique that prolongs the shelf life of many foods. Bombarding the food with a specified dose of gamma rays destroys bacteria, molds, insects, and any other parasites. Irradiation also slows down the ripening process and the sprouting of vegetables. Some countries only recommend the irradiation of certain types of food, such as poultry and prawns, to reduce the risk of food poisoning. Other countries prohibit irradiation and the import of any irradiated foods.

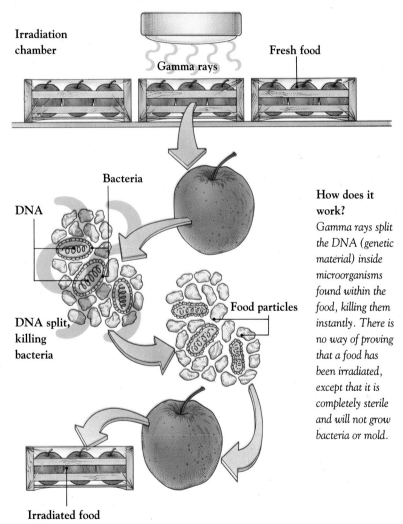

Irradiation chamber

Gamma rays

Fresh food

Bacteria

DNA

DNA split, killing bacteria

Food particles

Irradiated food

How does it work?
Gamma rays split the DNA (genetic material) inside microorganisms found within the food, killing them instantly. There is no way of proving that a food has been irradiated, except that it is completely sterile and will not grow bacteria or mold.

IS IRRADIATION SAFE?

Food that has been irradiated is not radioactive and radiation does not alter the flavor or appearance of most products. However, the process may destroy the vitamin content of some foods. The effect of irradiation on additives in food has not yet been fully established.

FOOD FOR LIFE

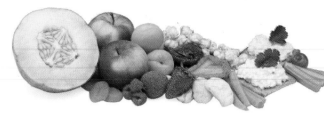

From birth through to old age, the food you eat is an important factor in keeping you fit and healthy.

A GOOD DIET IS an essential part of a healthy lifestyle. It is just as important to eat properly whether you are a growing child, a fully grown adult, a pregnant woman, or past retirement age. The nutrients in your diet keep your cells working properly and your tissues and organs well maintained and in good repair. If you neglect your diet, your health is likely to suffer.

Feeding your baby

Breast-feeding is best for your baby because it helps to protect against infection and bonds mother and infant. Nutritionally, however, both human milk and commercial formulas provide all your baby needs in the first few weeks of life. If you bottle-feed, take care not to over-feed your baby, otherwise there is a risk of him or her becoming over-weight. Formula milk is higher in fat and calories than breast milk.

Growing children

There is no nutritional or medical advantage to introducing solid foods before your child is four months old. Doctors recommend weaning babies onto solids once they are able to sit up with support and have good control of their head and neck. At around this time, your baby's ability to chew and swallow will be sufficiently developed and the digestive system mature enough to cope with foods other than breast or formula milk.

The first foods you give your baby should be bland, have a soft, moist texture, and be free of lumps. Do not add salt or sugar to your baby's food and introduce only one new food every 24 hours, in case it disagrees with your baby. A good first choice is a single grain cereal followed by pureed fruit or vegetables.

The key to establishing healthy eating habits for your children is to introduce many different types of food by the age of 12 months to help set the pattern for a diversified diet later in life. Do not force your children to eat foods they do not like or to eat more than they want to as it can cause obesity and eating problems.

A family affair

Eating is not just a way of consuming the nutrients that build cells and repair tissues, it is also an integral part of our social and family life. Healthy eating should be a pleasure.

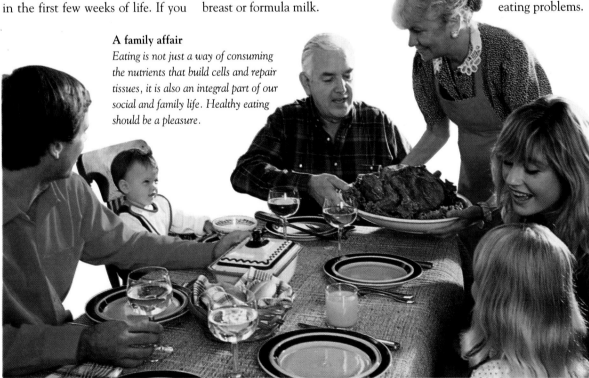

Pregnancy

Careful attention to diet is vital during pregnancy, both for the sake of the mother's health and the health of her baby. Ideally, to give all babies the best possible start in life, every woman should be eating a healthy diet even before becoming pregnant.

To provide for the growth of the baby and the placenta and to allow changes such as the formation of new tissue in the uterus and breasts to take place, nutritional requirements for calories, protein, vitamins, and minerals all increase.

How to balance your diet during pregnancy

Pregnant women should increase their energy intake by only about 300 Calories a day while they are pregnant. This increase should not just come from high-calorie, low-in-nutrient snacks, such as cakes and cookies. What is needed is an increased consumption of unrefined carbohydrates, such as fresh fruit and vegetables and whole grain breads and cereals which are high in fiber, vitamins, and minerals; as well as more low-fat, high-protein foods, like skimmed milk and low-fat cheese or yogurt which also contain calcium.

A woman of average height and weight should gain about 25-30 lbs (11-14 kg) during pregnancy. But, even if a pregnant woman puts on more weight than this, if she has been sticking to a healthy diet, all the excess should come off once the baby is born.

A healthy start
Breast milk is the ideal food for your baby. To be sure that your baby is getting the best, you must eat well yourself.

Breast-feeding

Nutritional requirements for energy, protein, vitamins, and minerals increase in women who are breast-feeding. Again, these increased needs can be met by eating a well-balanced diet. As your baby grows, the amount of milk consumed increases. For example, by the time your baby is four months old, your body needs an extra 500 Calories a day to produce enough milk. You will also need more of some vitamins and minerals, such as vitamin C and calcium. Remember to drink more to replace the fluid used in the production of breast milk.

Good eating habits for a lifetime

Every adult needs to eat a balanced, varied diet. Fresh fruit and vegetables, and whole grain breads and cereals will provide you with fibre and essential nutrients,

The right choice
Shopping for food involves more than just selecting what you want. You must also choose what is good for you: fresh foods are best, but reading the labels on processed foods will help you choose those without added salt, sugar, or saturated fats.

offering protection against heart disease and some cancers. Do not eat too much saturated fat as it increases the level of cholesterol in your blood, clogging your arteries.

As we age, our metabolism slows down. Older people also tend to be less active. Eating the same amount of food will therefore cause weight gain. The elderly need to reduce their calorie intake, particularly by cutting consumption of foods that are rich in saturated fats, to avoid becoming obese.

Much illness in old age is either brought on, or made worse, by eating poorly. Some elderly people live on crackers, soup, toast, and tea. These foods are easy to prepare but lacking in vitamins, minerals, and fiber. Meals on wheels, some useful kitchen aids and gadgets, or help with cooking and shopping can improve their diet.

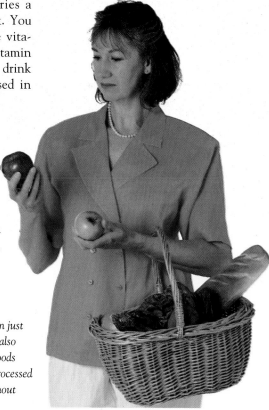

NUTRITION DURING
PREGNANCY AND BREAST-FEEDING

FROM THE MOMENT the fertilized egg implants into the wall of the uterus, your baby depends entirely on you for nourishment, so the nutritional state of your own body is very important.

After the first few weeks of pregnancy, you will need about 300 more Calories per day. There is also a need for additional protein throughout your pregnancy. These extra calories and protein provide for the normal growth of the fetus and

Eating a healthy diet from before you conceive until after you stop breast-feeding will give your baby the best possible start in life.

placenta. They are also used to lay down new tissues, for example in the breasts in preparation for feeding your baby.

Pregnancy and nutrient needs
Every mother-to-be needs more of specific vitamins and minerals. For example, almost twice as much

calcium is required during pregnancy while the baby's teeth and skeletal system are being formed.

To get extra calories, protein, and vitamins, without extra weight, you must make the most of what you eat. Low-fat protein sources, such as skimmed milk, cottage cheese, fish, and chicken add

GETTING THE MOST FROM YOUR FOOD

Eating a variety of fresh, unprocessed foods should ensure that you get all the nutrients you need during pregnancy.

The vitamins and minerals listed below are required in greater amounts to help in the growth and development of your baby.

NUTRIENT	FOOD SOURCES	FUNCTIONS
Calcium	Low-fat dairy products such as skimmed milk, fish with edible bones, and nuts.	Development of baby's bones and teeth.
Iron	Lean red meat, whole wheat bread, dried fruit, and green leafy vegetables. Iron tablets may be prescribed.	Formation of blood cells in mother and baby's circulation.
Vitamin C	Fresh fruit and vegetables.	Formation of strong, healthy placenta. Aids absorption of iron.
Folic acid	Green leafy vegetables, nuts, and whole wheat bread. A supplement may be prescribed.	Development of baby's nervous system.
Zinc	Lean meat, whole grain cereals, whole wheat bread, and seafood.	Growth of baby's tissues.

protein and calories to your diet, with little fat. Snack on nutritious foods like fresh fruit.

Constipation can be a problem, but do not try to solve it by adding bran to your diet. Bran can interfere with the absorption of essential nutrients. Instead, eat more fresh fruit and vegetables which are not only a good source of fiber, but full of vitamins and minerals too.

Nutrition and breast-feeding

To produce breast milk, your body requires extra calories. The quality of your milk depends on eating healthy foods. Ideally you will need to consume greater amounts of a number of vitamins and minerals, such as niacin, iron, riboflavin, zinc, thiamine, and vitamins A, C, and E. Also, you need to drink at least six pints of fluid a day while you are breast-feeding, to maintain your body's water balance.

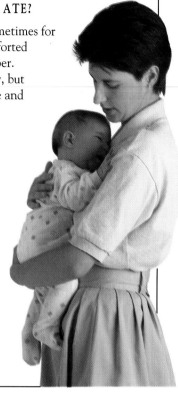

COLIC – WAS IT SOMETHING YOU ATE?

A baby with colic cries inconsolably, sometimes for more than an hour, and will not be comforted with a feed, a cuddle, or a change of diaper. During an attack, the baby looks healthy, but seems to be in pain, going red in the face and drawing up his or her legs.

Colic normally starts at around three weeks and continues until the baby is three to four months old. Attacks are typically more severe in the evening.

If you are still breast-feeding, and your baby is suffering from regular attacks of colic, you may be advised to cut out certain foods from your diet, for example:

- Milk and dairy foods – substitute soy bean products
- Eggs
- Citrus fruit
- Coffee – try drinking camomile tea
- Foods containing wheat products

FOODS TO AVOID

In the same way that essential nutrients from your food cross the placenta into your baby's bloodstream, so may other substances that can be potentially harmful, such as alcohol, caffeine, food poisoning bacteria, and excessive amounts of vitamin A.

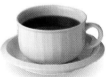

Caffeine
passes into breast milk and may make your baby irritable.

Liver
contains high levels of vitamin A which have been linked with miscarriage and birth defects.

Soft and blue-veined cheeses
may contain listeria, bacteria which can cause miscarriage, stillbirth, and meningitis.

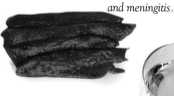

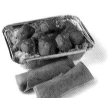

Leftover foods
that are not reheated properly may contain listeria and other food poisoning bacteria that could harm your baby.

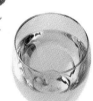

Alcohol,
even in tiny amounts, may cause birth defects or mental retardation, so it is better not to drink at all.

PREVENTING MORNING SICKNESS

Nausea and vomiting is a common problem in early pregnancy brought on by hormonal changes inside your body. Do not worry, it will not cause any harm to your baby, who will continue to take all the nourishment he or she needs. Check with your doctor before you take any anti-sickness drug, as drugs may pass through the placenta and affect your baby. Only rarely is morning sickness bad enough to need treatment in hospital. Self-help measures include:

- Eat small, regular meals.
- Suck hard candies if you feel sick.
- Drink ginger or mint teas.
- Avoid greasy foods.
- Do not go too long without eating.
- Try eating a piece of dry toast or a cracker before getting up.

FEEDING YOUR BABY

Milk, whether human or formula, is the fuel that makes your baby grow more quickly during the first year than at any other time.

By the age of six months, most babies will have doubled their birth weight. Whether you choose to breast-feed or bottle-feed, both human and formula milk provide the right nutrients for the first months of life, with just the right balance of carbohydrates, proteins, fats, vitamins, and minerals.

If your baby is born prematurely or has a low birth weight, additional nutrients may be required. Vitamins can be added to breast milk that has been expressed by the mother, before giving it to the baby; or formula milk can be enriched with extra vitamins. Ask your doctor if you need to do this.

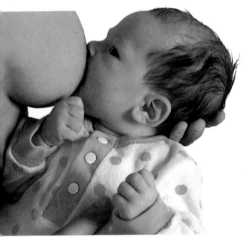

Latching on
Babies take the whole nipple into their mouths and "milk" the breast with their jaws, making their temples and ears move.

BREAST-FEEDING

Human milk provides the perfect balance of nutrients. It also contains antibodies from the mother: special proteins that protect the baby against gastrointestinal and respiratory infections and against allergies. Breast milk is always available – already sterile and at the right temperature. The physical contact between mother and baby also encourages bonding. Breast-fed babies are also less likely to become overweight due to excessive feeding. Mothers who breast-feed find it easier to return to their prepregnancy body weight.

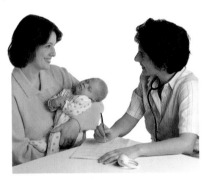

• Check with your doctor before taking any medication.
• Do not let a hungry baby cry as he or she will become distressed and unable to feed properly. Always offer your breast first when your baby cries.
• You may need a pillow on your lap to raise your baby's head to the right level.

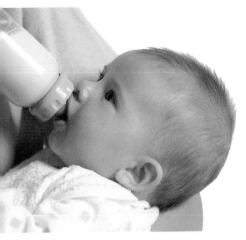

Giving a bottle
Cuddle your baby close to you in a semi-upright position: let your baby decide when he or she has had enough.

BOTTLE-FEEDING

Bottle-feeding lets you see how much your baby is drinking, which some mothers find reassuring.

Commercial formulas contain all the right nutrients in the right proportions. It is essential that the formula be made up according to the instructions on the packet. Both powder and water must be measured exactly. Do not pack the powder down; level it with a knife. Adding extra powder to the water is not good for your baby.

When bottle-feeding, always cuddle and talk to the baby. This is especially important if the mother herself is not feeding the baby.

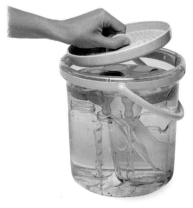

• Bacteria thrive in milk. Clean and sterilize all equipment between feedings.
• Make up the bottle following the instructions on the packet exactly.
• Do not add milk powder, cereal, sugar, or baby rusks to a formula.

FEEDING PROBLEMS

- **Sore or cracked nipples**. Wash nipples with water, not soap, which can dry out the skin. Try an emollient cream, an antiseptic spray, or a nipple shield.
- **Mastitis**. If your breast is inflamed and painful, you may have an infection. Antibiotics will stop an abscess forming. You can usually continue feeding.

- **Blocked milk duct**. A hard, tender red lump may be a blocked milk duct. Bathe your breast in hot water, massage the lump gently, and then try to give a feeding. If it does not clear, see your doctor.
- **Vomiting**. Regurgitation of a little milk is normal. See your doctor if a lot of milk is brought up after most feedings.

- **Poor feeding**. If you are worried that your baby is not getting enough milk, weigh him or her every two or three days.
- **Prolonged crying after a feed**. Ask your doctor or health visitor for advice if your baby cries after a feeding. It may be colic.
- **Engorgement**. Express excess milk if your breasts feel hard and painfully full.

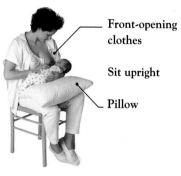

Front-opening clothes

Sit upright

Pillow

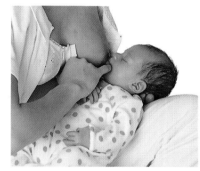

- Wear loose, front-opening clothes or two-piece outfits with tops you can pull up. A nursing bra can give support.
- Sit in an upright position with your back well-supported during a feeding.
- Relax your shoulders.
- Allow 10 minutes per breast. Milk at the end of a feeding has more calories.

- To take your baby off the breast, put your finger between mouth and breast.
- Use the other breast first the next time you feed your baby.
- Increase your fluid and calorie intake while you are breast-feeding.
- Do not breast-feed lying down. You might fall asleep and roll onto the baby.

HOW TO STOP BREAST-FEEDING

Your body's system of milk production takes time to wind down, so you need to stop feeding gradually to allow your body time to adjust.

- Drop one feed at a time; leave three days before dropping the next.
- Do not stop breast-feeding abruptly, unless you really have to.
- Try not to express to relieve the full feeling; expressing just stimulates milk production. Your milk will be gradually reabsorbed over the following few days.

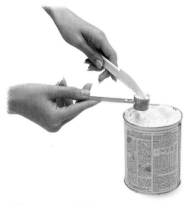

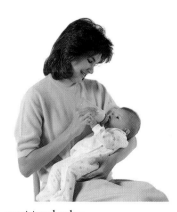

COW'S MILK

Untreated cow's milk is unsuitable for babies because it contains high concentrations of minerals, such as potassium and sodium, which the baby's immature kidneys would find difficult to process. It also contains a form of protein that babies cannot digest, which provides less nutrients than the protein found in human and formula milks. Cow's milk has little carbohydrate. It can be introduced gradually from nine months, unless there is a history of asthma, eczema, or allergies.

- Do not overfeed your baby. Every 24 hours, give your baby about 2½ fl oz of milk per 1lb of body weight (150 ml per kg).
- Do not warm formulas in the microwave. This may alter their

nutritional value.
- Discard leftover milk after a feeding.
- Do not tilt the bottle too much as the baby may choke. The hole in the nipple should not be too small or the baby will have to suck too hard.

FEEDING A GROWING CHILD

Establish healthy eating habits by offering the right foods at the right time and keeping meal times relaxed and happy.

HEALTHY FOODS FOR CHILDREN

• Give your child a varied diet with lots of fresh foods.
• Avoid too many processed foods, which are high in fat and sugar.
• Do not add salt, sugar, or spices to your child's food.
• Offer healthy snacks between meals, not sweets or cookies.
• If you give your child sweets, opt for those that can be eaten quickly and offer them at the end of a meal.
• Serve diluted fruit juices or water at meal times.
• Provide skimmed milk or water to drink between meals, not sweetened drinks that encourage tooth decay.

WHEN YOUR BABY is around six months old, start by offering three to four tablespoons of savory food. Only give more when, and if, that is eaten. Finish by trying about two tablespoons of pudding. Do not worry if your baby eats very little on some days, as long as he or she continues to put on weight.

Once your child is eating the same foods as the rest of the family, offer a variety of foods during the week. Never force your child to eat anything he or she does not like or to finish everything on the plate.

Avoiding feeding problems
The secret of avoiding problems at meal times is for you to try and remain relaxed, patient, and friendly.

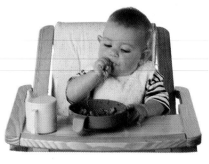

Only the best
Home-made is best, but if you do buy baby foods be sure they do not contain sugar (dextrose or sucrose) or salt.

Letting your child join you at the table from an early age teaches important social skills, even if the noise and mess give you indigestion. If your child finds meal times a stimulating and entertaining experience, you are much less likely to encounter feeding problems in the future.

Spending a long time preparing a meal just for your child can make you feel upset if it is refused. Keep children's meals simple and do not force your child to eat any particular food. Just try something different the next time. The key to a healthy diet is variety; fresh fruit and vegetables, milk, bread, and cereals should easily provide all the necessary nutrients.

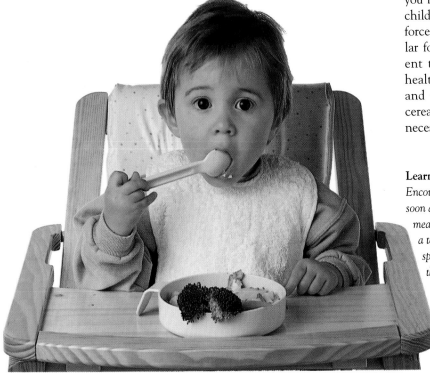

Learning to use a spoon
Encourage your baby to use a spoon as soon as he or she wants to, even if the meal does take a lot longer and makes a terrible mess. You can go on offering spoonfuls, while your baby plays with the food or holds another spoon.

Never try to persuade your child to eat more than he or she wants. A child who is growing normally is eating enough. Rewarding your child for eating something he or she does not like is unwise because it is likely to make your child become difficult about eating other foods or trying new tastes.

What about snacks?

Children burn up a lot of calories as a result of being active all day, so they often ask for something to eat between meals. It is better to offer nutritious snacks such as carrot sticks, fruit, or raisins, rather than ice cream, cookies, or sweets, which are high in sugar.

NUTS

You should never give a young child whole nuts to eat – particularly peanuts. Children can very easily choke on a small piece of the nut or even inhale it, which can cause a severe type of pneumonia.

THE FIRST TWELVE MONTHS

Begin offering adult food at three to six months. Try each new food on its own, then wait 24 hours to see how your child reacts. If it causes diarrhea, sickness, or a rash, avoid that food for a few months. It is normal to see a little undigested food in the diaper.

Moisten pureed, mashed, or minced foods with boiled water, breast or formula milk, or cooking liquid. Never add salt, sugar, or spices – your baby will not mind the bland taste. Cows' milk is not recommended for children under nine months, due to the risk of allergy.

4 – 6 months
Pureed or sieved foods which are bland, smooth, and free of any lumps are best. Wash and peel fruit and vegetables; remove pits and string; boil or steam.

6 – 8 months
Introduce foods that are minced or mashed to the texture of cottage cheese. Moisten with breast or formula milk, boiled water, or liquid from the cooking. Trim all visible fat and skin from meat or fish, then grill or poach, and mince. Boil eggs for at least seven minutes, and mash. Start finger foods.

8 – 10 months
Introduce chunkier textures. Chop up food rather than mashing or mincing. Give small pieces of stewed meat. Finger foods such as apple, peach, and apricot improve feeding skills. Hard foods like celery or carrots aid teething.

10 – 12 months
Your child is now eating most foods, chopped up into manageable pieces. Remove the skin from tomatoes. Do not add salt or spices to the food – salt your own at the table. Offer new foods one at a time – this will let your child experience new tastes and textures.

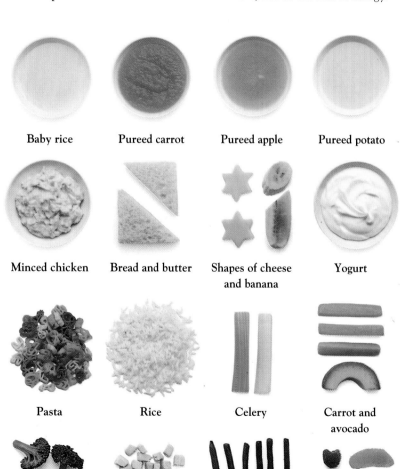

Baby rice   Pureed carrot   Pureed apple   Pureed potato

Minced chicken   Bread and butter   Shapes of cheese and banana   Yogurt

Pasta   Rice   Celery   Carrot and avocado

Steamed broccoli   Chicken   Green beans   Fresh fruit

HEALTHY EATING IN LATER LIFE

LIKE OTHER TYPES of machine, the human body begins to work less efficiently as it gets older. But health problems are not an inevitable part of aging. Adapting your eating habits to compensate for the changes in your body that occur as a normal part of growing older can help you stay fit and well.

Changes in metabolism

Many people put on weight as they age because of a natural reduction in their basal metabolic rate, the energy used by the body to maintain all the vital body functions. Your basal metabolic rate will normally be about one quarter less at

One important way of avoiding illness as you grow older is to continue to eat a healthy diet.

age 75 than it would have been in your mid-twenties, so less energy is burned when you are at rest as you age. Weigh yourself regularly. If you are gaining or losing weight for no reason, see your doctor.

To avoid putting on weight, you should reduce your daily intake of calories or, better still, increase your level of physical activity to burn off those excess calories. But many elderly people do not adjust their calorie intake, even if they

become less active after retirement. Obesity is a common problem among the elderly as a result.

Nutrient deficiency

The diets of some older people are lacking in both variety and balance. Because it is difficult to get to the shops, there is a tendency to stock up on processed and canned products instead of buying fresh foods regularly. Lack of motivation or some form of physical disability,

SIMPLE STEPS TO A HEALTHIER DIET

Healthy eating can begin at any age, but it is especially important for older people. A poor diet can cause vitamin deficiencies or even general malnutrition, which

increases the risk of illness. The healthiest diet contains lots of fresh fruit and vegetables, whole grain bread, cereals, and pasta, a moderate amount of protein, and a small amount of fat.

- Eat plenty of fresh fruit and lightly cooked vegetables.
- Choose unrefined starchy foods, such as whole grain bread and cereals, brown rice, and potatoes.
- Avoid processed foods, which contain a lot of fat or sugar.
- Pick low-fat dairy products. They provide just as many vitamins and minerals, but much less saturated fat.
- Eat fish and poultry – they are rich in protein and low in saturated fat.
- Cut down on fried foods and use vegetable oils, rather than butter or lard in your cooking.
- Drink at least 8 cups of fluid a day. This will help prevent constipation.

Variety is the spice of life
Turn to some of the many cookbooks that feature health-conscious recipes for help in changing your diet.

such as arthritis, are other reasons why an elderly person may rely too heavily on convenience foods.

Although lack of money is sometimes blamed, a balanced diet containing lots of fresh foods should actually cost less than processed and convenience foods. The problem is often a practical one of who is going to buy, prepare, and cook a meal for an elderly person, who cannot, or will not, do it.

Improving your diet

Eating a balanced and varied diet is even more important as you age. Avoid processed foods containing added fat or sugar. Unrefined foods, like fruit, vegetables, brown rice, potatoes, and whole grain bread are a valuable source of fiber, vitamins, and minerals. They prevent constipation which is a common problem in the elderly. Drinking plenty of fluids will help keep your bowel functioning normally.

COMMON NUTRIENT DEFICIENCIES IN THE ELDERLY

Nutrient deficiency can lead to anemia and other deficiency diseases. Calcium deficiency is a common problem which leads to osteoporosis, but it cannot be corrected in later life by eating calcium-rich foods. The risk of osteoporosis is influenced by the diet eaten before the age of 35.

NUTRIENT	CAUSE	CURING THE DEFICIENCY
Vitamin C	Lack of fresh fruit and vegetables.	Eat more fresh fruit and vegetables.
Vitamin D	Lack of sunlight if housebound.	Eat oily fish (sardines, herring, and tuna), eggs, and margarine.
Iron	Impaired absorption, due to aging of the digestive system. Anemia.	Eat liver, meat, fish, whole grain cereals, and green leafy vegetables.
Thiamine	Increased requirement with aging.	Choose whole grain cereals, whole wheat bread, brown rice, liver, fish, beans, and nuts.

MAKING FOOD PREPARATION EASIER

The majority of older people do not need kitchen aids. For others, however, even such simple gadgets as large-handled cutlery can ensure their continued ability to live independent lives.

Arthritis is one common ailment that can make opening jars and turning on taps difficult, if not impossible. Specially designed gadgets can help with many such tasks in the kitchen.

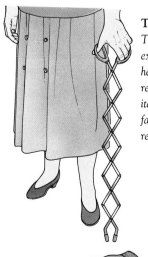

Tongs
These extending tongs help in the retrieval of any item that has fallen out of reach.

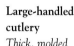

Tap turner
This device helps people grip and turn on taps more easily.

Large-handled cutlery
Thick, molded handles on different items of cutlery make them easier to hold and manipulate.

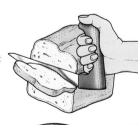

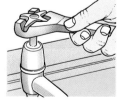

Jar opener
Stubborn lids can be opened more easily with a specially designed jar opener.

Can opener
Everyday objects like can openers can be adapted for use by the elderly.

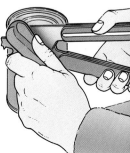

FOOD AND GOOD HEALTH

All the evidence suggests that diet does influence your health, even preventing heart disease and some cancers; it is therefore wise to make sure that your diet is low in fats and sugar and high in fiber.

THERE IS NO DOUBT at all that poor eating habits can harm your health. Studies comparing the incidence of various diseases among different populations that have their own characteristic diets have established that a number of medical conditions are associated with eating too much, or too little, of certain types of food.

What is a healthy diet?
A healthy diet promotes good health and reduces the risk of contracting any diet-related diseases. It contains the widest possible variety of natural foods and provides a good balance of carbohydrates, fats, protein, fiber, vitamins, and minerals. In addition, the number of calories in a healthy diet should not normally exceed the amount of energy expended, which should then keep body weight relatively constant. Obesity puts people at greater risk of suffering from a stroke, diabetes, coronary heart disease, and osteoarthritis.

How diet can prevent disease
In developed countries, deficiency diseases such as scurvy, rickets, and beri-beri are extremely rare. Dietary problems in the Western world do not usually come from a lack of essential nutrients but from overconsumption of food. The pendulum has swung the other way and many common disorders are the result of consuming more food than you need, or too much of the wrong sorts of food.

Is your family eating a healthy diet?
To give your family a healthy diet, extend the range of foods they eat to include more fresh fruit and vegetables, whole grain breads, and nuts. Try to cut down on those foods that are high in calories and low in essential nutrients, such as cookies, cakes, soft drinks, and alcohol.

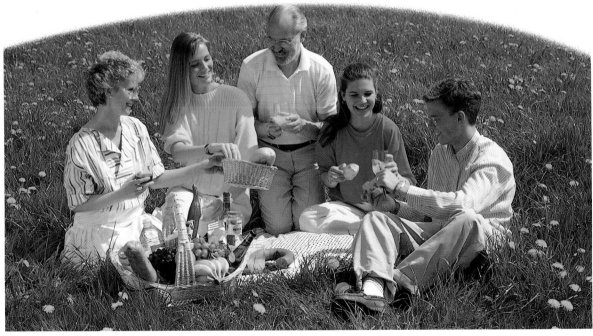

In the West, however, a number of conditions do still exist that are caused by the lack of a particular nutrient. The high incidence of osteoporosis in women after menopause would certainly be reduced in the future if young women increased their consumption of calcium-rich foods, such as sardines or other fish with edible bones and dairy products, particularly while they are pregnant or breast-feeding.

Diet and cancer

Comparing the various types and rates of cancer in different populations in different countries around the world suggests that diet is a crucial factor. Too much fat may lead to the development of cancer of the bowel and of the breast, while moldy foods are suspected of being a cause of cancer in the liver and the esophagus.

The role of fiber

Fiber is not an essential nutrient, but it does play an important role in preventing many disorders. The lack of fiber in the typical Western diet is a major contributory factor not only in many digestive disorders, such as hemorrhoids, constipation, and diverticulosis, but also in more serious conditions like coronary heart disease, bowel cancer, diabetes, and obesity.

Setting a balance

The occasional unhealthy meal is not going to hurt you. It is your regular diet that determines the state of your health. You are at risk of developing a number of serious medical problems if you consistently consume excessive amounts of fats, particularly saturated fats, and refined carbohydrates; if you exceed your daily energy requirements; or if your diet is lacking in vital elements such as fiber.

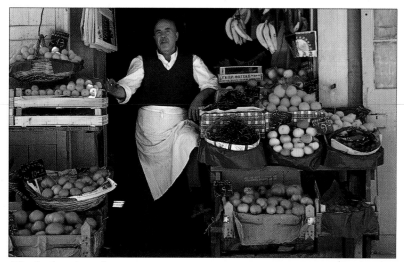

The freshest ingredients
Fruit, vegetables, and fish are central to the Mediterranean diet. They ensure that it is high in vitamins, minerals, and fiber, but also low in fat and sugar.

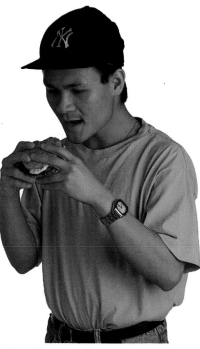

Your diet can influence your future health
Our fast-food culture encourages a high incidence of certain diet-related diseases. Foods that are high in saturated fats or refined sugar and low in fiber, increase the risk of obesity, heart disease, and cancer of the bowel.

THE MEDITERRANEAN DIET

The Mediterranean diet comes highly recommended both by nutritionists and doctors. This is because the typical dishes contain a perfect balance of protein, fats, and carbohydrates, with a good supply of fiber and essential vitamins and minerals.

• Protein sources, which include fish and other seafoods and lean meats such as chicken, goat, and veal, all contain low amounts of saturated fat.
• Cooking is done mainly in vegetable oil, while mayonnaise and salad dressings are prepared using olive oil. Much of the fat in the Mediterranean diet is therefore unsaturated and will not raise blood cholesterol levels.
• Very little carbohydrate is eaten in the form of refined sugar. Most of it comes from unrefined starchy foods such as rice, pasta, dried beans, potatoes, and lentils, which are rich in fiber and essential nutrients.
• Large amounts of fresh fruit and vegetables are eaten in the typical Mediterranean diet. This boosts the daily consumption of vitamins, minerals, and fiber.

EATING FOR A HEALTHY HEART

Heart disease accounts for about one third of all adult deaths, but dietary changes would help prevent it.

ONE OF THE MAIN reasons why Americans have a much higher incidence of heart disease than the populations living in most other countries around the world is our unhealthy diet. Most deaths from heart disease are the result of coronary heart disease, a condition in which deposits of fat build up on the lining of the arteries that supply blood to the heart muscle.

Studies comparing the rates of heart disease between countries with different eating habits show clearly that those people who eat a high-fat, low-fiber diet have a much greater risk of developing coronary heart disease.

Public education can change an unhealthy diet. Many Americans have altered their diets in response to the threat of heart disease. They have reduced their consumption of saturated fats and increased their intake of fiber. The result has been a dramatic decline in the incidence of coronary heart disease.

Dangers of nutrient deficiency

In developing countries, most diet-related heart problems are caused by extreme malnutrition. For example, thiamine-deficient diets may cause beri-beri, a condition which sometimes results in enlargement of the heart and failure of its normal pumping action.

Heart disease that is caused by a nutritional deficiency is rare in the US. Anorexia nervosa, however, may lead to death due to cardiac arrest, as a result of damage to the heart muscle through starvation.

Death rates due to heart disease
For each country, the death rate is shown for three time periods: 1960 to 1964, 1970 to 1974, and 1980 to 1984. They have been adjusted to allow for the differing spectrum of ages and are quoted as a figure per 100,000 of the population.

HEART DISEASE AROUND THE WORLD

Although death rates from heart disease have fallen over the last 20 years, it is still the number one killer worldwide. Compared to Japan, Costa Rica, Italy, and Uruguay, death rates in the US, UK, Finland, and Australia are high – perhaps due to excess saturated fat in the diet. US death rates have fallen steeply recently due to changes in diet.

KEY

| | 1960 – 64 | | 1970 – 74 | | 1980 – 84 |

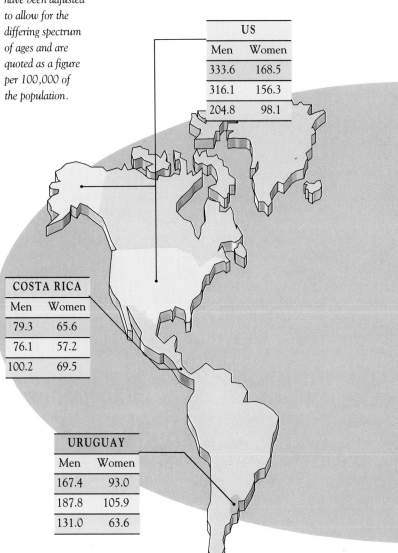

US	
Men	Women
333.6	168.5
316.1	156.3
204.8	98.1

COSTA RICA	
Men	Women
79.3	65.6
76.1	57.2
100.2	69.5

URUGUAY	
Men	Women
167.4	93.0
187.8	105.9
131.0	63.6

DIETARY FATS AND OILS

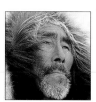

Eskimos. Even though Eskimos eat more fat in their diet than any other population around the world, they have a very low incidence of coronary heart disease. This is because most of the fat they eat comes from fish and seal blubber, which are polyunsaturated. The advantage of polyunsaturated fish oils is that they have a protective effect on the circulation. They lower the level of harmful cholesterol in the blood and reduce the tendency of blood to form clots. These actions help to keep the walls of the arteries clear, including those that supply blood to the heart muscle.

Britons. The populations in Northern Europe, including Britain, eat a lot of fat in their daily diet. However, in contrast to the Eskimo diet, most of this fat is saturated. The fat in the British diet comes mainly from red meats, dairy produce, and processed foods. Saturated fats are harmful because they encourage the build-up of fatty deposits on the walls of arteries around the body by raising the level of cholesterol in the blood. Cutting down the total consumption of fat, and substituting polyunsaturated for saturated fats where possible, is far healthier for your heart.

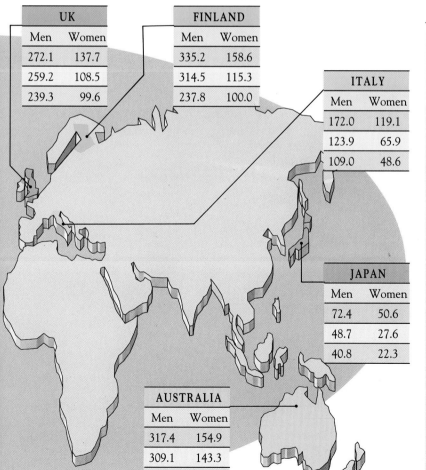

UK	
Men	Women
272.1	137.7
259.2	108.5
239.3	99.6

FINLAND	
Men	Women
335.2	158.6
314.5	115.3
237.8	100.0

ITALY	
Men	Women
172.0	119.1
123.9	65.9
109.0	48.6

JAPAN	
Men	Women
72.4	50.6
48.7	27.6
40.8	22.3

AUSTRALIA	
Men	Women
317.4	154.9
309.1	143.3
215.1	98.2

EATING TO PROTECT YOUR HEART

- **Eat more fiber**. It can be found in whole grain cereals and breads, fresh fruit and vegetables, dried beans, peas, and lentils. Fiber reduces the amount of fat and cholesterol you absorb while digesting fatty foods.
- **Eat less saturated fats**. Cut down on fatty foods, choosing lean meats and polyunsaturated vegetable oils such as olive oil. Eat more fish and poultry, and switch to skimmed milk and low-fat dairy products.
- **Cut down on fats and sugar**. Avoid fats and highly refined sugary foods, such as ice cream, cookies, cakes, and many processed products.
- **Keep your weight down**. Obesity is known to increase your risk of coronary heart disease.
- **Eat only four eggs a week**. They are high in cholesterol.
- **Reduce your salt intake**. It may raise your blood pressure, which in turn increases your risk of developing coronary heart disease.

EATING FOR A HEALTHY DIGESTIVE SYSTEM

FOR MOST OF our history, human beings have lived as hunter-gatherers, eating a diet of cereals, nuts, berries, roots, and occasionally fish and meat. Our stomachs and intestines are designed to digest this type of diet.

The more closely the food we eat resembles the diet of primitive man, the fewer digestive disorders we will experience. Since dairy farming only arrived comparatively recently in the human era, our bodies do not function well on a diet that relies heavily on cows' milk, butter, and cheese.

The major difference between the modern diet and that of our

Most digestive disorders are the result of unhealthy eating habits; common causes include not eating enough fiber, eating too fast, and simply overeating.

ancestors is in the amount of fiber it contains. We eat much less today.

The benefits of fiber

Lack of fiber in the diet is the most common reason for constipation. Fiber consists of those parts of a plant which pass directly through your intestine without being digested and absorbed. It adds bulk to your feces, thus encouraging

efficient bowel function. Increase your fiber consumption by eating more fruit, raw and green leafy vegetables, whole grain bread and cereals, and dried beans which will both prevent and treat constipation.

An inadequate intake of fiber-rich foods is thought to contribute to many other digestive disorders. In diverticulosis, for example, an abnormal build-up of pressure in

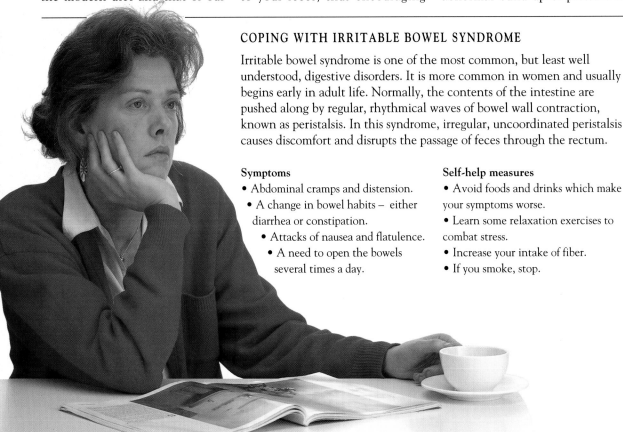

COPING WITH IRRITABLE BOWEL SYNDROME

Irritable bowel syndrome is one of the most common, but least well understood, digestive disorders. It is more common in women and usually begins early in adult life. Normally, the contents of the intestine are pushed along by regular, rhythmical waves of bowel wall contraction, known as peristalsis. In this syndrome, irregular, uncoordinated peristalsis causes discomfort and disrupts the passage of feces through the rectum.

Symptoms
- Abdominal cramps and distension.
- A change in bowel habits – either diarrhea or constipation.
- Attacks of nausea and flatulence.
- A need to open the bowels several times a day.

Self-help measures
- Avoid foods and drinks which make your symptoms worse.
- Learn some relaxation exercises to combat stress.
- Increase your intake of fiber.
- If you smoke, stop.

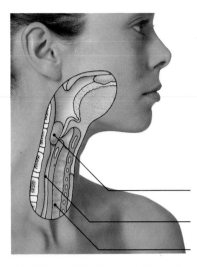

SWALLOWING

When you swallow, the muscles at the entrance to the trachea tighten, closing the opening. The food is propelled by muscular contraction down the esophagus into the stomach.

Tongue

Food

Esophagus

Trachea (windpipe)

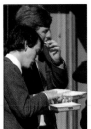

Eating on the run *makes digestion difficult because much of the blood that normally flows to your stomach and intestines during digestion is diverted to your muscles. Rushing your meals, eating on the move, or exercising after eating puts you at greater risk of digestive disorders such as recurrent heartburn, chronic indigestion, or a peptic ulcer.*

PREVENTING INDIGESTION

• Eat slowly and make sure you chew your food properly.
• Relax at meal times – do not try to eat on the move.
• Allow yourself at least half an hour's rest after a meal.
• Always avoid eating a large meal late at night.
• Do not drink too many carbonated drinks, including fizzy water. They introduce gas into the digestive tract.
• When beginning a high-fiber diet, build up your fiber intake gradually to avoid any discomfort or flatulence.

the bowel is the most probable cause of damage to the bowel wall, where small pouches form in the lining of the colon. Fiber, by binding water during digestion, softens up the feces, making them easier to pass, and thus helps to prevent this excessive rise in pressure inside the colon.

Fiber may prevent appendicitis and hemorrhoids (piles). Small, hard pellets of feces can block the tiny opening into the appendix, causing appendicitis; while the increased effort required to expel a hard bowel motion often leads to the development of hemorrhoids.

A sudden increase in the amount of fiber in your diet can cause abdominal cramps and flatulence. Build up your intake slowly over several weeks, to ensure that your bowel has time to adapt.

Maintaining your water balance is vital

Water is an important part of your diet. About 60 percent of your body is made up of water and many bodily processes require water to function normally. During the passage of waste products along the intestine, toward the rectum, water is drawn in from the surrounding blood vessels, softening the feces and making them easier to pass.

There is a continuous loss of water from your body in urine and sweat, as moisture in the air you breathe out, and, in small amounts, in the feces.

This lost water is replaced by drinking and eating. Many foods, like fruit and vegetables, contain water. Water is also formed inside the body by the metabolism of carbohydrates, fats, and proteins.

When to see your doctor

If there is a change in your normal bowel habits that continues for more than two weeks, you should visit your doctor for a check-up. You may need tests to exclude a more serious bowel disorder. If you suffer from constipation, your doctor can prescribe a bulk laxative to help regulate your bowel action. If you are experiencing cramping pain, you might be given a drug to relax the spasm in your bowel wall.

Drink more water
You should drink at least eight glasses of water a day. If you do not drink enough water, you may become constipated.

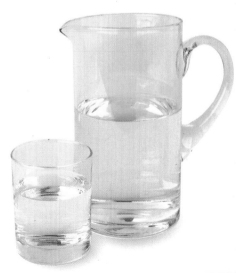

PREVENTING TOOTH DECAY

Tooth enamel is the hardest substance in your body, but it can be eroded to cause tooth decay.

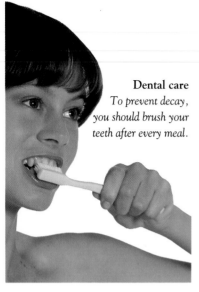

Dental care
To prevent decay, you should brush your teeth after every meal.

TOOTH DECAY IS one of the most common diseases. Anyone who eats a typical Western diet, which is high in sugar, is likely to have at least some tooth decay.

Sugar deposits form around your teeth and gum line. Bacteria that live in your mouth act upon them, releasing acids. These acids erode tooth enamel to cause decay.

As a result of tooth decay, about 10 percent of adults in the US have lost all their natural teeth.

The health of children's teeth, however, has improved greatly over the last 15 years due to better dental hygiene and the widespread use of fluoride toothpastes.

After you have eaten something sweet, your teeth are attacked for up to an hour by acids. You can fight tooth decay by limiting sugary foods to mealtimes, snacking on fresh fruit or raw vegetables, and by cleaning your teeth immediately after every meal.

THE CAUSE OF TOOTH DECAY

Dental plaque, a sticky coating that forms on and between teeth, is the primary cause of tooth decay. It consists of food particles, mucus, and bacteria. Sugar within this plaque is broken down into acids, which, if they remain in contact with the teeth, gradually erode the enamel surfaces to form cavities.

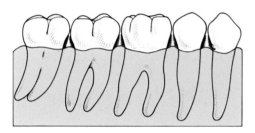

1 Plaque forms mainly between the teeth and along the gum line where it surrounds each individual tooth.

SYMPTOMS OF TOOTH DECAY

- There may be no symptoms in the early stages.
- Toothache – often brought on by consuming something sweet, very hot, or very cold.
- Unpleasant taste in the mouth.
- Bad breath.

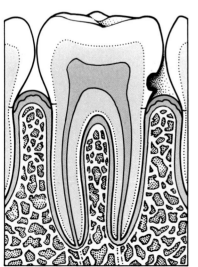

2 Acids, produced by the activity of mouth bacteria on the plaque that has not been removed by brushing and flossing, erode tooth enamel to form cavities.

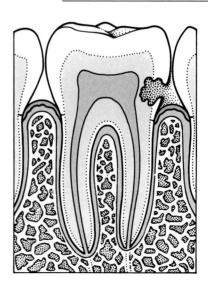

3 If this early decay is not treated, the acids continue to eat slowly through the tooth enamel to expose the underlying dentine.

Nutrients for healthy teeth

To develop strong, healthy teeth, your diet must provide adequate amounts of six essential nutrients: calcium, phosphorus, magnesium, vitamins C and D, and fluoride. If you eat a varied and balanced diet, containing foods from all the major groups, including bread and cereals, dairy produce, fruit and vegetables, grains and beans, you will be taking in more than enough of the first five nutrients on this list.

Fluoride, which strengthens your tooth enamel, making it more resistant to acid attack, is found in seafood. The amount of fluoride in your diet will vary depending on the level of this mineral in your water supply, and in the soil in which your vegetables have been grown. In some parts of the country where fluoride levels are low, supplements for children may be recommended by dentists.

Children and sweet drinks

Do not let young children use a bottle of fruit juice or any other sweet drink as a comforter for more than a few minutes. If the sugary liquid bathes the gums or teeth for long, there is a high risk of developing badly decayed teeth.

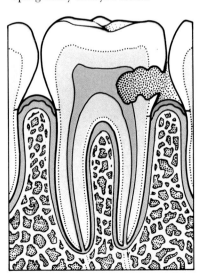

4 Dentine contains minute canals which allow bacteria inside the cavity to spread down into the pulp at the center of the tooth. If this cavity is not cleared and filled by a dentist, the infection will eventually kill the tooth, and an abscess may form.

FOODS TO AVOID

To help prevent tooth decay, you should try to limit your daily intake of highly refined sugar-rich foods, such as sweets, cookies, cakes, jams, and processed fruit and vegetables that contain added sugar.

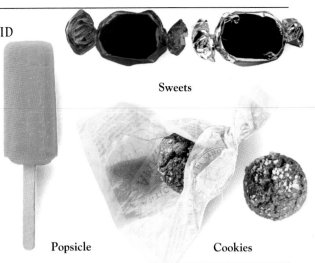

Sweets

Popsicle

Cookies

FOODS TO EAT

If you cannot clean your teeth after every meal, eat cheese as this can neutralize acid formation. Crisp foods such as celery and apples are often recommended to freshen up your teeth, but they are not very effective in cleaning off deposits of sugar.

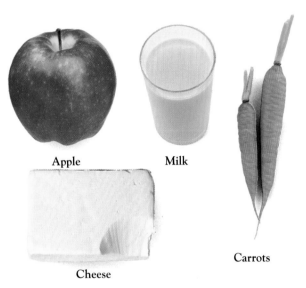

Apple

Milk

Cheese

Carrots

FLUORIDATION OF WATER

Because fluoride strengthens tooth enamel, a fluoride supplement is sometimes added to tap water. Fluoridation of water is thought to have been one of the most influential factors in the reduction of the incidence of tooth decay that has occurred over the last 15 years, particularly in children's teeth.

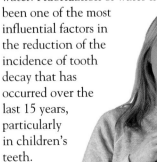

REDUCING THE RISK OF CANCER

Dietary habits account for up to 35 percent of cancer-related deaths in developed countries.

SUSPECTED CANCER CAUSERS

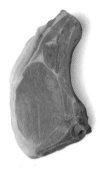

Fatty foods *are linked to bowel and breast cancer. The precise mechanism is still not clear, but some link with a high fat diet is certain.*

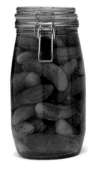

Pickled foods *and other highly acidic foods have been linked to the development of stomach cancer.*

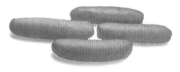

Nitrites and nitrates *are used to preserve meat and may be converted inside the stomach to potentially cancer-causing chemicals called nitrosamines. Vitamin C is now added to these foods to reduce the risk.*

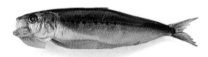

Salt-cured meat and fish *are thought to be the cause of the high incidence of throat cancer in places that still use this method of preservation for many foods.*

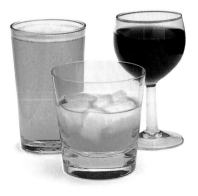

Alcohol *consumption can put you at risk of developing cancers of the mouth, throat, esophagus, stomach, liver, and bowel if you drink too much. It is not known whether it is the alcohol, or another ingredient, that does the damage. Alcohol is especially toxic when combined with smoking cigarettes, pipes, or cigars.*

PREVENTING CANCER

Cancer specialists have now published a number of dietary recommendations based on the results of their studies:

• Fat should provide 30 percent, or less, of the daily calorie intake.
• Daily fiber consumption should gradually be increased to between 20 and 30 grams.
• Fresh fruit and vegetables should be eaten every day to ensure a good supply of vitamins and minerals.
• Alcoholic drinks should only be consumed in moderation.
• Smoked, nitrate-cured, and salted foods should not be eaten regularly.
• Body weight should be kept within normal limits.

POPULATION STUDIES have shown a relationship between specific dietary habits and the incidence of some cancers. The evidence that certain foods, and food contaminants, may cause cancer is mainly circumstantial. But the link is strong enough to suggest that dietary changes could reduce the risk of developing some cancers.

Few food substances can cause cancer directly. The methods of preserving and preparing foods, and how much fat and fiber you eat, do however seem to influence your chances of avoiding cancer.

Fat and fiber

In countries, such as Japan, where fat consumption is low, the incidence of breast and bowel cancer is much lower than in countries where a lot of fat is eaten, such as the UK and US. The children of Japanese immigrants to the US lose their protection against breast and bowel cancer, presumably as a result of eating a Western diet.

However, this does not prove conclusively that fat causes cancer. Many other factors may be involved. High-fat diets also tend to be low in fiber, so it may be a lack of fiber that causes the development of these cancers. Eating less fat and more fiber is good for your heart and it may well protect you against cancer, too.

Obesity

People who are 40 percent or more over their ideal weight are twice as likely to die of certain cancers. This may not be directly due to obesity; socioeconomic and environmental factors may be responsible. But maintaining your body weight within normal limits could be one way of protecting yourself.

CANCER PREVENTERS

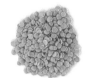

Fiber *reduces the risk of developing bowel cancer – perhaps by speeding up the passage of faeces through the bowel. Whole grain breads and cereals, dried peas and beans, and fresh fruit and vegetables are high in fiber.*

Vitamin E, *like selenium and vitamins A and C, is thought to help prevent cancer by neutralizing the damaging effects of oxidizing substances in the body. Good sources include nuts, vegetable oils, meat, green leafy vegetables, and cereals.*

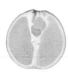

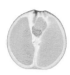

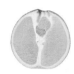

Vitamin C *may help prevent cancer, especially of the esophagus and stomach, by stopping cancer-causing substances from being formed. Vitamin C is found in fresh fruit and vegetables, but it may be a different ingredient which protects against cancer.*

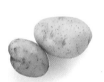

Selenium *is found in fish, shellfish, meat, whole grain cereals, and dairy products. It may prevent cancers caused by damage to cells from oxidizing substances released inside the body.*

Cruciferous vegetables, *such as cauliflower, cabbage, Brussels sprouts, and turnips, may reduce the risk of digestive and respiratory tract cancers, probably because they contain Vitamin A.*

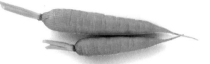

Vitamin A *curbs cancer by a direct action on the cells, preventing them from changing to a cancerous state. However, too much vitamin A can be harmful, especially during pregnancy.*

CANCER RISK DUE TO DIET

Type of cancer

90%	Colon
	Rectum
	Stomach
50%	Breast
	Gall bladder
	Pancreas Uterus (endometrium)
20%	Bladder Larynx
	Cervix Mouth
	Lung Esophagus Throat
10%	
	Other cancers

Estimated percentage of risk attributed to dietary factors

Although many of the links between food and cancer are not scientifically proven, or fully understood, making certain simple changes to your diet provides an opportunity to reduce your risk of developing some types of cancer.

EATING FOR HEALTHY BONES

Every bone is a living tissue, which needs a variety of nutrients from your diet to maintain its strength and resilience.

THE BONES OF THE human skeleton provide a rigid framework to support the hundreds of muscles which move different parts of the body. They also protect internal organs, such as the heart and lungs. The nutrients used in the growth of new bone, and the replacement of old bone, include vitamins A, C, and D, and the minerals calcium, phosphorus, magnesium, fluoride, and copper.

Osteoporosis causes the internal structure of bones to weaken, making them more susceptible to fractures. It increases the chances of a fracture after a fall, which is why older people often break their wrists or hips. To protect your bones against osteoporosis you must build up the strength of your skeleton while you are young. One good

Normal bone

Structure of normal bone
This cross section shows the densely packed structural units of bone.

Artery

Femur

BONE

A living tissue

Bones are living structures which consist of a collagen scaffolding, on which a mineral matrix, containing mainly calcium, is deposited. Each bone is made up of several layers: a thin, membranous outer surface that has a network of blood vessels and nerves running through it; a hard, dense shell, known as compact or cortical bone; and a central cavity, that in some bones contains spongy material, in which bone marrow is found. The dense shell of cortical bone is formed out of columns of bone cells, some of which are responsible for breaking down old bone, others for building up new bone. This constant turnover of bone tissue, called remodeling, is important for the growth, repair, and maintenance of bone. The bone-forming cells need calcium, phosphorus, vitamin D, and small quantities of other nutrients to function efficiently.

CALCIUM-RICH FOODS

Milk and most dairy products, fish with edible bones (sardines and canned salmon), green leafy vegetables, citrus fruit, nuts, and dried peas and beans all contain calcium. Skimmed or low-fat milk has as much calcium as whole milk, but less saturated fat.

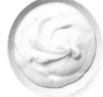

Yogurt

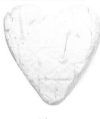

Cheese

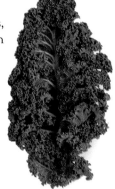

Kale

way to strengthen your bones is to get regular exercise. Any form of physical activity that puts your whole body weight through your joints will be beneficial.

However, in addition to regular exercise, it is essential that you eat a diet which provides adequate amounts of calcium. Your body is continuously using up calcium for a number of different cell activities, including the growth and mainte-nance of healthy bone tissue. Your daily diet therefore needs to supply sufficient amounts of this mineral. It is important to remember that the recommended dietary allowance for calcium increases for women during pregnancy and when they are breast-feeding.

Anyone who has taken regular exercise and consumed sufficient calcium throughout their life, is much less likely to develop osteo-porosis with increasing age.

BONE LOSS WITH AGE

Everyone loses bone density, and so bone strength, as they age. Women lose bone strength faster after menopause, when the protective effects of estrogen are lost. Black women, whose bones are denser to begin with, are less likely to suffer from osteoporosis.

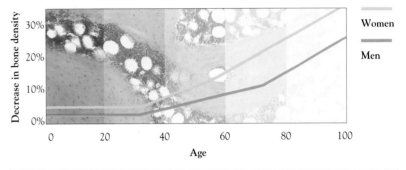

OSTEOPOROSIS

Unhealthy bone

Osteoporosis reduces the density of affected bones, making them more fragile and easily fractured. The canals between the columns of bone cells enlarge, and spaces appear among the collagen fibers that make up the bone's framework. The affected bone becomes lighter and weaker. The risk of osteoporosis increases with age: almost everyone over 55 has at least some bone loss. Women are especially vulnerable after menopause when the ovaries stop producing the female hormone estrogen that had helped maintain bone strength.

Osteoporosis
Numerous gaps form inside the bone: areas where protein and calcium have been reabsorbed faster than new bone can be laid down.

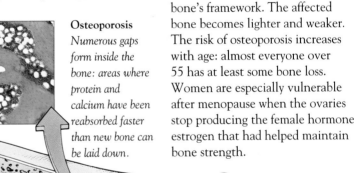

Vein   **Osteoporotic bone**

HOW TO HELP PREVENT OSTEOPOROSIS

• Eat lots of calcium-rich foods.
• Get regular exercise.
• Some women may benefit from having hormone replacement therapy for a few years after menopause.
• If you smoke, stop. Smoking causes early menopause, so reducing bone density. Cut down on alcohol and caffeine: they can weaken bones.

Milk   **Sardines**

FOOD POISONING

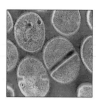

Staphylococci
*may get into food
when an uncovered
wound touches it
during preparation.*

Bacillus cereus *is
found in raw rice.
Boiling will not
destroy its spores.
Refrigerate so
toxins do not form
in leftover rice.*

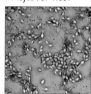

**Clostridium
botulinum** *occurs
when food is not
sterilized properly
during canning. It
harms the nervous
system and may
cause death.*

Salmonella
*bacteria are very
common and are
found in poultry
and eggs.*

F OOD POISONING IS due to eating
food or drinking water that is
contaminated with bacteria, viruses, molds, chemicals, or toxins.
Symptoms include nausea, vomiting, diarrhea and abdominal
cramps. In most cases symptoms
clear up as rapidly as they appear.

Food may be contaminated before you purchase it (particularly
seafood and poultry) or it may be
contaminated during cooking and
storage (foods which are most at
risk are those that are prepared
many hours before being eaten).
Raw or lightly cooked eggs may be
a source of salmonella. Soft cheese,
ready-prepared salads, and cook-
chill foods may be contaminated
with listeria which is particularly
dangerous for the very young and
the very old. Pregnant women with
this infection may lose their babies.

Identifying the cause

Your doctor can carry out tests to
find out what the source was. The
public health department should be
informed so that faulty food preparation or storage in the offending
restaurant, shop, or home can be
rectified. Careless food hygiene in
the kitchen is often the cause of
food contamination.

Diagnostic tests include sending
samples of feces and vomit to the
laboratory for tests to detect viruses
and bacteria. Any remaining
suspect food will be examined for
contamination in the same way.

Treating your symptoms

No solid food or milk should be
eaten until the diarrhea and vomiting have stopped. Drink plenty of
clear fluids to avoid dehydration. A
special sugar and salt rehydration
mixture, that is available from the
pharmacist, can replace lost body

salts and provide a source of energy.
Once the symptoms clear up, eat a
light meal, like soup and dry toast.

Occasionally, when diarrhea and
vomiting is severe or prolonged,
intravenous fluids may have to be
given in hospital.

High-risk foods include poultry, eggs, seafood, and undercooked meat.

> **WARNING**
> Contaminated
> food may still
> look, taste, and
> smell normal.

SALAD BARS AND FOOD BUFFETS

High standards of hygiene are required if salad bars
and buffets are not to become breeding grounds for
bacteria. Contamination can occur before the food
is laid out or from other customers.

Inadequate refrigeration
*Food left standing for long periods should
be well-chilled to stop bacteria multiplying.*

Faulty design
*Screens should prevent dust, flies, fungal
spores, and bacteria in the air from settling
on food. Customers should not reach
across uncovered food to serve themselves.*

Bad positioning
*To prevent temperature changes, food
must not be near doors, under rotating
fans, or in direct sunlight.*

Dirty serving equipment
Keep utensils out of food and off the floor.

Stale food
Throw away stale leftover food.

KITCHEN HYGIENE

- Store raw meat away from all other types of food.
- Clean utensils and cutting boards thoroughly with soap
and very hot water after preparing raw meat.
- Wash fresh fruit and vegetables in cold, running water.
- Never use food from containers that are leaking,
bulging, or damaged.

SYMPTOMS OF FOOD POISONING

Each type of food poisoning has its own characteristic symptom pattern; how ill you become depends on how heavily the food was contaminated.

CAUSE	SYMPTOMS	ONSET
Chemical poisoning	Diarrhea and vomiting	Within 30 mins.
Staphylococcal toxins	Vomiting	1 to 6 hours
Bacillus cereus	Diarrhea and vomiting	2 to 14 hours
Clostridium perfringens	Abdominal cramps	6 to 12 hours
Clostridium botulinum (botulism)	Difficulty speaking, blurred vision, and paralysis	12 to 36 hours
Salmonella organisms	Diarrhea and vomiting	8 to 48 hours
Viruses	Diarrhea and vomiting	12 to 48 hours
Shigella organisms	Diarrhea and abdominal cramps	2 to 3 days
Campylobacteria	Diarrhea	2 to 6 days
Listeria monocytogenes	Influenza-like symptoms	7 to 30 days

Shigella *are the result of fecal contamination, either from flies or from hands left unwashed after using the toilet.*

Campylobacteria *is found in contaminated beef, chicken, water, and milk.*

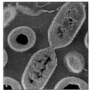

Listeria monocytogenes *are found in soil and water and causes illness when lots of the bacteria are consumed, for example in blue-veined cheese and unwashed ready-packed vegetables.*

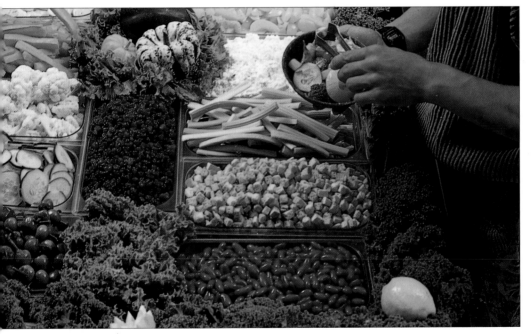

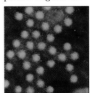

Norwalk virus *is found in shellfish that have been feeding in heavily polluted waters.*

- Keep refrigerator temperatures below 41°F (5°C); freezer temperatures below 0°F (–18°C).
- Thaw frozen meat or poultry completely before you cook it.
- Eat meat as soon as it is cooked. Cover up leftovers; cool; refrigerate within 90 minutes.
- Reheat meat quickly and thoroughly.
- To preserve food, sterilize it in a pressure cooker at 250°F (120°C) for 30 minutes.
- Put fish in the coldest part of the refrigerator.
- Keep egg dishes in the refrigerator.
- Always wash your hands before touching any food and after handling raw meat. Cover any cut or sore on your hand with a waterproof dressing.

MYTHS AND REALITIES

Cutting through the hype about diet is a difficult task when every week seems to bring a new fad or myth.

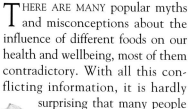

THERE ARE MANY popular myths and misconceptions about the influence of different foods on our health and wellbeing, most of them contradictory. With all this conflicting information, it is hardly surprising that many people are confused about which foods are good or bad. Learning about diet and nutrition will help you tell fact from fiction.

Here are a few of the common myths about food. Many of these myths can be explained by our desire to discover miracle cures for common ailments, or by our need to justify eating certain foods because they are "good for you."

Are oysters an aphrodisiac?

No substance has ever been scientifically proven to increase sexual drive or enhance sexual performance. Over the centuries, however, various substances such as ginger, ginseng, and oysters have become known as aphrodisiacs. This is due more to the power of suggestion than to any physical effect they might have. So if you believe that oysters will help your love life, they might just do so.

Can carrots help you see in the dark?

If you already eat a well-balanced diet, eating more carrots will not make any difference to how well you see in the dark. The myth may have sprung up because night blindness is one of the complications resulting from a deficiency of vitamin A and carrots are a good source of this vitamin. Only people who are deficient in vitamin A could possibly benefit from eating mounds of carrots.

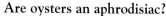

Does eating fish make you more intelligent?

Although fish is acknowledged as a highly nutritious food – rich in protein, vitamins, and minerals, and low in saturated fats – it does not help brain function any more than other sources of protein, either vegetable or animal. This myth may have evolved as a parental strategy to persuade reluctant children to eat certain foods because they were thought to be very good for them.

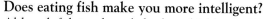

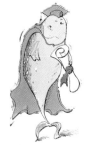

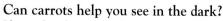

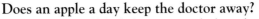

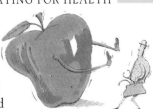

Does an apple a day keep the doctor away?

An apple – like all fresh fruit – is an ideal snack, providing fiber, vitamins, and minerals, without too many extra calories. An apple contains about three grams of fiber, three milligrams of vitamin C, and small amounts of iron, thiamine, and niacin. It provides around 40 Calories, and with its high water content contributes to your daily intake of fluid. Many years ago an apple a day would have helped prevent scurvy, which was then common due to a lack of vitamin C. However, eating an apple every day cannot guarantee a life free from the need for medical treatment!

Is brown sugar better for you than white?

Brown sugar is not as highly refined as white sugar. This means that brown sugar contains fiber, vitamins, and minerals which are lost during the processing of white sugar. But the amounts of these different nutrients are tiny, and brown sugar, like white, has a lot of calories, so it is not an essential part of a healthy diet. Other "brown" foods are healthier. Brown rice and whole grain bread provide significantly more nutrients and fiber than the more highly refined white bread and polished white rice.

Does spinach make you strong?

Spinach is a good source of vitamins A and C, and also of the minerals iron and calcium; but it is no more nutritious than other green leafy vegetables. The myth stems from a parental desire for children to eat vitamin-rich vegetables. Cartoons, showing a muscular sailor-hero magically growing stronger by swallowing the contents of a can of spinach, help feed the myth.

Are snacks between meals bad for you?

There is no harm in eating the occasional snack, as long as you choose healthy foods. The problem with the usual snack foods, like cakes, potato chips, cookies, chocolate, and ice cream, is that they are rich in calories, with large amounts of fats, sugars, and salt. If you want a snack, it is much better to munch on a piece of fresh fruit or a raw vegetable. In addition to filling yourself up, you will take in essential vitamins, minerals, and fiber, but not too many extra calories.

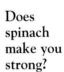

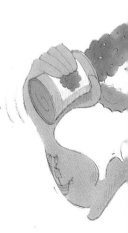

Burning up calories
Just changing your diet is not likely to produce permanent weight-loss. You must also increase the amount you exercise.

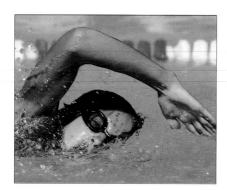

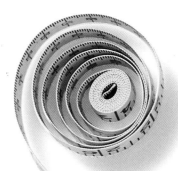

Vital statistics
If you combine a healthier diet with more exercise you will tone your muscles and lose weight as well.

Too much fat?
The skin fold test is a quick way of finding out whether you need to lose weight. If you can pinch more than 1 in (2 cm) you need to take action.

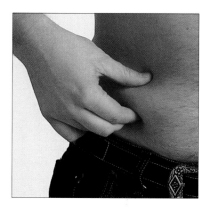

Monitor your weight
By weighing yourself once a week you can see whether your weight is stable or not. If you notice an increase you can take action before serious problems occur.

CHAPTER THREE

WATCHING YOUR WEIGHT

IN MOST DEVELOPED countries, the principal dietary disorder is not a deficiency of essential nutrients, but rather a surplus of body fat. This is caused by a combination of overeating and not exercising enough to burn off excess calories. In the US, over one-third of all adults weigh too much and overweight is becoming a serious heatlh problem. Obesity can lead to many serious health problems – people who are overweight are much more likely to suffer from heart disease, diabetes, and some cancers.

It is all too easy to eat too much and to exercise too little, causing you to gain excess weight gradually over the years. Your body weight will only remain stable if the energy content of the food you eat is in balance with the energy needs of your body. If you take in more calories than you need, or if you start doing less exercise, you will gain weight. To maintain a healthy weight, you must learn to eat and exercise wisely.

Problems of obesity
Seriously overweight people have less energy and are also more prone to developing disorders such as high blood pressure and osteoarthritis.

A healthy diet
The occasional treat does no harm but the best way to avoid weight-gain is to eat plenty of low-fat, high-fiber foods. Beware of processed foods – they often have added sugars and are therefore high in calories.

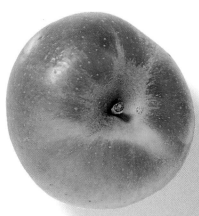

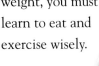

ARE YOU OVERWEIGHT?

At least 34 percent of the American population are known to weigh more than is healthy for their height and their age.

FAT SHOULD ACCOUNT for about 15 to 20 percent of body weight in healthy young adult men and 20 to 25 percent in healthy young adult women. These proportions will increase slightly with age. A greater level of body fat is considered unnecessary and unhealthy.

Way too much

Many people in the Western world carry excess fat and are overweight. It is thought that five percent of the population in this country are more than just overweight – they are obese. You are classed as being obese if you weigh 20 percent over your ideal maximum weight.

An accurate measure of obesity is given by your Body Mass Index (BMI). This figure is calculated as

SKIN FOLD TEST

To assess roughly how much body fat you are carrying, try pinching a fold of skin between your thumb and index finger. Take care not to include any muscle

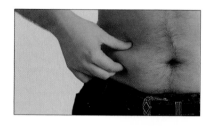

Skin fold test
Men and women should have similar levels of fat around their waists, making this the ideal place to try the test.

Places to pinch
You can also try the skin fold test on the front of your upper arms or the back of your shoulder blades.

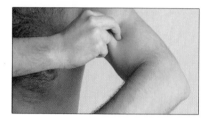

Where do men store fat?
Men and women store deposits of fat under the skin all over the body. The shaded areas on this figure indicate where fat is most likely to build up on a man. Unlike women, men tend to accumulate fat as an abdominal paunch.

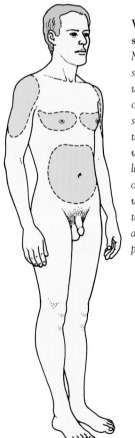

CHECK YOUR WEIGHT

First choose the appropriate chart (male or female). Next locate your height measurement on one side of the graph and your weight on the top or bottom of the graph. Trace along both of these lines and note

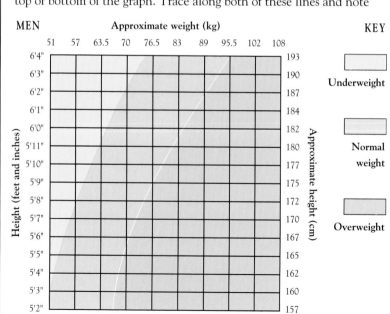

MEN — Approximate weight (kg)

51 57 63.5 70 76.5 83 89 95.5 102 108

Height (feet and inches): 6'4", 6'3", 6'2", 6'1", 6'0", 5'11", 5'10", 5'9", 5'8", 5'7", 5'6", 5'5", 5'4", 5'3", 5'2"

Approximate height (cm): 193, 190, 187, 184, 182, 180, 177, 175, 172, 170, 167, 165, 162, 160, 157

Weight (pounds): 112 126 140 154 168 182 196 210 224 238

KEY

Underweight

Normal weight

Overweight

tissue in the pinch. If you can pinch more than just one inch of fat, you would definitely benefit from losing some weight.

Overall body fat
Skin callipers record skin fold thickness. They allow you to calculate an overall percentage of fat.

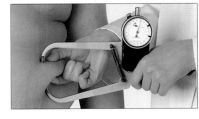

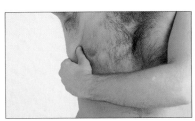

Less fat
If you go on a diet or increase your level of exercise, take the skin fold test every week to check your fat-loss.

Weight divided by Height squared. For both men and women, a BMI figure of between 20 and 25 is healthy – if it is over 30 you are seriously endangering your health.

Know your ideal body weight

Everyone should be aware of the body weight best suited to their height, age, and physique. By keeping your weight around this level, your body will be healthier, work more efficiently, and look better.

The tables shown below let you assess whether your current weight is appropriate for your height and sex. They have a wide normal weight range to allow for factors which govern body weight that are beyond your control, such as age and variations in overall build.

WEIGHT PROBLEMS

Apart from carrying excess fat, there are other warning signs that you are overweight:

• Frequent breathlessness.
• Feeling of heaviness.
• Getting easily overheated.
• Aching joints in the lower back, hips, and knees.

where they intersect. The area in which the lines cross reveals whether you are underweight, normal weight, or overweight. If your weight is 20 percent above the top of the normal range you are obese.

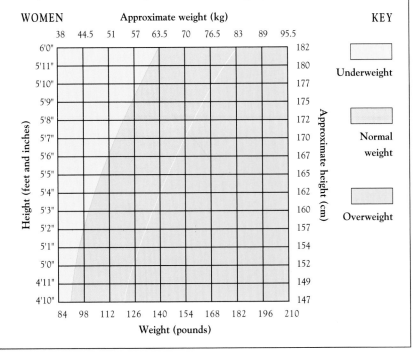

WOMEN   Approximate weight (kg)

	38	44.5	51	57	63.5	70	76.5	83	89	95.5

Height (feet and inches): 6'0", 5'11", 5'10", 5'9", 5'8", 5'7", 5'6", 5'5", 5'4", 5'3", 5'2", 5'1", 5'0", 4'11", 4'10"

Approximate height (cm): 182, 180, 177, 175, 172, 170, 167, 165, 162, 160, 157, 154, 152, 149, 147

Weight (pounds): 84, 98, 112, 126, 140, 154, 168, 182, 196, 210

KEY

Underweight

Normal weight

Overweight

Where do women store fat?
Like men, women build up fat deposits under the skin all over the body, notably around the top of the arms, the abdomen, and the buttocks. Women, however, also accumulate fat deposits under the skin of the breasts and around their hips and thighs.

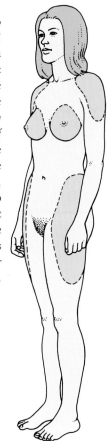

CAUSES OF WEIGHT GAIN

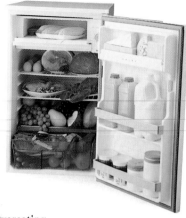

IF YOU WEIGH TOO much, answer the questions set out below and find out what could lie at the root of this problem. Medical disorders are rarely the cause. Most people who are overweight have simply taken in more calories than they use up as energy.

These people eat more than their bodies need. It is not, however, the amount eaten in terms of bulk, but rather the type of food, that causes the weight problem.

The most common cause of weight gain is simply eating more food than your body needs.

Grazing or bingeing?

If you are overweight, consuming frequent small meals – sometimes called grazing – is the best way to control your weight. The foods you eat should have a high nutrient

Overeating

Eating calorie-rich foods high in fat and refined carbohydrates, that contribute little to the overall nutritional value of a meal, will cause weight gain.

Q *Do you eat more when you are under a great deal of stress or as a way of making yourself feel less anxious or depressed?*

Many people resort to "comfort eating" to avoid confronting emotionally difficult or stressful situations. In some cases, eating helps the individual deal with excessive demands; in others, it is just a means of overcoming boredom.

Try to find other ways to improve your state of mind. Exercise may relieve stress, anxiety, and depression; it will also burn off excess calories. Taking up meditation or a new relaxing hobby may also help.

Q *Have you been putting on weight gradually as you have grown older?*

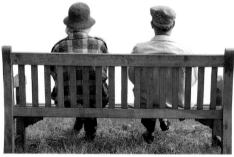

Elderly people have lower energy requirements than when they were younger because they have a lower basal metabolic rate and often exercise less.

To avoid gaining weight as you grow older you must cut your intake of calories or exercise more often, or both. You can raise your basal metabolic rate by exercising vigorously at least three times a week.

Q *Have you been taking any medication recently?*

A number of drugs, particularly steroids and the contraceptive pill, may cause a gradual increase in body weight.

Talk to your doctor about your weight gain. You may need to lower your dosage or take a different drug. If that is not possible, you may have to reduce your calorie intake or exercise more frequently in order to keep your weight down.

Q *Have you become overweight since you took up a less physically demanding job or gave up playing a particular sport?*

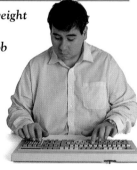

Failure to match your calorie intake to your lifestyle is another common cause of weight gain.

Modify your diet by reducing your calorie intake or take up some form of regular physical activity to prevent this energy surplus.

content and should not add up to an excessive number of calories. The "grazer" is less likely to feel hungry because there is just a short interval between meals, which makes high-calorie snacks such as cakes and cookies less tempting.

Studies have shown that when the same number of calories are eaten during the day in the form of three or more meals of moderate size, rather than one or two larger meals, more calories are given off as body heat. If you fast for most of the day, your body will receive warning signals telling it to try and conserve energy in response to the temporary absence of food.

Basal metabolic rate

Energy requirements are set partly by your basal metabolic rate and partly by your level of physical activity. The basal metabolic rate is the amount of energy needed to maintain vital body functions such as breathing, temperature, and heartbeat at rest.

While most people have a similar basal metabolic rate, some have inherited an abnormally slow metabolism. These people, sometimes called "underburners," do not need as many calories to satisfy their daily energy needs. If they eat the same foods as someone of the same age, sex, weight, and lifestyle who has a normal metabolism, they are likely to put on weight.

At the other end of the scale there are "overburners," people whose metabolisms are higher than normal. They can consume larger amounts of calories than normal without excessive weight gain.

Q *Are other members of your family overweight?*

The tendency to be overweight does seem to run in families. However, while it is thought that genetic factors do play a part in the development of obesity, it may also be due to families sharing the same unhealthy eating and exercise habits or to a combination of all three factors.

Anybody who has a family history of weight problems needs to make an extra effort to ensure that they eat sensibly and keep to a regular exercise routine.

Q *Did you put on weight after you gave up smoking?*

Giving up smoking can cause a weight gain of a few pounds, partly because eating can act as a substitute for having a cigarette in your mouth and partly because nicotine artificially raises your normal metabolic rate.

Putting on a small amount of weight is far less harmful than continuing to smoke. To minimize this weight gain, try to snack only on healthy low-calorie foods such as fruit, yogurt, or air-popped popcorn. Exercising more will also help.

Q *Since you started gaining weight, have you noticed any other symptoms of ill-health?*

Occasionally weight gain occurs because of an underlying medical problem. A number of hormonal disorders can lead to weight problems. For example, one in every 100 cases of obesity is in fact due to an underactive thyroid gland which has caused the body's metabolism to slow down.

Consult your doctor if, in addition to being overweight, you have any other symptoms, such as dry skin, hair loss, lethargy, muscle cramps, or feeling cold.

Q *Did your weight gain persist after having a baby?*

Body fat laid down during pregnancy may remain after the birth of the baby if you continue taking in extra calories, or if you put on too much weight while pregnant.

Exercising gently and eating foods that are low in fat and sugar, but high in unrefined carbohydrates, protein, and fiber will enable most women to return to their pre-pregnancy weight. Breast-feeding is helpful because milk production helps use up fat stores.

RISKS OF OBESITY

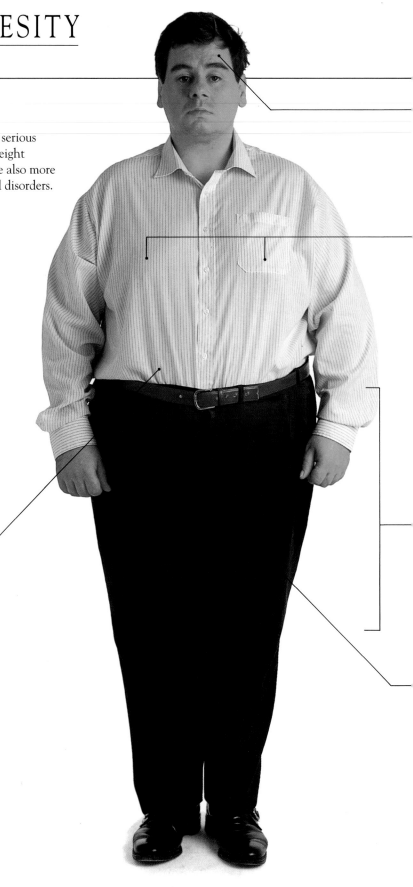

HOW CAN OBESITY DAMAGE YOUR HEALTH?

Over a period of time, being obese is a serious hazard to your health. Seriously overweight people tend to have less energy and are also more vulnerable to a wide variety of medical disorders.

High blood pressure

Men and women who are very overweight are more likely to die from complications caused by high blood pressure than people of comparable age whose weight is within the normal range. Even a moderate reduction in weight can significantly lower abnormally raised blood pressure.

High blood cholesterol

Seriously overweight people have a greater chance of having high blood cholesterol. This high level is thought to be the result of eating too much saturated fat which is turned into cholesterol in the liver.

Gallstones

Because obese people have an increased level of cholesterol production inside their liver, larger amounts are released into the bile. This cholesterol is more likely to crystallize in the gallbladder and bile ducts to form gallstones.

Cancer risk

Recent population studies have shown that the more overweight that men become, the more they risk suffering from cancer of the colon, rectum, and prostate gland. Similarly, obese women increase their risk of developing cancer of the breast, uterus, and cervix. These findings are still being analyzed and await final confirmation.

Stroke
A stroke happens when the blood supply to the brain is damaged. Strokes are twice as likely to occur in obese people because they often have a high level of blood cholesterol or high blood pressure.

Breathlessness
Obesity commonly causes breathlessness during exertion and in severe cases even when at rest. This is partly because excess weight interferes with free movement of the diaphragm and partly because it increases the workload on the heart.

Back pain
Very overweight people commonly suffer from persistent or recurrent back pain. This is because the upper part of the body is heavy and the abdominal muscles that support this area tend to lack tone, putting pressure on the lower part of the spine.

Osteoarthritis
The joint stiffness, pain, and swelling associated with osteoarthritis may be made worse by obesity. Extra weight places more strain on the joints in the lower spine and legs. Losing this weight can slow down the rate of deterioration and can even help alleviate the symptoms.

Skin problems
Obese people are vulnerable to skin chafing and fungal infections in areas where there are folds of skin rubbing together, for example, in the groin.

Varicose veins
Obesity increases the risk of developing varicose veins. Lack of exercise can also make varicose veins worse.

Men and women who are seriously overweight have a greater risk of developing heart disease, diabetes, and some types of cancer.

THE INCREASE IN mortality among people who are obese is due mainly to circulatory diseases, such as coronary heart disease, high blood pressure, and stroke, and also to complications from the presence of diabetes.

Life expectancy and obesity

 A person who is more than 40 percent over the desirable weight for his or her age and height has twice the risk of dying of coronary heart disease. Being more than 20 to 30 percent over the ideal weight means that a person is about three times more likely to die of diabetic complications.

Heart disease in the obese

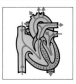 There are numerous reasons why people who are overweight are more likely to develop coronary heart disease and therefore suffer from angina and heart attacks. The more overweight you are, the more likely you are to have high blood pressure, diabetes, and raised levels of blood cholesterol. You are also less likely to undertake any form of strenuous exercise. All these factors increase the risk of coronary heart disease.

The risk to your heart seems to depend in part on where the excess fat is stored. For reasons that are not yet fully understood, if fat is concentrated around the abdominal region there is a higher risk of heart disease than if it is stored around the hips and thighs.

Diabetes in the obese

 Obese individuals are far more likely to suffer from non-insulin-dependent (maturity onset) diabetes than other people.

Insulin controls the uptake of glucose (sugar) from the blood into body cells. Putting on weight may result in the normal supply of insulin becoming insufficient to cope with the increased demand from tissues which now contain more cells. Glucose uptake is impaired and blood glucose levels rise.

Losing excess weight, and thus reducing the number of body cells, may restore this balance and avoid the need for drug treatment.

MONITORING YOUR HEALTH
Essential check-ups for the seriously overweight

If you are obese and unable to lose the excess pounds through dieting and exercise, you have an increased risk of developing a number of medical disorders. Make sure you have the following health checks:

• **Blood pressure** – have this measured at least every two years.
• **Urine or blood glucose** – get this tested at least every three years.
• **Blood cholesterol** – check your level at least every five years.

HOW TO LOSE WEIGHT

Positive changes in diet and lifestyle will lead to weight loss for most people.

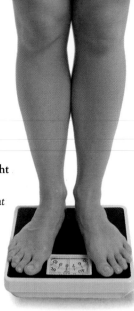

TACKLING THE problem of eating too much is as difficult for some people as beating an addiction to drugs or alcohol. Obese people seem to have a greater urge to eat and find losing weight harder than those who are less overweight.

The best way to achieve a safe and permanent reduction in weight is through lifestyle changes that include a regular program of exercise and a reduction in the number of calories in your diet. The diet that you choose should be one that you can continue to follow for life, not just until you have achieved your target weight.

Weight-loss cycle

Long-term weight control is far more important than your initial success in losing weight. Unfortunately, many dieters quickly return to their former eating and exercise habits once they have reached their desired weight. They often end up weighing more than they did before they started their diet.

Some experts now believe that continually repeating this cycle of weight-loss followed by weight-gain may be more damaging to your health than remaining overweight all the time.

The right weight
Many people set their target weight too low. Choose the weight that is right for you, not one that is a struggle to maintain.

EXERCISE IS VITAL

To reduce your weight, try to exercise vigorously at least three times a week. Physical activity burns up calories and increases your basal metabolic rate (the number of calories used by your body at rest). Loosening up, stretching, and strengthening exercises will trim off fat and also tone up your muscles.

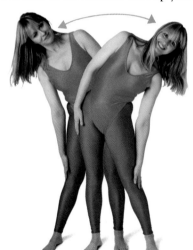

Sideways bends
Stand upright, with your feet slightly apart and arms down by your sides. First bend to one side and then to the other. Repeat 10 times.

Sideways leg raises
Lie on your side with your head supported in your hand. Raise and lower your leg 12 inches from the ground. Repeat 10 times, then turn over and exercise the other leg.

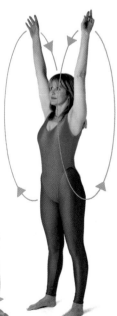

Arm rotations
Stand with your feet slightly apart and arms down by your sides. Rotate your arms from your shoulders, 10 times forward and 10 times backward.

TIPS ON LOSING WEIGHT

- Set yourself a realistic target – two or three pounds a week is ideal.
- Choose a varied, balanced diet, rich in fiber and low in fat and highly refined carbohydrates. Always opt for low-calorie snacks.
- Eat three meals of moderate size each day and do not skip meals.
- Avoid eating late in the evening.
- Eat slowly, use a smaller plate, and avoid watching TV while you eat.
- Avoid alcohol and sugary drinks that are high in calories. Choose low-calorie drinks or water instead.
- Join a weight-loss organization if you think it will keep you motivated.

HOW SAFE ARE POPULAR WEIGHT-LOSS DIETS?

The fact that no single diet is universally successful is reflected in the wide variety of diets recommended by doctors and nutritionists and by the large number of popular diet books on sale. Here is a brief summary of the composition, advantages and disadvantages, effectiveness, and safety of some of these diets.

TYPE	COMPOSITION	ADVANTAGES AND DISADVANTAGES	EFFECTIVENESS AND SAFETY
One dimensional	A single food or type of food, such as an all-fruit diet or a yogurt-only diet.	No advantages. Hunger, boredom, and bowel problems are common.	Not recommended. Causes loss of muscle protein and body water. Some form of nutritional deficiency is inevitable.
High-fiber diet	A variety of fiber-rich foods, such as fresh fruit and vegetables, whole grains, and nuts.	Helps satisfy the appetite without too many calories. Too much fiber can cause wind and indigestion.	A safe way to lose weight, as long as a variety of fiber-rich foods are eaten.
Very low-calorie, specially formulated, liquid diet (less than 500 Calories a day)	A liquid made from soy flour and low-fat milk solids that is rich in protein.	Does not teach sensible eating habits. Side effects are common. May aggravate metabolic disorders. Medical supervision is essential.	May lead to loss of muscle tissue, but can be helpful for extremely obese people when other diets have failed.
Low-carbohydrate, high-protein diet	Little or no carbohydrate, small amounts of protein-rich foods. Calories unrestricted.	Monotonous, unpalatable, nutritionally unbalanced. High in fat. Little if any body fat is lost.	Potentially harmful due to loss of body fluid and tissue protein.
Balanced, calorie-controlled diet	Wide variety of nutritious, low-fat foods, within a calorie-controlled menu.	Most people will lose weight if they keep to between 1,200 and 1,500 Calories a day, in addition to a program of regular exercise.	Highly recommended. Teaches healthy eating habits which can then be maintained when the calorie-controlled diet is over.

EXTREME MEASURES TO AID WEIGHT-LOSS

Diet Pills

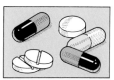

Only take diet pills under reputable medical supervision.
• **Appetite suppressants** – must be combined with a healthy diet, exercise, and counselling.
• **Stimulant appetite suppressants** – can only be taken for a short time, can cause dependence, and may be dangerous if you have heart disease, high blood pressure, diabetes, glaucoma, thyroid disease, or kidney problems.
• **Diuretics and laxatives** – do not help lose body fat.

Medical intervention

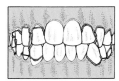

Radical procedures are only performed when obesity is life threatening and conventional measures have not worked. They are only used as a last resort by people who are either twice their ideal weight or more than 100 lb (45 kg) overweight. Measures include:
• **Jaw wiring** – restricts food intake.
• **Stomach stapling** – reduces stomach size.
• **Intestinal bypass** – prevents the absorption of food.

AVOIDING WEIGHT GAIN

If your calorie intake exceeds your energy and body maintenance requirements, you will gain weight.

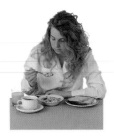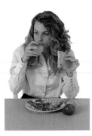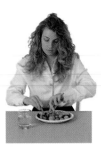

How often should you eat? *Do not miss meals to control your weight. Your body will function best on three healthy meals a day.*

THE PRINCIPAL DIETARY problem for sedentary people living in developed countries is that daily food consumption almost always exceeds what is required to satisfy the body's energy demands. This surplus food is converted into fat and leads to weight gain.

How much should you eat?
Your body needs food for warmth, for building and repairing tissues, and for energy to maintain vital physical and chemical functions. Energy requirements can vary a great deal. Some people have a slow metabolism and require less energy from food to keep their body running. If you have inherited this type of metabolism, you need a stricter calorie-controlled diet to avoid putting on weight.

However, for the majority of healthy people, daily calorie needs lie close to an average value which is calculated from age and level of physical activity, as shown in the table below.

Control your weight
To achieve a balance of calorie input and energy output and therefore avoid putting on weight, you need to learn which foods are good for you and which should only be eaten in

AVERAGE DAILY CALORIE REQUIREMENTS

Calories provide a measure of how much energy your food contains. Study the tables below (Men ♂ and Women ♀) and find out how many calories you should be eating each day, at every stage of your life.

♂ AGE	LIFESTYLE	CALORIES / DAY
18 – 35 years	●	2,500
	○	3,000
	●	3,500
36 – 55 years	●	2,400
	○	2,800
	●	3,400
56+ years	●	2,200
	○	2,500

♀ AGE	LIFESTYLE	CALORIES / DAY
18 – 55 years	●	1,900
	○	2,150
	●	2,500
	Pregnant	2,400
	Breast-feeding	2,800
56+ years	●	1,700
	○	2,000

KEY ● Inactive ○ Active ● Very active

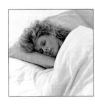

Sleeping *uses 65 Calories per hour.*

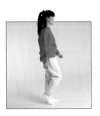

Walking *will burn up 250 Calories per hour.*

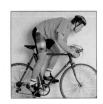

Steady cycling *uses over 300 Calories per hour.*

moderation. Eating plenty of fresh fruit and vegetables is an easy way of improving your diet. They are full of nutrients, low in calories, and are very filling. You should avoid foods that are high in calories and fats, such as convenience foods and cakes.

Weigh yourself regularly. This will help you monitor whether you are successfully balancing your energy intake with your energy needs. If your weight increases you should simply reduce your calorie intake and start getting more exercise.

The exercise factor

Physical activity helps you avoid putting on weight by burning up calories. It also raises your basal metabolic rate, thereby increasing the number of calories your body will burn up when you are at rest.

CHOOSING FOODS WISELY

It is easy to reduce the number of calories in your diet. You do not always need to cut down on the bulk of the food you are eating. Balance is the key to success – simply choose from a wide variety of natural foods.

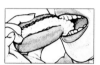

- **Increase your fiber consumption**. Fiber-rich complex carbohydrates, such as whole grain products, fresh fruit and vegetables, dried beans, peas, and brown rice, are low in calories and rich in vitamins and minerals. Fiber is filling and also reduces your absorption of cholesterol and glucose.

- **Avoid refined carbohydrates**. These foods are often much higher in calories and are nearly always lower in vitamins and minerals. White flour, white bread, polished rice, and products which have added sugar are all highly refined.

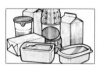

- **Cut down on saturated fats**. Choose low-fat dairy products and eat lean meat. When you cook, use vegetable oils such as sunflower and safflower. Rather than frying, try grilling your food. Cut down on convenience foods like cookies, pastries, and cakes – they are rich in invisible fats. Pound for pound, fats contain more than twice the calories of carbohydrates or proteins.

CHILDREN AND OBESITY

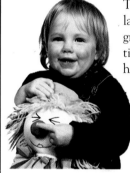

The rate at which body fat is laid down during childhood growth is highly variable. At times your child may appear to have too much body fat, but this is usually only a temporary "overshoot." At birth, body fat makes up around 15 percent of body weight. This may increase to as much as 26 percent by six months of age and then decrease as the child becomes more mobile. By six years of age a child has about 15 percent body fat; just before puberty this may be as high as 20 percent. After puberty, young women average 25 percent and young men have only 13 percent of their weight as body fat.

It is important to take steps to prevent your children becoming overweight. Overweight children and teenagers risk becoming obese adults.

CHECK YOUR CHILD'S WEIGHT

- If you bottle-feed, do not force your baby to take more than he or she wants.
- Delay starting solid foods until four months of age.
- Do not insist that your child clears the plate.
- Do not offer food as a reward for good behavior.
- Offer healthy snacks, not sweets and cookies.
- Do not set a bad example. Encourage the whole family to cut down on their intake of fatty foods and convenience foods which have added sugar.
- Encourage your child to get more exercise.

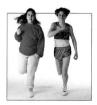

Slow running or jogging *can use as many as 400 Calories per hour.*

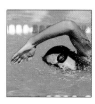

Swimming *at only a moderate pace will burn up over 500 Calories per hour.*

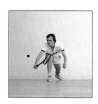

Squash *burns up at least 650 Calories per hour.*

EATING DISORDERS

Anorexia nervosa afflicts roughly one in every 2000 adolescent boys and one in every 100 teenage girls.

ALTHOUGH MANY TEENAGERS go through a phase of excessive dieting, only a few develop a serious eating disorder like anorexia nervosa, often known as the "dieter's disease," or bulimia nervosa.

Anorexics suffer from a psychological or behavioral disorder in which they refuse to eat properly, believing that they are overweight. No matter how thin and ill they become, they continue to follow a strict starvation diet.

Causes of anorexia nervosa
Although many suggestions have been put forward to explain the problem, the causes of this highly complex condition are still under debate. Some doctors believe that these obsessional behavior patterns are due to an unwillingness of the adolescent child to become a sexually mature adult. Anorexics may see strict dieting as their only way of imposing control over their lives and what they see as an uncertain and frightening future.

Other specialists have suggested that there could be a medical cause for anorexia nervosa. Perhaps the hypothalamus – a gland that controls functions such as hunger, thirst, and sexual activity – could be at fault in some way. Or there may be a serious psychological problem, such as depression, schizophrenia, or even a simple phobia about putting on weight.

Fear of food
To an anorexic food is the cause of all their problems. They believe that if they could only weigh less these problems would simply disappear.

Treatment of anorexia nervosa
Severe anorexia nervosa is best treated in hospital. Unless a careful watch is kept, the individual will avoid eating by hiding or throwing away food. Treatment may vary, but it will usually include a closely controlled feeding program, in conjunction with individual psychotherapy or family therapy, to help resolve personal and family conflicts. Medication may be prescribed if there are any signs of an underlying mental illness.

Once the target weight gain has been achieved, the anorexic will usually be allowed to go home. The

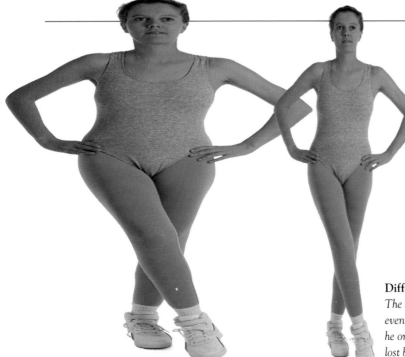

DISTORTED SELF-IMAGE
The underlying problem of anorexia nervosa lies in an abnormal perception of the body's size and shape. This has been made worse by general attitudes in our society that equate attractiveness with a thin rather than a curvaceous figure. Believing themselves to be overweight, anorexics exist on a starvation diet. Even when they are severely emaciated they perceive their body as being fat.

Different points of view
The anorexic victim does not see a slim, or even underweight, body in the mirror – all he or she sees is excess fat which must be lost by dieting.

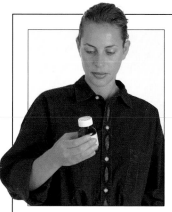

BULIMIA NERVOSA

Bulimia nervosa is most commonly found in young adult women who have been treated for anorexia nervosa in the past. They develop a constant craving for food, but still fear becoming fat. Sufferers binge on huge amounts of food and then induce vomiting or take diuretics and laxatives. Treatment for bulimia is the same as for anorexia nervosa. Eating habits are supervised and, where appropriate, psychotherapy and antidepressant drugs are used. Although most bulimics appear to be of normal weight, or only slightly underweight, this constant bingeing and purging can cause a number of complications:

- Dehydration.
- Repeated vomiting of stomach acids can corrode the teeth, making them rough and sharp.
- Muscle cramps and weakness as a result of potassium depletion.
- Compulsive eating patterns can lead to severe mental distress.

WARNING SIGNS OF AN EATING DISORDER

It can be difficult to distinguish between an ordinary diet and the start of an eating disorder. Both trigger a progressive loss of weight but the anorexic may try to disguise this by wearing baggy clothes. There are, however, many other warning signs. Physical problems may include excessive fatigue, difficulty sleeping, constipation, dry skin and brittle nails, the growth of fine downy hair over the cheeks, neck, forearms, and legs, and female sufferers may find that their periods stop. Psychological signs include a preoccupation with food, obsessive exercising and overactivity, and secretive and defensive behavior.

family will be counseled on how to monitor progress and how to spot the warning signs of a relapse.

Future prospects

It is a mistake to think that this condition has been cured as soon as a normal body weight has been restored. About half of all patients treated for anorexia nervosa need to receive regular counseling over several years. The slightest stress can trigger a relapse.

Between 5 and 10 percent of anorexics actually die as a result of their condition. These deaths are generally suicides. Some anorexics do, however, starve themselves to death. Complications that can prove fatal include infection, dehydration, and heart failure due to changes in blood chemistry.

Seeing the specialist
Having decided on a target weight and started a controlled feeding program, the specialist will try to help resolve any underlying emotional conflicts.

WHEN TO SEEK MEDICAL HELP

Anorexia nervosa cannot be treated simply by urging or forcing the sufferer to eat sensibly. The anorexic will just devise increasingly ingenious methods to give the appearance of eating normally. Expert treatment is needed as soon as possible because as the condition progresses it becomes more and more difficult to treat successfully. If your child seems to be dieting excessively and displays any of the eating disorder warning signs, consult your doctor without delay.

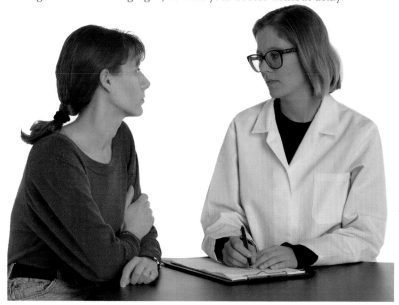

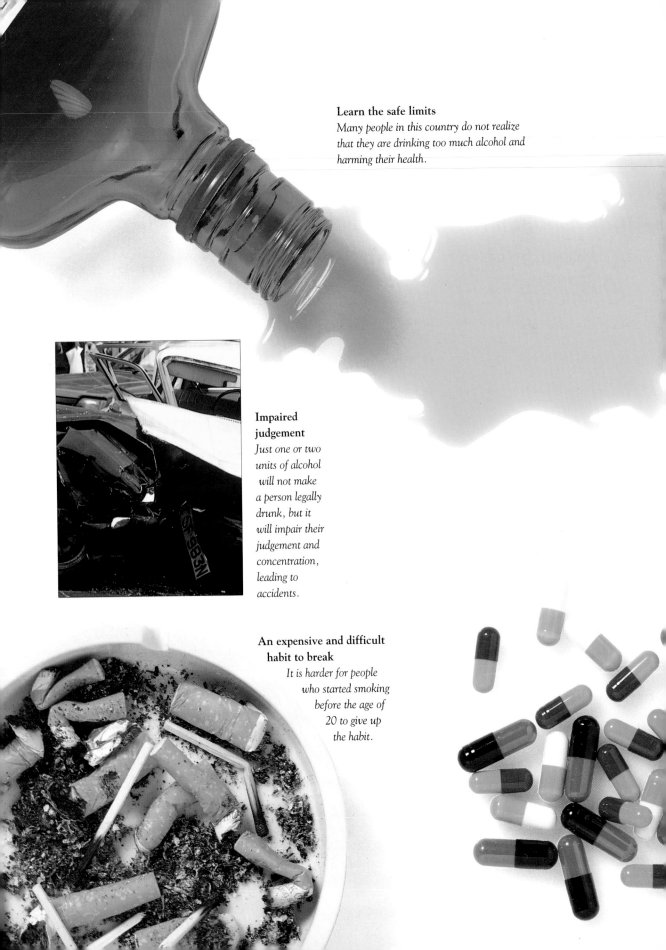

Learn the safe limits
Many people in this country do not realize that they are drinking too much alcohol and harming their health.

Impaired judgement
Just one or two units of alcohol will not make a person legally drunk, but it will impair their judgement and concentration, leading to accidents.

An expensive and difficult habit to break
It is harder for people who started smoking before the age of 20 to give up the habit.

CHAPTER FOUR

Cocaine
Made from coca leaves, overdose of this hallucinogenic drug can lead to cardiac arrest.

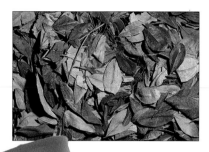

ALCOHOL, SMOKING, AND DRUG ABUSE

THE MOST WIDELY used and abused drugs are not illegal substances like heroin and cocaine but the readily available, and usually legal, stimulants: alcohol, tobacco, and caffeine.

Cigarette smoking is the most common cause of illness and premature death in the West, due primarily to cancer and heart disease. But most smokers continue their unhealthy habit despite the fact they know that giving up would immediately improve both their life expectancy and their quality of life.

Overconsumption of alcohol is a major health hazard which adds to many of society's problems, contributing to about one third of road traffic accidents, as well as to antisocial behavior, crime, divorce, and loss of productivity due to ill-health.

Smoking and drinking are hard habits to break because nicotine and alcohol are addictive. Smokers often cannot kick the habit even though they know that cigarettes increase their risks of becoming ill or dying young. Most drinkers are aware that overindulgence can have unpleasant consequences, but many have either become dependent on alcohol or just do not realize how destructive regular alcohol abuse can be to their physical and mental health. Yet with help and determination, both smoking and alcohol abuse can be stopped.

The dangers of smoking
Over the age of 16 smoking is legal – but it is not sensible. Smoking increases your risk of suffering from a heart attack, a stroke, and many types of cancer, particularly cancer of the lungs.

Addiction to prescribed drugs
Taking tranquillizers for more than two weeks can cause physical dependence.

SETTING A SAFE LIMIT

THE MORE YOU drink, and the more often you drink, the greater the risk that your internal organs will be damaged by alcohol, and that you may become dependent on it. Although these risks are closely linked to the amount you drink, a susceptibility to alcohol problems can be inherited. The children of problem drinkers or alcoholics would be well advised not to drink at all. Women can tolerate less alcohol than men partly because they are usually smaller.

Alcohol in your bloodstream

The way alcohol influences you depends on the level of alcohol in your blood. The level rises more quickly if you gulp a drink because your body has less time to distribute it to different tissues and to start metabolizing it. Drinks that have a high alcohol concentration, such as spirits, are absorbed more rapidly, causing a higher alcohol level.

Your blood alcohol increases with each drink. It takes about one hour to get rid of the alcohol from one drink. After drinking heavily late into the night, you will still have some alcohol in your bloodstream the next morning. Food slows down alcohol absorption, so drinking with a meal will result in a lower peak blood alcohol level.

As many as 1.5 million people in this country are harming their health with alcohol; 7 million are drinking more than the recommended limits.

Getting help

If you want to cut down but are not able to, then you are truly alcohol-dependent. Most alcoholics refuse to admit that they have a problem.

If you, or someone close to you, is drinking too much, seek help. Talk to your family doctor or visit Alcoholics Anonymous.

In severe cases, hospitalization and medication may be required to control withdrawal symptoms. Psychotherapy or a drug that creates unpleasant reactions if taken with any alcohol may be used.

WHAT IS A UNIT OF ALCOHOL?

To make it easier to record your intake of alcohol, a system has been devised which allows for the different alcohol content of different drinks. Alcohol consumption is now measured in units: each unit is roughly equivalent to eight grams of alcohol. The following drinks contain on average one unit of alcohol: half a pint of beer, one glass of table wine, one small glass of sherry, or one single shot of spirits.

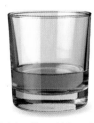 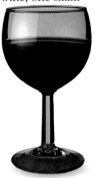 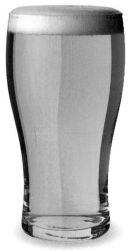

Spirits *like whisky, gin, vodka, and brandy contain between 30 and 40 percent alcohol. Home measures may be more generous, with three or four units per glass.*

Wine *contains about 10 percent alcohol. Fortified wines (sherry or port) contain up to twice as much alcohol, so a smaller glass is equivalent to one unit.*

Beer or lager *contains around 3.5 percent by volume of alcohol, but real ales and extra-strength lagers can contain nearly twice as much alcohol.*

TEENAGE DRINKING

Youngsters may turn to alcohol to help them cope with the problems of adolescence. But it can interfere with their ability to deal with difficult emotions. Some parents think that alcohol is better than other drugs or that teenagers should learn sensible drinking by having a glass with the rest of the family, but drinking can become a dangerous habit. Teenagers who drink regularly may become dependent. Your doctor can help if you think your teenager has a drink problem.

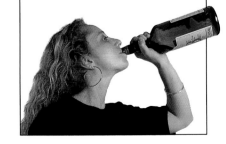

ARE YOU DRINKING TOO MUCH?

Alcohol has become a socially acceptable drug, with millions of people in this country regularly drinking at least once or twice a week. However, it is important to remember that alcohol is still a drug, and a potentially addictive one. There is a very fine line dividing the moderate social drinker from those people who have become dependent on alcohol, or who are damaging their health as a result of drinking too much.

Answer the following questions to assess your drinking habits. The more YES responses you give, the more likely it is you are developing a drinking problem or have one already and need professional help.

 Do you often have a drink when you are alone, either in a bar or at home?

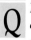 *Do you get into arguments at home after you have had a few drinks?*

 Do you continue drinking after your friends have said they have had enough?

 At a party, if your glass is empty, do you always go in search of another drink?

 Do you feel uncomfortable if you go a whole day without having any alcohol?

 Do you drink as a way of relaxing or winding down at the end of the day?

 Are you sometimes unable to remember things that happened when you have been drinking?

 Have you ever had to take time off work or miss an appointment because of your excessive drinking?

 Do you ever have the shakes, or find yourself craving a drink, when you wake up in the morning?

DRINKING IN MODERATION

• **Have two alcohol-free days a week**. You may have to avoid the places you normally have a drink, and the friends you usually drink with, on those days.

• **Choose low-alcohol or non-alcoholic drinks**. There are numerous brands on the market. Many taste just as good as their alcoholic equivalents.

• **Cut down**. Learn to say no to friends who ask you to have just one more. Buy your own drinks, drink at your own pace, and do not drink more than you intended.

• **Start with a thirst quencher**. When you go out, make your first drink a soft drink. Later, dilute your drinks to slow down your alcohol intake by adding a mixer like tonic or soda water.

• **Slow down**. Put your glass down between sips.

• **Record your units per day**. This will help you to identify when and where most of your drinking takes place, and to begin to cut down.

SAFE LIMITS

Drinking in moderation is unlikely to harm your health. The risks from alcohol rise steadily in proportion to the amount you consume. Monitor your weekly intake of alcohol and keep it below a maximum of 21 units for men and 14 units for women. The limits are lower for women partly because they tend to be smaller and partly because their bodies contain more fat, in which alcohol will not dissolve. The same quantity of alcohol therefore produces a higher concentration in a woman's bloodstream. Everyone should drink much less than the maximum limits and aim for at least two alcohol-free days per week.

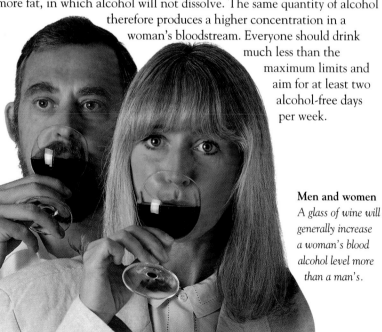

Men and women
A glass of wine will generally increase a woman's blood alcohol level more than a man's.

THE DANGERS OF ALCOHOL

Drinking to excess is not only dangerous in the short term, but on a regular basis it may seriously damage your health.

EVERYONE KNOWS that the heavy drinker damages his or her health and risks having accidents on the road, at home, and at work. Heavy drinking is also a major cause of vagrancy, antisocial behavior, and violence in the home, as well as of the breakdown of personal relationships.

Many people, however, drink regularly but never become drunk, violent, or argumentative and so assume that their drinking is not harming them. They are deluding themselves. Regular consumption of substantial amounts of alcohol may damage the liver, the heart, and the brain. If a high alcohol intake is maintained for many years, permanent damage to these organs is inevitable. Alcohol abuse can also cause a number of different types of cancer.

The risks to your physical health from alcohol depend on how much you drink, not how much it affects your behavior. Drinking regularly gets your body used to alcohol so that it takes a lot more to produce the same effects. A heavy drinker can drink a lot without appearing drunk. Someone who "can hold their drink" is therefore at greater risk than someone who can only drink one or two glasses before becoming affected.

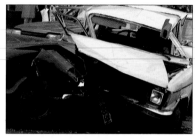

Drinking and driving
The blood alcohol level of one third of drivers who are killed is over the legal limit. Even a little alcohol will impair your judgement, concentration, and driving skills, so do not drink if you are driving.

DEATH DUE TO ALCOHOLIC LIVER CIRRHOSIS

Comparing death rates due to alcoholic cirrhosis of the liver and the annual per capita consumption of alcohol in different countries shows a clear link between the amount of alcohol being drunk and the number of reported cases of cirrhosis.

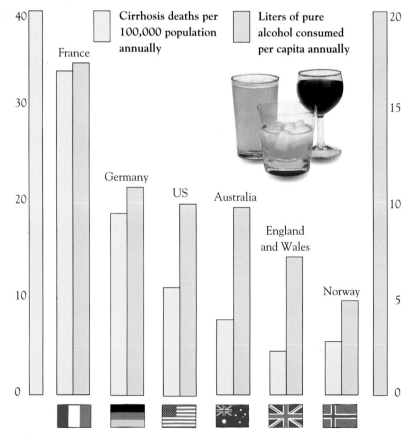

Cirrhosis deaths per 100,000 population annually

Liters of pure alcohol consumed per capita annually

France

Germany

US

Australia

England and Wales

Norway

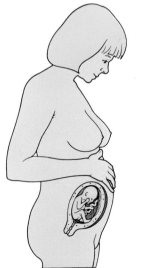

Alcohol and pregnancy
Heavy drinking during pregnancy may cause fetal alcohol syndrome, where the baby is born mentally retarded and with a variety of other serious birth defects. Even small amounts of alcohol increase this risk, so it is better to abstain completely.

LONG-TERM DAMAGE

Persistent heavy drinking may damage many different body tissues, resulting in a number of serious diseases.

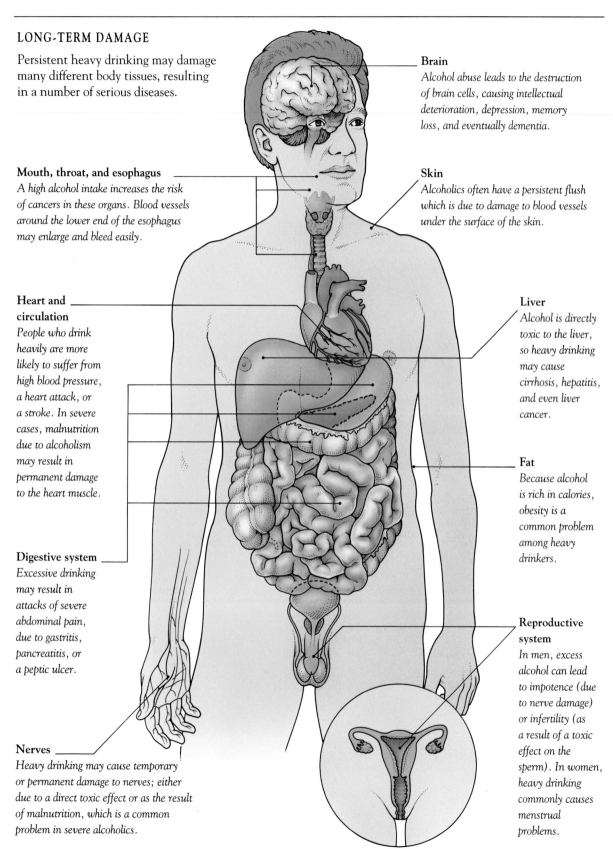

Brain
Alcohol abuse leads to the destruction of brain cells, causing intellectual deterioration, depression, memory loss, and eventually dementia.

Mouth, throat, and esophagus
A high alcohol intake increases the risk of cancers in these organs. Blood vessels around the lower end of the esophagus may enlarge and bleed easily.

Skin
Alcoholics often have a persistent flush which is due to damage to blood vessels under the surface of the skin.

Heart and circulation
People who drink heavily are more likely to suffer from high blood pressure, a heart attack, or a stroke. In severe cases, malnutrition due to alcoholism may result in permanent damage to the heart muscle.

Liver
Alcohol is directly toxic to the liver, so heavy drinking may cause cirrhosis, hepatitis, and even liver cancer.

Fat
Because alcohol is rich in calories, obesity is a common problem among heavy drinkers.

Digestive system
Excessive drinking may result in attacks of severe abdominal pain, due to gastritis, pancreatitis, or a peptic ulcer.

Reproductive system
In men, excess alcohol can lead to impotence (due to nerve damage) or infertility (as a result of a toxic effect on the sperm). In women, heavy drinking commonly causes menstrual problems.

Nerves
Heavy drinking may cause temporary or permanent damage to nerves; either due to a direct toxic effect or as the result of malnutrition, which is a common problem in severe alcoholics.

THE RISKS OF SMOKING

SINCE THE 1950's, when the health risks of smoking were first studied, smoking has been directly linked with cancers of the lung, mouth, throat, esophagus, larynx, and bladder. Smokers are also suspected of having a higher risk of contracting cancers of the kidney, pancreas, and stomach.

Although most people are fully aware of the increased cancer risk from smoking, there are numerous other smoking-related conditions that are less well known. Smokers have a much greater chance of suffering from a heart attack or a stroke. Women who smoke are likely to have an earlier menopause, which inevitably increases their risk of developing osteoporosis.

In addition to the typical smoker's cough, many smokers go on to develop chronic bronchitis and emphysema which can severely limit their ability to get exercise. Just walking a few yards may cause shortness of breath and even respiratory distress.

Smoking in pregnancy
Miscarriage, stillbirth, and premature or low birth weight babies are more common among smokers because nicotine restricts the amounts of oxygen and nutrients that reach the fetus. There is also an increased risk of sudden infant death syndrome, lung problems, and some fetal abnormalities among infants whose mothers smoked during pregnancy.

Are low-tar and low-nicotine brands less hazardous?
There is no safe cigarette. Smokers compensate for the reduced tar and nicotine in some brands by puffing harder and longer, smoking more, and inhaling more deeply.

Inhaling cigarette smoke is a major health risk: 85 per cent of lung cancers stem from smoking.

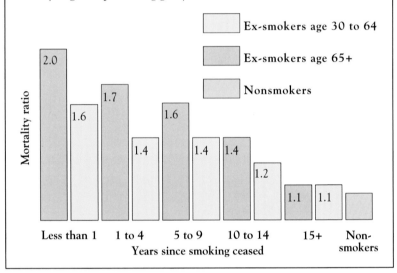

DECREASING MORTALITY RISK IN EX-SMOKERS

As soon as you give up smoking, you lower your risk of dying from smoking-related diseases. This bar chart shows how the mortality ratio (the number of times more likely it is that an ex-smoker will die in any one year than a lifelong nonsmoker) reduces as the years since you gave up smoking go by.

Ex-smokers age 30 to 64

Ex-smokers age 65+

Nonsmokers

Mortality ratio

| Less than 1 | 1 to 4 | 5 to 9 | 10 to 14 | 15+ | Non-smokers |

2.0 — 1.6 — 1.7 — 1.4 — 1.6 — 1.4 — 1.4 — 1.2 — 1.1 — 1.1

Years since smoking ceased

HOW DOES SMOKING CAUSE LUNG CANCER?

Smoking cigarettes is the main cause of lung cancer. The more cigarettes smoked per day, and the lower the age at which smoking started, the greater the risk of contracting lung cancer. Pipe and cigar smokers do

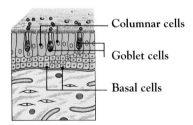

Columnar cells

Goblet cells

Basal cells

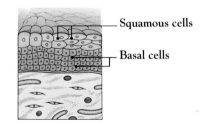

Squamous cells

Basal cells

1 Most types of lung cancer develop in the wall of one of the large airways (the bronchi). The linings of these bronchi are made up of basal cells; goblet cells, which produce mucus; and tall columnar cells, which are covered by fine hairs (cilia).

2 Regular smoking leads to changes in the structure and function of all these cells. Columnar cells lose their cilia, and become progressively more flattened, to form the squamous type of cell, similar to those found in the skin.

SYMPTOMS OF SMOKING-RELATED DISEASES

The symptoms described here are more common among smokers. A number of these symptoms will improve quickly once you stop smoking. Continuing to smoke will only aggravate them.

Breathlessness and wheezing
Smoking impairs lung capacity and can result in difficulty breathing during exertion. Chronic bronchitis and emphysema, which both cause shortness of breath and wheezing, are common problems in smokers, and can be extremely disabling.

Indigestion
Recurrent attacks of abdominal pain, with nausea, vomiting, and belching, may be due to gastritis or a peptic ulcer, aggravated or brought on by smoking.

Blood in urine
The appearance of blood in your urine may be a symptom of bladder or kidney cancer, both of which are more likely to develop in smokers.

White or red patches in your mouth
These symptoms may be the result of early cancerous changes and should be reported immediately to your doctor or dentist.

Coughing
A persistent cough in a smoker may be due to chronic bronchitis, emphysema, or occasionally lung cancer.

Chest pain
Smoking is a major risk factor in coronary heart disease which causes chest pain brought on by exercise (angina) and heart attacks. Persistent chest pain is also occasionally a symptom of lung cancer.

Circulation problems
Cramping pains in your legs, brought on by walking, are a warning symptom of impaired circulation and are usually the result of smoking. Unless you stop smoking, leg ulcers and gangrene may develop, requiring major surgery.

---

have a reduced risk compared with cigarette smokers, but because they still inhale tobacco smoke they have a much higher risk than people who do not smoke at all.

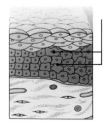

Basal cells become cancerous

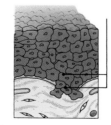

Multipyling cancer cells break through basilar membrane

3 *New cells formed in the basal layer replace those damaged or killed by tobacco smoke, but they too may be affected by chemicals in the smoke. When basal cells multiply quickly, some of them may transform into cancer cells.*

4 *Cancer cells grow and divide rapidly to replace healthy cells in the basal layer. The developing cancer may then block the air passage or may break through the membrane beneath to spread into the deeper tissues of the lung.*

PASSIVE SMOKING

Breathing in the smoke from other people's cigarettes is known as passive smoking. Smoke from burning tobacco contains even more nicotine, tar, and carbon monoxide than that inhaled by the smoker. Nonsmokers who are regularly exposed to tobacco smoke increase their risk of cancer by 10 to 30 percent. Young children whose parents smoke are more likely to develop bronchitis and asthma.

How to Stop Smoking

I T IS NEVER TOO late to give up smoking. No matter how long you have smoked, the risk of developing a smoking-related disease like chronic bronchitis or suffering from a heart attack, decreases as soon as you give up. After five years of not smoking, the risk of premature death from these diseases is almost halved; after around 15 years, the ex-smoker has about the same risk as a nonsmoker.

Although nearly four out of five smokers say they would like to give up, only about one quarter of those who try actually manage to do so. Motivation is the key factor in successfully quitting smoking.

If you stop smoking, will you put on weight?

Some people do put on a few extra pounds when they give up smoking, partly because their appetite

Every day you do not smoke is an investment toward your future health.

increases and partly because of a change in their body's metabolism. However, being overweight is not as bad for your health as smoking. You can keep your weight under control by nibbling on healthy snacks such as air-popped popcorn and fresh fruit between meals. By eating sensibly, you can limit your weight gain to about 5 lb (2.5 kg).

Why do you smoke?

To help you stop smoking, it is worthwhile to think carefully about the reasons why you smoke. Once you have assessed your smoking habits, you can find out what type of smoker you are. Then you stand a much greater chance of successfully breaking your habit.

The nicotine addict

If you are addicted to nicotine, you will begin to feel restless and crave another cigarette within a few minutes of putting out your last one. These withdrawal symptoms, which may also include headaches, anxiety, and irritability, make it more difficult to quit. If you suffer from these symptoms, a prescription for nicotine chewing gum from your doctor can help. Prolonged use of nicotine gum can occasionally be habit-forming, but it will not damage your health as much as the inhalation of carbon monoxide, tar, and other toxic substances from cigarettes.

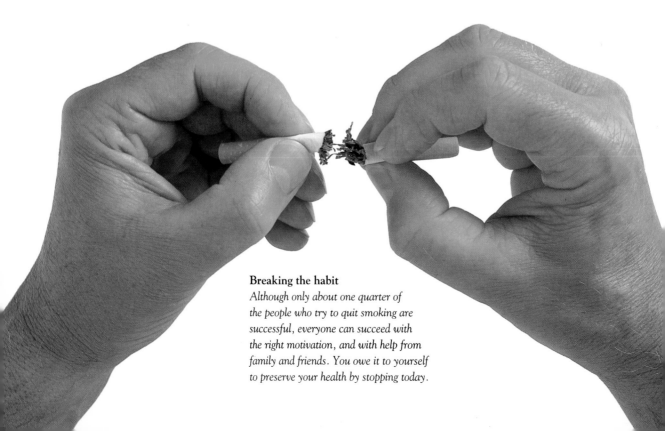

Breaking the habit
Although only about one quarter of the people who try to quit smoking are successful, everyone can succeed with the right motivation, and with help from family and friends. You owe it to yourself to preserve your health by stopping today.

The habitual smoker

To break the habit, you must disrupt your daily routine, avoiding situations in which you will want to smoke. If you usually have a cigarette right after a meal, then get up from the table and pour yourself a drink of water.

Smoking to relax

If you smoke simply as a way of relieving tension, try some other ways of coping with the stresses in your life, such as taking up some form of physical activity, or doing a relaxation exercise.

The social smoker

If several of your friends smoke, you may need to avoid them for the first few weeks until you have built up your resistance to the temptation to smoke. Practice looking in the mirror and saying, "No thanks, I don't smoke." You should also avoid going to those places where you would normally smoke, such as a bar.

Smoking to occupy your hands and mouth

Many smokers turn to food instead of a cigarette as something to do with their hands and mouth. Choose some other simple activity such as playing with worry beads or chewing sugar-free gum.

Smoking to alleviate boredom

If you smoke when you are bored and have nothing else to do, take up a hobby or sport. Exercising will also help you shed any weight gained after you quit.

RELAXING WITHOUT CIGARETTES

To stop feeling tense and anxious when you go without a cigarette for a few hours, try a relaxation exercise:

To rest your body
Tighten up the muscles in each part of your body in turn, starting with your feet, and working up to your face and scalp. Hold each group of muscles tight for a count of 10; then let them relax.

To calm your mind
Sit in a quiet room, close your eyes, empty your mind, and listen to your breathing. Count each breath until you reach 50. Then, sit quietly for a while thinking of nothing in particular. Any time your mind wanders, start counting again.

HOW TO GIVE UP

- You must really want to stop. Make a list of all your reasons for trying to quit and choose a relaxed, stress-free day to start. Alternatively, you could begin on a day you feel ill.
- Stop altogether, not gradually. Do not be tempted to take another puff.
- Ask those close to you for help. You could even give up with a friend.
- Throw away cigarettes and lighters and avoid people and places where you are tempted to smoke.
- Cut down on chocolate, red meat, tea, coffee, and alcohol: they can make you crave a cigarette. Eat healthy foods and sip water instead.
- Take up an exercise or hobby.
- Buy yourself a treat with the money you would have spent on cigarettes.
- Try hypnosis or acupuncture.

CHILDREN AND SMOKING

Many children smoke. They may be attracted by the desire to appear mature, pressure from their friends, or the need to disguise their shyness or awkwardness in social situations. Glossy ads can also influence children. Although cigarettes are no longer promoted on television, a number of sporting events are still being sponsored by tobacco companies.

It is even harder for those who started before the age of 20 to give up smoking than for those who took up the habit when they were older.

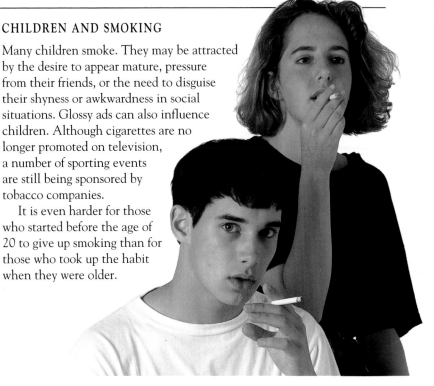

DRUG ABUSE

DRUG ABUSE IS the improper use of any drug, for purposes other than those for which it is normally prescribed or recommended. Addiction to a drug of abuse includes psychological dependence, where the individual feels intense craving or emotional distress when that drug is no longer being taken; and physical dependence, where stopping the drug causes unpleasant withdrawal symptoms.

Dependence on any type of drug is likely to lead to various physical, psychological, social, and financial problems. Not all drug dependence involves illegal drugs; many thousands of people are dependent on alcohol, nicotine, and caffeine. Certain prescription drugs may also cause dependence. They include barbiturates, corticosteroids, and the benzodiazepine tranquillizers, such as diazepam.

The risks from drug abuse include toxic side effects, accidents while under the influence, and the likelihood of developing a habit.

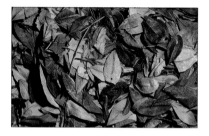

Cocaine *comes from the leaves of the coca plant. It is a stimulant, causing heightened sensations and even hallucinations. Effects include dilated pupils, trembling, and insomnia. Regular inhaling, or snorting, may damage the nose. Overdose can cause seizures and cardiac arrest. Long-term use will cause psychological dependence.*

Heroin and morphine *are powerful painkillers, used medically to treat severe pain, such as in cancer. They are abused because they replace feelings of anxiety and depression by contentment and intense wellbeing. Effects include lethargy, mood swings, and slurred speech. Regular abuse leads to physical dependence, with an unpleasant withdrawal reaction if they are stopped suddenly.*

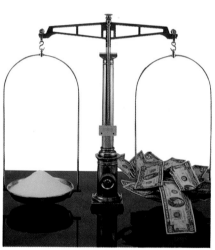

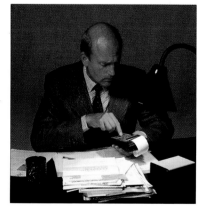

Amphetamines *are stimulants, which, because they suppress appetite, were once commonly prescribed to help people lose weight. They are abused because of their ability to induce feelings of excitement and energy; and to overcome the effects of fatigue or lack of sleep. Physical effects include dilated pupils, trembling, diarrhea, and insomnia. Regular use can cause delusions or violent behavior.*

Marijuana *comes from the flowering tops and dried leaves of the Indian hemp plant Cannabis Sativa. It causes feelings of relaxation and heightened perception. Physical effects include a dry mouth, increased appetite, slight clumsiness, and mild reddening of the eyes. Prolonged, regular use may cause depression and apathy.*

ALCOHOL, SMOKING, AND DRUG ABUSE

Benzodiazepine *tranquillizer drugs are used to treat anxiety and insomnia and are abused for their relaxing effects. Diazepam is one example. Regular use for more than two weeks may cause physical dependence. Doctors usually only prescribe them for short periods, and in a low dosage. After long-term use, the dose must be reduced gradually to prevent withdrawal symptoms.*

Barbiturates *are sedative drugs prescribed for epilepsy, and occasionally for insomnia. They are abused because of their relaxing, calming effect. Physical effects include slurred speech, loss of coordination and balance, and drowsiness. Regular use leads to physical dependence, with an unpleasant withdrawal reaction if they are stopped suddenly.*

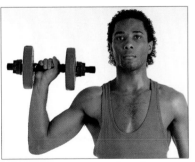

Anabolic steroids *are abused by some athletes to help them develop their muscle strength and bulk. Because they speed up muscle recovery, anabolic steroids allow a more demanding training schedule. They are banned in all competitive sports, not just because they give an unfair advantage, but also due to the serious side effects they can cause, such as liver damage and infertility.*

Solvents *are volatile substances, such as glue and cleaning fluids. When inhaled they cause hallucinations and feelings of wellbeing. Effects include dilated pupils, flushing, and confusion. Regular abuse may lead to inflammation and sores around the mouth and nose. Permanent brain, liver, or kidney damage is possible, as well as asphyxia while actually inhaling.*

CHILDREN AND DRUG ABUSE

Warning signs that a child may be abusing drugs:

• Periods of drowsiness and lethargy, alternating with hyperactivity and euphoria.
• A change in appetite.
• Marked mood swings and changes in personality.
• Unusually small or large pupils, and heavy eyelids.
• Confusion, slurred speech, and irrational behavior.
• Bouts of shivering.
• Soreness around the nose and constant sniffing.
• Unsteadiness and poor coordination.

General points to keep in mind:

• Be careful when accusing a child of drug abuse. Many teenagers go through natural phases of moodiness, irritability, or withdrawn behavior.
• It is important to warn your child about drugs.
• If you do suspect a problem, offer support rather than confrontation, and visit your family doctor.

LSD *is a powerful hallucinogenic drug. It is unpredictable; the hallucinations may be pleasant or terrifying. Effects include dilated pupils, sweating, trembling, and altered behavior. A single dose may cause repeated episodes of mental disturbance. A few people have died under the influence of the drug, for example by believing they can fly and stepping out of windows.*

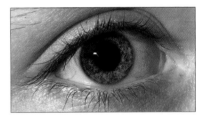

COMING OFF DRUGS

• Your doctor, or groups like Release or Samaritans, should be able to refer you to a drug rehabilitation center.
• Reducing your dosage over several weeks, under medical supervision, can minimize withdrawal symptoms.
• Heroin addiction is sometimes treated by abrupt abstinence and the use of methadone, a painkiller, to relieve the withdrawal symptoms.
• Psychotherapy may be advised.
• Moving to a new environment and breaking with drug-taking friends may reduce the risk of readdiction.
• Self-help groups can help maintain the motivation to stay off drugs.

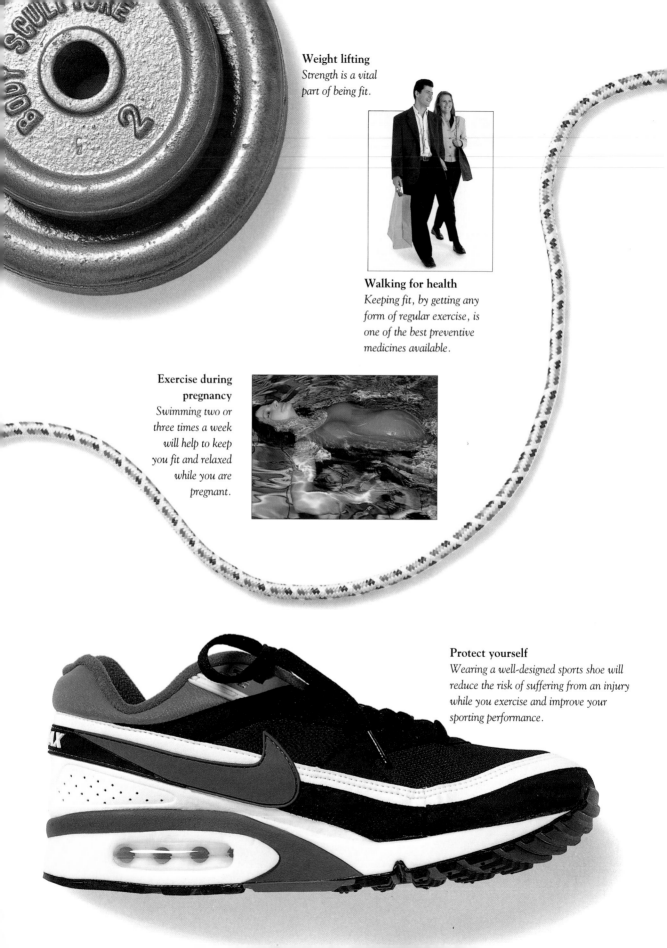

Weight lifting
Strength is a vital part of being fit.

Walking for health
Keeping fit, by getting any form of regular exercise, is one of the best preventive medicines available.

Exercise during pregnancy
Swimming two or three times a week will help to keep you fit and relaxed while you are pregnant.

Protect yourself
Wearing a well-designed sports shoe will reduce the risk of suffering from an injury while you exercise and improve your sporting performance.

CHAPTER FIVE

FIT FOR LIFE

A simple and effective exercise
Skipping rope is not just for the young; it can be enjoyed at any age. Like all forms of aerobic exercise, it makes your heart and lungs fitter.

How to start
The first step to becoming fitter is to choose an exercise you will enjoy and that is suitable for your level of fitness.

Check your pulse rate
Your level of fitness can be assessed roughly by taking your pulse. If you count more than 100 beats per minute when you are at rest, you may have a problem and should therefore consult a doctor.

EVEN THOUGH MOST people know that fitness is important, they may not know what fitness really means. It is not the same as athletic excellence.

Fitness is simply the ability to cope with the physical workload of everyday activities, while still having energy in reserve to meet any sudden unexpected demands. The average adult should be able to carry heavy shopping, dig the garden, or run for the bus, without becoming breathless and exhausted.

Unfortunately, many people think they are fit when they are not. Just because you are rarely ill, does not necessarily mean that you are in good shape physically. The only way to stay fit is to exercise vigorously, at least three times a week.

Although you probably know that exercise is good for your health, like many people, you may think that exercise is not for you. The list of excuses for not exercising is endless: too busy, too tired, or too out of condition. But the benefits you will get from exercise far outweigh the effort it takes.

Exercise will make your heart and lungs more efficient and your muscles stronger, as well as improving your figure and posture and enhancing your sense of wellbeing. You will also feel more relaxed, sleep better, and be able to deal more effectively with day-to-day stresses. By continuing to stay active throughout your life, you are likely to live longer and stay in good health. The habit of exercising regularly will keep you fit for life.

THE BENEFITS OF EXERCISE

HAVING AN EXERCISE routine as a regular feature of your normal day-to-day lifestyle is probably the most positive step you can take to keep yourself fitter and healthier over the years ahead. Your heart, lungs, circulation, muscles, bones, joints, and even your state of mind will all benefit from undertaking frequent physical activity. Exercise brings about both short and long-term benefits, it improves the overall efficiency of your body, and helps to fight off disease. If your job is not physically demanding you should take up a sport in your free time. This will help to ensure that you stay active.

Exercising just two or three times a week for periods of only 20 minutes will help keep you fit for life.

MODERATE EXERCISE IMPROVES YOUR LIFE SPAN

Life expectancy is significantly higher for people who are classified as being of medium fitness than for those who are unfit.

In a recent study, the physical fitness levels of 13,344 volunteers were measured using a treadmill. The participants were classified into five categories, ranging from the least fit in group one, through the medium fit in groups two and three, to the highest levels of fitness in groups four and five. Each group's death rates were then monitored, over a number of years.

Results revealed that the death rate for the unfit people in group one was more than double the figure for people of medium fitness. There was a further reduction in the death rate between the medium and high fitness groups, but this was not as dramatic.

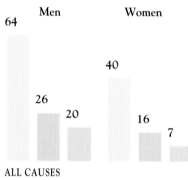

Men   Women

ALL CAUSES

CARDIOVASCULAR DISEASE

CANCER

Deaths per 10,000 people per year

EXERCISE PROTECTS AGAINST DISEASE

• **Relieves back pain**. Exercises that keep spinal and abdominal muscles strong improve your posture and may prevent back pain.

• **Fights obesity**. Regular exercise, in combination with a balanced diet, helps you keep control of your weight. Obesity increases your risk of developing many diseases including diabetes, heart disease, and gallstones.

• **Decreases cancer risk**. Research has confirmed that a poor level of fitness can increase your risk of developing some types of cancer.

• **Combats anxiety and depression**. Frequent exercise can enhance your self-esteem and make you feel brighter and more relaxed.

KEY

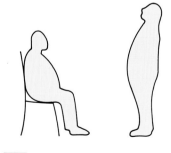
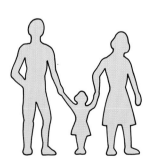
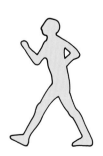
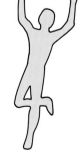

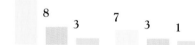

☐ Group 1 – low fitness   ☐ Groups 2 and 3 – medium fitness   ☐ Groups 4 and 5 – high fitness

IMPROVING YOUR HEALTH
Regular exercise

Infrequent bouts of intense physical activity are of little long-term benefit to your health. It is much more important that you persevere with a regular exercise routine. If you do not, all the benefits will be lost as your fitness begins to deteriorate.

- **Strengthens bones**. Regular moderate exercise strengthens your bones by increasing their mineral content, thereby reducing the risk of developing osteoporosis later in life. Osteoporosis causes bones to become progressively thinner, which makes them more fragile and vulnerable to fracture.

- **Reduces your risk of heart disease**. Exercise helps to prevent obesity, high cholesterol levels, and high blood pressure.

- **Alleviates menstrual disorders**. Some women have found that exercise reduces premenstrual symptoms and eases period pain.

- **Helps you sleep**. Exercise encourages deep sleep, as long as you allow at least an hour between exercising and retiring to bed.

MUSCLE CHANGES

Regular exercise aids muscle efficiency by causing the small blood vessels which supply oxygen to the muscles to multiply. Exercise also increases the size and number of mitochondria (energy-producing power units) within the muscle cells. The mitochondria use this extra oxygen to produce more energy.

LONG-TERM BENEFITS OF EXERCISE

Exercise over a long period of time will increase the efficiency of many organs within your body.

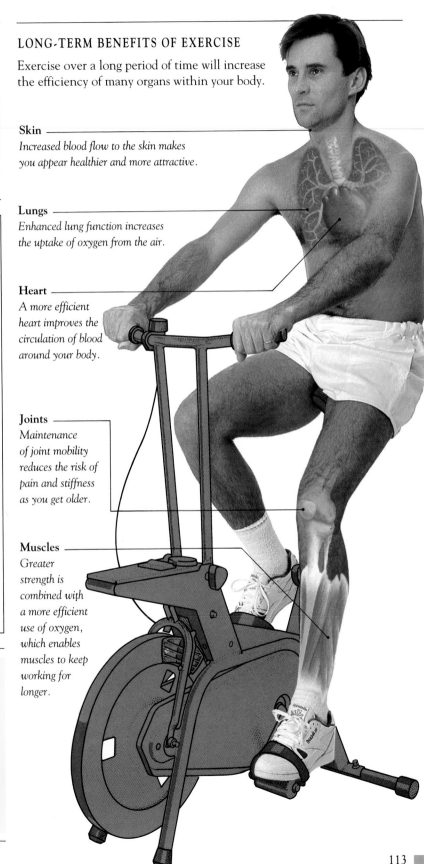

Skin
Increased blood flow to the skin makes you appear healthier and more attractive.

Lungs
Enhanced lung function increases the uptake of oxygen from the air.

Heart
A more efficient heart improves the circulation of blood around your body.

Joints
Maintenance of joint mobility reduces the risk of pain and stiffness as you get older.

Muscles
Greater strength is combined with a more efficient use of oxygen, which enables muscles to keep working for longer.

EXERCISE AND THE HEALTHY HEART

Regular exercise encourages your heart to work more efficiently.

THE MUSCLE FIBERS in the walls that surround the chambers of the heart thicken and strengthen in response to regular energetic exercise. As the heart of a physically fit person is strong, it is able to pump a much larger volume of blood with each beat, both during exercise and while at rest.

Because fitness produces a more powerful and efficient heart, a relatively slow heartbeat is able to pump the required volume of blood around the body while at rest. Many of the world's top athletes have a resting pulse of only 40 beats per minute. In contrast, someone who is very much out of condition may have a pulse as high as 90 to 100 beats per minute.

Another sign of a fit heart is that the pulse rate rapidly returns to normal after vigorous exercise. In someone who exer-

cises regularly, the pulse generally returns to the resting level within one minute. A person who is not used to strenuous physical activity may take four or five minutes to return to normal.

If you take more than a few minutes to recover from energetic exercise, or suffer from prolonged palpitations, see your doctor.

Activity promotes good health

Regular, vigorous activity decreases the risk of suffering from pain in the heart (angina) or having a heart attack.

Exercise protects against heart disease by "flushing through" the arteries which supply the heart muscle. Fatty material from cholesterol might otherwise "clog-up" these arteries. If they become completely blocked it could cause a heart attack. Exercise also prevents obesity, which could lead to high blood pressure and diabetes.

Powering your way to fitness
A healthy heart normally pumps up to 9 pints (5 liters) of blood around the body in a minute and beats 60 to 70 times a minute. During intense exertion, the volume of blood pumped around the body may reach 54 pints (30 liters) a minute and the heart rate can speed up to 200 beats per minute.

WHERE DOES THE BLOOD GO?

Muscles require very little energy when they are at rest. Much of the blood being pumped around the circulation is therefore diverted to other tissues, for example to the digestive system to help with the absorption of nutrients from food.

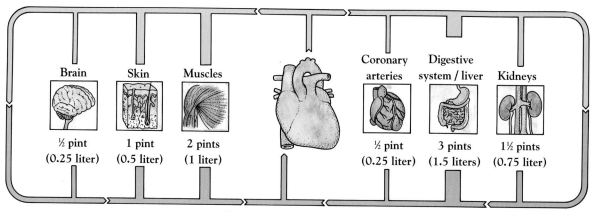

Brain	Skin	Muscles		Coronary arteries	Digestive system / liver	Kidneys
½ pint (0.25 liter)	1 pint (0.5 liter)	2 pints (1 liter)		½ pint (0.25 liter)	3 pints (1.5 liters)	1½ pints (0.75 liter)

Blood flow (per minute) at rest

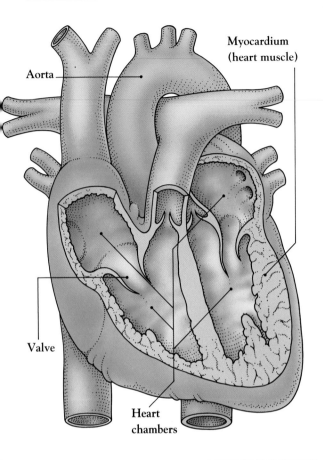

Aorta

Myocardium
(heart muscle)

Valve

Heart
chambers

EXERCISE AND A CHANGE OF HEART

Regular exercise improves the efficiency of the heart, both at rest and during exercise. This improvement in the performance of the heart occurs as the result of changes inside its muscle wall.

• Muscle fibers become stronger and thicker to produce a more powerful contraction.
• Blood vessels in the muscles proliferate, improving the supply of oxygen and nutrients to the muscle cells.

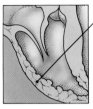

Heart wall of a
sedentary person

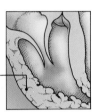

Heart wall of a
person who
exercises often

HEART RATE AND EXERCISE

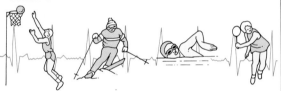

Age 15
145 beats
per minute

Age 30
133 beats
per minute

Age 45
120 beats
per minute

Age 60
110 beats
per minute

Vigorous exercise will increase the speed and the overall strength of your heartbeat. After just a few minutes of energetic exercise, your pulse should be close to the recommended target value for your age, as shown above.

During strenuous exercise, the blood is pumped faster around the body to supply the muscles more efficiently. This extremely large volume of blood supplies the muscles with all the extra oxygen and nutrients needed to provide energy for sustained and vigorous contraction.

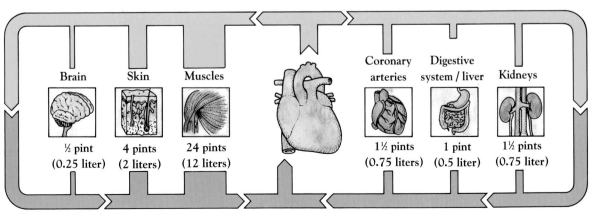

Brain	Skin	Muscles		Coronary arteries	Digestive system / liver	Kidneys
½ pint (0.25 liter)	4 pints (2 liters)	24 pints (12 liters)		1½ pints (0.75 liters)	1 pint (0.5 liter)	1½ pints (0.75 liter)

Blood flow (per minute) during exercise

WHAT IS FITNESS?

Fitness is simply the ability to carry out normal daily activities, without becoming unduly exhausted or breathless.

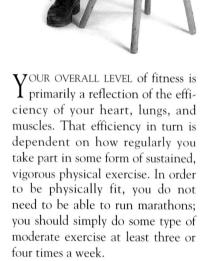

Y OUR OVERALL LEVEL of fitness is primarily a reflection of the efficiency of your heart, lungs, and muscles. That efficiency in turn is dependent on how regularly you take part in some form of sustained, vigorous physical exercise. In order to be physically fit, you do not need to be able to run marathons; you should simply do some type of moderate exercise at least three or four times a week.

Components of fitness

Physical fitness is made up of three distinct elements: strength, flexibility, and endurance. Each type of sport or physical activity can be rated according to the amount of these three elements required to perform it.

All three fitness components are needed to some extent in every sport. However, in gymnastics, for instance, a high level of flexibility is more important than endurance,

Helping you enjoy life
Improving your endurance, strength, and flexibility will help you in your daily life as well as while you are exercising.

as each gym exercise routine only lasts a minute or so, while in long-distance running, endurance is by far the most important factor.

Strength

At least one quarter, or even as much as one half, of your body weight is made up of muscle tissue. This muscle tissue provides you with your strength, which is simply the ability to exert enough muscular force to push, pull, lift, or carry a heavy load.

Your body contains around 400 muscles, which are attached to your skeleton by tendons. All your body's movements are controlled by contracting or relaxing specific groups of muscles.

Flexibility

Flexibility is your ability to bend, stretch, or twist through a full range of movements. A good level of flexibility is dependent on your joints, muscles, and tendons being able to move easily. It is important in all sports and physical activities, but particularly those where you need to be agile, such as skiing, gymnastics, and judo. Women in their late teens are generally the most flexible group of people.

FITNESS FACT

At rest, a fit heart can pump 25 percent, and during exercise 50 percent, more blood than an unfit heart.

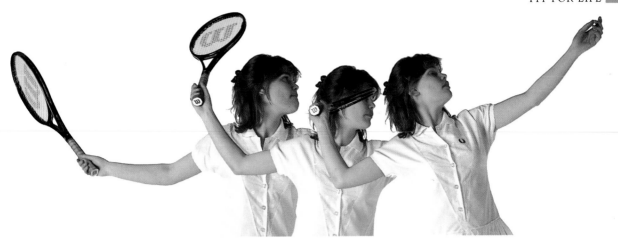

Being flexible decreases your risk of suffering a sprain or strain, because supple, elastic tissues are better able to absorb the shock of sudden or rapid movements. People with tight back and leg muscles are more likely to suffer from back pain and stiffness after exertion.

Endurance

Endurance is the ability to exercise at a steady rate, without a rest, for a long period of time. It is dependent on the efficiency and performance of your heart, lungs, and muscles. Low endurance may result in muscle fatigue and poor coordination. To improve your overall endurance you need to exercise vigorously for a period of at least 20 minutes, three times a week.

There is no perfect exercise, but any energetic activity will improve your level of fitness. To succeed in your quest for health you must find a sport that you enjoy, otherwise you are unlikely to exercise enough. Ideally this activity should enhance your strength, your flexibility, and your endurance.

KEY

S Strength   **F** Flexibility   **E** Endurance

● High   ● Medium   ○ Low

Are you fit enough for tennis?

To play tennis competitively you need a high level of all three components of fitness. Strength is required to hit a powerful serve. Flexibility in the shoulder and elbow are essential for an efficient technique, in both serving and stroke play, in order to minimize your risk of injury. Endurance helps prevent fatigue and muscle cramps.

ELEMENTS OF FITNESS NEEDED FOR VARIOUS PHYSICAL ACTIVITIES

The chart below lists a wide range of popular sports, plus a few everyday activities, and rates them according to the levels of strength, flexibility, and endurance they normally require. However, it is important to realize that the exact demands made by these activities will depend, at least partly, on how vigorously you perform them.

ACTIVITY	S	F	E
Basketball	Low	Low	High
Dancing	Low	Medium	Low
Gardening	Low	Low	Low
Golf	Low	Low	Low
Housework	Medium	Low	High
Running, long-distance	Medium	Low	High
Soccer	Low	Low	High
Squash	Medium	Medium	High
Swimming	Medium	Low	High
Tennis	Medium	Medium	Medium
Walking	Low	Low	Low
Weightlifting	Medium	Low	Low

AEROBIC EXERCISES

Aerobic exercises improve your health by making your heart and lungs fitter.

AEROBIC EXERCISE IS any form of physical activity that can be performed without a break for at least 12 minutes. The muscles can keep working because they receive a constant supply of oxygen, while the energy they need is provided from the body's stores of glucose (sugar), glycogen (starch), and fat.

The heart and the lungs have to work harder to increase the amount of oxygen-rich blood circulating around the body to the muscles. Because the muscles are not being pushed too hard, there is sufficient oxygen to meet their demands. As a result, the muscle cells tire slowly, and the exercise can be carried on for a long period.

Aerobic exercises are the best type of activity for increasing your general level of fitness, particularly the performance and efficiency of your heart, lungs, and muscles. It is an essential part of any balanced physical fitness program.

MONITORING YOUR PROGRESS
How to become fitter

• Start slowly, and gradually build up your endurance over a few weeks.
• Exercise until your heart beats faster and you are short of breath, not until you are spent and breathless.
• Exercise continuously for at least 20 minutes three times a week.
• Increase either the time or the distance by around 10 percent a week. If you feel uncomfortable, ease off a little until your fitness improves.

Jogging
You should be able to walk briskly for two miles, without any difficulty, before you attempt to go jogging. Alternate jogging and walking in 110 yard (100 m) stretches at first. As you improve, gradually increase the time you jog until you are jogging the whole way.

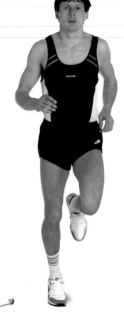

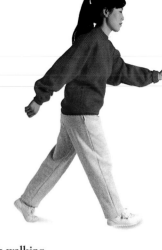

Brisk walking
At first, walking only a short distance may make you breathless and tired. However, once your fitness improves you should be able to walk farther, and for a longer time. You should take at least three brisk half-hour walks each week, unless of course you are doing some other aerobic activities as well.

Cross-country skiing
In some countries, where there is snow on the ground for much of the year, cross-country skiing is a popular aerobic activity. It is a demanding sport that works the muscles in the shoulders, back, chest, and abdomen.

Swimming
Swimming is an excellent aerobic activity. Gradually decrease the frequency of the breaks you take to get your breath back. Aim to swim continuously, at a steady pace, for 20 minutes. Alternate days of swimming with rest days to give your muscles time to recover.

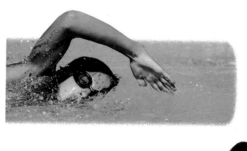

Rowing
Rowing improves your overall strength and endurance. Rowing machines allow this excellent aerobic exercise to be performed in the privacy of your own home.

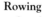

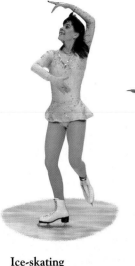

Ice-skating
If you are able to skate energetically, without falling over every few minutes on the ice, then you can use this sport to keep fit.

Jumping Rope
Jumping rope is convenient, once the technique is mastered. It may be easier to keep going for the full 20 minutes by alternating it with jogging on the spot. So as not to jar your joints, only raise your feet around 4 in (10 cm) off the ground.

Cycling
Cycling is an enjoyable aerobic activity. A good way to incorporate it into your daily routine is to cycle to the store or to work if possible. Be sure to wear reflectors and a proper safety helmet.

Aerobic dancing
In "aerobics" every part of the body can be exercised to music. To reduce the risk of jarring joints, it is best to do aerobics on a floor made of hardwood laid over a cushion of air. At home, these exercises should be carried out on a cushioned exercise mat.

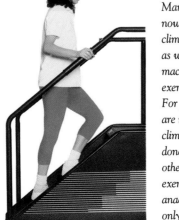

Stair-climbing
Many health clubs now provide stair-climbing machines, as well as rowing machines and exercise bicycles. For people who are unfit, stair-climbing must be done very slowly, otherwise the exercise becomes anaerobic and can only be done for a short period.

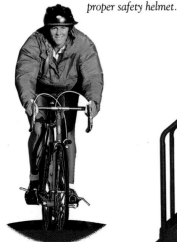

FITNESS FACT

Sports such as tennis and squash involve periods of intense effort, during which muscles are being forced to work anaerobically. This is why these activities are not ideal for improving heart and lung fitness.

ANAEROBIC EXERCISE

Anaerobic exercises consist of short, sharp bursts of intense muscle activity, during which the blood supply does not provide as much oxygen as the muscles need. The 110 yard (100 m) sprint is one such activity.

Lacking oxygen, the muscles have to use other "anaerobic" chemical processes to release the energy they require. These anaerobic reactions also produce lactic acid, which builds up rapidly in the muscles to cause fatigue, a heavy sensation, and even cramp. Anaerobic exercise cannot be continued for long, and so will not improve the fitness of the heart and lungs. It is therefore not an essential part of your fitness schedule.

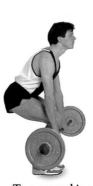

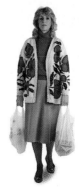

Two anaerobic activities
Weightlifting and carrying heavy shopping are both anaerobic exercises. Lactic acid builds up in your muscles, causing discomfort.

WALKING FOR FITNESS

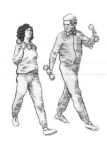

Walking with weights
Some walkers fasten weights to their arms, legs, or even around their waists. This strengthens specific groups of muscles while they are walking, as well as making their heart and lungs work harder.

Throughout the 20th century everyone living in the Western world has become increasingly dependent on the motor car. With every passing decade people have needed to walk less each day. Only relatively recently have the full benefits of exercise for long-term health been realized. Now, the simple pleasures of walking are becoming popular once again.

The main appeal of walking is that it is a type of aerobic exercise that almost everyone can easily incorporate into their daily routine. It is sociable, enjoyable for people of all ages, and only carries a slight risk of injury. This impressive list of advantages has encouraged a growing number of people to regularly take a brisk walk to try and improve their overall fitness level.

Whatever your age, whatever your level of fitness, walking is a simple and effective form of exercise.

The long-term benefits derived from this relaxing, yet not too strenuous, form of exercise are great. Regular walks will slowly improve your heartbeat, endurance, and all-around level of fitness. They will help to protect you from disorders such as osteoporosis, cancer, and heart disease. Walking will also enhance your figure and help you lose weight.

A family outing
A good way to involve the whole family in exercise is to organize a walk through the park or around a local scenic spot. If your children learn to associate exercise with fun they are likely to continue this healthy habit throughout the whole of their lives.

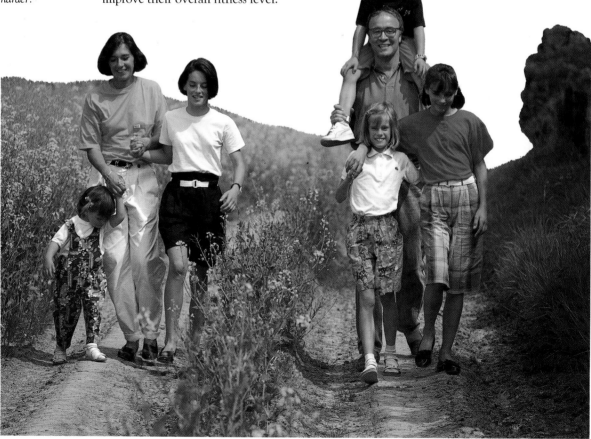

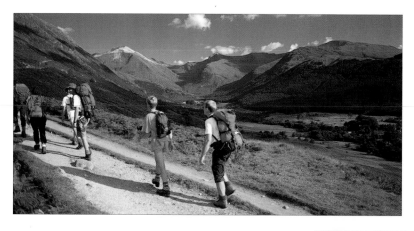

Hiking clubs

Joining your local hiking club can provide the motivation to walk regularly. Look for details in the local paper or library, or ask your council for the names and addresses of any such organizations. These groups are not just for mountain-climbing fitness fanatics. Ordinary people can join in too. There will usually be sections which cater specifically for senior citizens and young people. These guided walks will soon increase both your level of fitness and your circle of friends.

Window shopping

Many people enjoy walking around their local shopping center; it provides an opportunity to window shop and socialize.
The modern shopping center, with covered walkways, provides the whole family with an opportunity to exercise in comfort and safety.

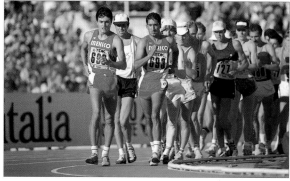

Race walking

Real walking enthusiasts, who have built up their fitness over a long period of time and developed a correct and efficient technique, can compete against other fast walkers.

PUT ON YOUR WALKING SHOES

- Start at a slow pace and be careful to build up your speed and distance gradually.
- Walk fast enough to become a little breathless and slightly tired, but never leave yourself gasping for air or completely exhausted.
- Leave the car at home if you need to mail a letter or visit local shops.
- Walk at least part of the way to and from your place of work.
- Take the whole family out walking on the weekend or in the long summer evenings.
- Aim to walk about 2 miles (3 km), at least three times a week. An adult should take around 30 minutes to complete this distance.
- Once your walking fitness has improved, you can start climbing a few hills.

STRENGTH EXERCISES

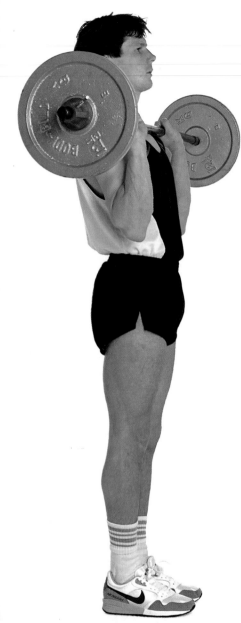

Any exercise that improves the condition of your muscles will make day-to-day tasks easier to manage.

YOUR BODY CONTAINS hundreds of muscles and it is possible to strengthen every single one. Strength exercises can be simply divided into two separate types: dynamic, where the muscle actually changes in length, and isometric, where the muscle contracts but does not shorten.

Benefits of strength exercises

If your muscles are weak you will find many routine activities, like shopping, housework, and gardening, have become a struggle. People who have allowed their spinal and abdominal muscles to become out of condition are more vulnerable to episodes of back pain due to injury. Regular exercise will help solve all these problems. Improving your muscle strength will make it easier

NOT FOR EVERYONE

Isometric muscle exercises tend to raise blood pressure, so have your blood pressure checked before you attempt them. People who have had a stroke or any heart condition are advised to avoid these exercises and choose stretching exercises instead.

for you to carry, lift, push, or pull heavy loads, and will enhance your ability in any sporting activity that requires strength.

Dynamic exercises

These muscle exercises are further subdivided into isotonic, in which the length of the muscle changes while its tension remains roughly constant, and isokinetic, in which special equipment is used to vary the mechanical resistance to movement, so that the tension in the muscle can be varied in many different positions.

The most effective and safest form of dynamic muscle exercise consists of repeated movements

Lifting heavy weights
It is not necessary to lift heavy weights in order to increase the strength and tone of your muscles. The only reason for ever using a heavy set of weights is when you deliberately wish to build up your muscle bulk. This kind of exercise is anaerobic (see p119) and will rapidly cause a build-up in lactic acid, so you will only be able to perform a few repetitions. To avoid a muscle or tendon injury, you should seek expert advice on how to lift safely.

Lifting small weights
Multiple repetitions, using small weights, improve muscle strength and tone, without dramatically increasing muscle bulk. Start with light weights, so that you can complete eight repetitions. Build up to 12 gradually, over a 60-second period, and then try a slightly heavier load.

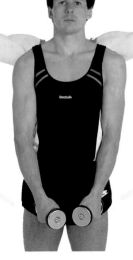

• Holding the weights at the furthest point from the center of the movement, breathe out, and hold for two seconds. Do not rush the exercise.

• Exercise one group of muscles, then rest these for five minutes and work on another group. Repeat three times.

against a force. This need not be a weight – a modern gym apparatus lets you work against springs, hydraulic valves, and elastic tubing. Dynamic exercises should be started under the supervision of an instructor, who can recommend exercises to work each specific group of muscles and make sure that you carry out the movements correctly, thus reducing your risk of injury.

Isometric exercises

Any exercise that makes a muscle contract without changing its length, so that there is no visible movement of that part of the body, is known as an isometric muscle-strengthening exercise. This can be achieved by using one part of your body to resist the movement of another part or by holding one of your limbs away from your body, against the pull of gravity.

BENEFITS OF EXERCISING ISOMETRICALLY

Isometric exercises, which can be done by holding your muscles against the pull of gravity, are a useful way of increasing muscle strength without using equipment such as weights or a multigym. They are not recommended for people with hypertension because they tend to raise the blood pressure.

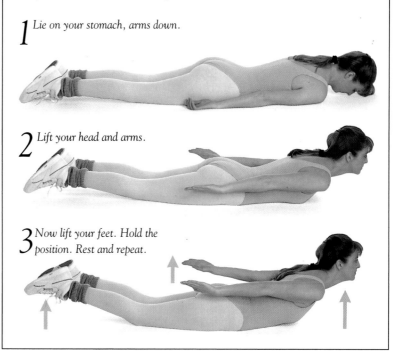

1 Lie on your stomach, arms down.

2 Lift your head and arms.

3 Now lift your feet. Hold the position. Rest and repeat.

Step-ups

This exercise strengthens the calf muscles and the quadriceps at the front of your thighs. Move each foot alternately up onto the step, making sure you straighten your knee.

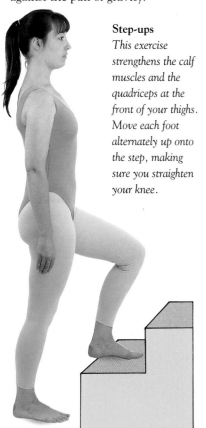

SAFETY TIPS

• Always stretch your muscles before doing any strength exercises. This will warm them up, reducing the risk of suffering from a strain or tear.

• Strength exercises may cause a burning discomfort in the muscles being worked. Stop at once if you suffer any sharp or piercing pain.

• Exercises with heavy weights are not recommended for children under the age of 14. Up to the age of 20 the skeleton is still growing and is more vulnerable to injury.

Sit-ups

Sit-ups strengthen your abdominal muscles. Always do them with your knees bent and your hands reaching to at least mid-thigh.

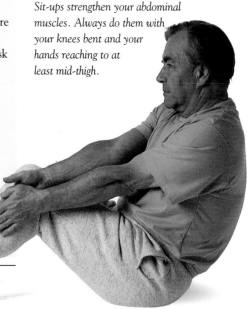

FLEXIBILITY EXERCISES

Stretching exercises are simple and can be started by anyone at any time in their life.

As A FORM OF physical exercise stretching is enjoyable, easy, and safe. It helps maintain and also improve the flexibility of numerous different parts of your body. To achieve the best results, you should perform a wide range of muscle-stretching exercises on a regular basis. Frequency, not intensity, of practice is the key factor to achieving a fit and flexible body.

The most important muscle stretches involve your shoulders, your chest, the lower part of your back, the front of your hips, the front and back of your thighs, and your calf muscles. Be patient with all these different stretches; it can take several weeks before you begin to notice much improvement in your flexibility.

Stretching exercises enhance your ability in any sport where flexibility is particularly important, for example in swimming or gymnastics. In addition, the more flexible you become, the less chance you have of straining or tearing a muscle during any form of activity.

Many people find that these gentle exercises, as part of a daily routine, can prevent minor aches and pains. Regular stretching can also improve your posture, which can help prevent backache.

Ideal warm-up exercises

A range of flexibility exercises should also be carried out before and after any energetic physical activity, to help you warm up and cool down. They are particularly important if you are attempting a muscle-strengthening exercise routine, as this type of training tends to tighten and shorten muscles. Neglecting warm-up exercises will increase your risk of injury.

Chest stretches
Stand with your arms raised above your head, hands together and elbows straight. Lean backwards slowly so that your lower back arches.

• *This exercise stretches the muscles across your chest and abdomen.*
• *Stop if the stretch causes pain in the lower back.*

Abdominal stretches
Kneel in an upright position and slowly lean backwards. Arch your spine and keep your knees bent at a right angle.

• *This movement stretches the muscles at the front of your abdomen and thighs.*
• *Only lean back as far as you find comfortable. As you become more flexible you will find that you are able to reach progressively further back.*

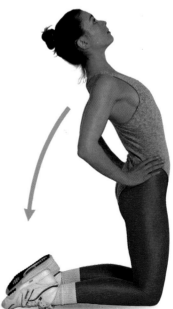
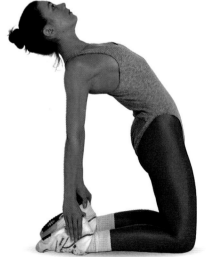

124

HOW TO STRETCH SAFELY

• Always wear comfortable, loose-fitting clothing.
• Warm up with simple loosening-up exercises before you begin to stretch.
• Stretch to the point where you feel a pull; hold this pull for a count of 10.
• Do not bounce or jerk while stretching – you may strain a muscle.
• Never force the stretch so that it becomes painful.
• If you stretch to music, avoid tunes with a strong beat as they might encourage you to bounce.
• Stretch the muscles on both sides of your body equally.

Shoulder stretches

Stand with your legs apart, one arm above your head and the other down by your side. Gently lean over toward the arm by your side.

• *This movement stretches the muscles down the side of your shoulder and trunk.*
• *Having held the position for a count of 10, repeat on the opposite side with your other arm raised.*

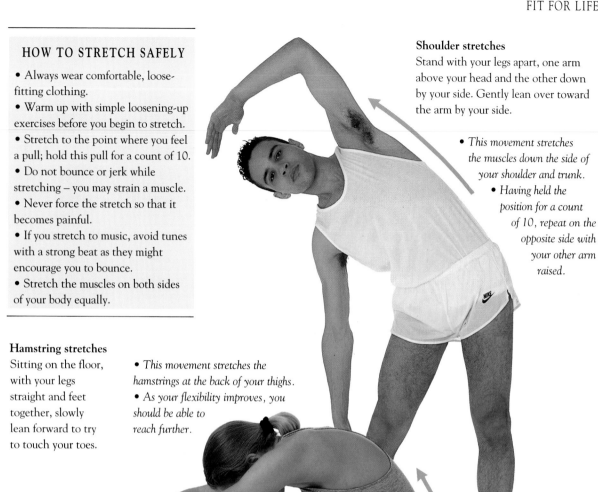

Hamstring stretches

Sitting on the floor, with your legs straight and feet together, slowly lean forward to try to touch your toes.

• *This movement stretches the hamstrings at the back of your thighs.*
• *As your flexibility improves, you should be able to reach further.*

Back stretches

Lie on your back, with legs bent, knees together, and feet flat on the floor. Move your knees as far as you can to the left, repeat to the right. Then, starting in the same initial position, push your lower back down into the floor. Gently arch your back up, raising your buttocks and your back off the ground.

• *Both these movements improve the flexibility of your lower spine and pelvis.*
• *Stop stretching if they cause or aggravate any pain in your lower back.*

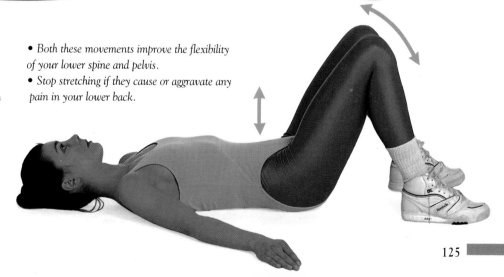

EXERCISE IS FOR EVERYONE

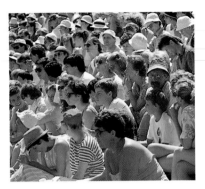

Spectator sports
Many people enjoy watching all kinds of sports, but it would be better for their health if they participated instead.

Whether you are young or old, male or female, in good health or suffering from a chronic medical problem, your health would benefit from some form of regular exercise.

EVEN THOUGH THE physical and psychological benefits of exercise are widely accepted, there are still many people whose health, fitness, and peace of mind are being undermined because they do not exercise regularly.

Starting a habit for life

Even very young children who are naturally and spontaneously active sometimes do not get enough exercise. Early in childhood, bad habits become established. Television has an incredibly strong pulling power. The average teenager watches three hours of programs everyday and even more on weekends.

Many young people develop a negative image of exercise from the way it was presented to them as children. They see exercise as a chore, and acquire an aversion to all types of physical activity, that will last for the rest of their lives.

Lazy, inactive children are likely to grow up into lazy, inactive adults, who are overweight and unhealthy as a result. It is therefore important that children learn to associate physical activity with having fun. A child who exercises regularly will benefit in many ways. Children need exercise to develop strong, healthy bones and muscles, to maximize the efficiency of their heart and lungs, and to enhance their flexibility, coordination, balance, and speed.

Exercise in pregnancy

Exercising regularly can enable women to enjoy pregnancy and childbirth more. Pregnant women who have kept themselves fit and active are much less likely to

Wheelchair athletes
Even a severe disability need not be a barrier to reaching an extremely high level of fitness.

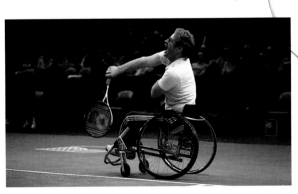

Jumping Rope
This excellent form of aerobic exercise is not just for children. Regular jumping will soon improve anyone's fitness.

develop problems, such as excessive weight gain and varicose veins. They are also better able to deal with the physical exertion of labor. It is never too late to start improving your fitness, but to gain the most benefit from being fit while pregnant it is best to start eating a better diet, losing excess weight, and exercising long before you become pregnant, as part of your preparation for starting a family.

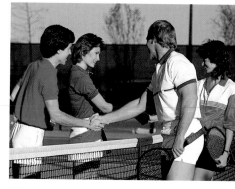

Watching your weight
Regular exercise is useful for anyone who is at all overweight. Many people set out to shed their excess weight just by going on a slimming diet. They may not realize that even low intensity physical activities, such as walking or swimming at a gentle pace, could burn off extra calories. Regular physical activity raises your basal metabolic rate, so that your body uses up more calories, even when you are resting or asleep.

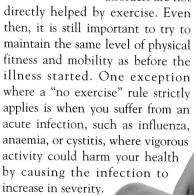

Exercise classes
Exercising in a group can provide you with the motivation to become fitter.

Exercise for a lifetime
Although the search for the secret of how we can slow down the aging process and stay younger for longer still eludes doctors and scientists, there is a lot to be gained by staying active all our lives.

Regular exercise slows down the natural degeneration of muscles, tendons, ligaments, bones, and joints. It maintains muscle strength, joint flexibility, balance, and coordination, keeping people mobile and independent.

Exercise and chronic illness
Anyone who develops a chronic medical disorder should attempt to remain at least as active as they were before. For numerous conditions, such as arthritis, back pain, diabetes, high blood pressure, and some heart disorders, regular exercise under guidance from a doctor can reduce the severity of the symptoms, lower the risk of complications, and slow down the progress of the disease.

A number of disorders are not directly helped by exercise. Even then, it is still important to try to maintain the same level of physical fitness and mobility as before the illness started. One exception where a "no exercise" rule strictly applies is when you suffer from an acute infection, such as influenza, anaemia, or cystitis, where vigorous activity could harm your health by causing the infection to increase in severity.

Mixed doubles
Making sport a part of your social life, perhaps by playing tennis with friends, will help you get fit painlessly.

Keeping supple during pregnancy
Sitting cross-legged on the floor improves blood flow to the lower part of your body, straightens your back, and makes your back and pelvis more flexible.

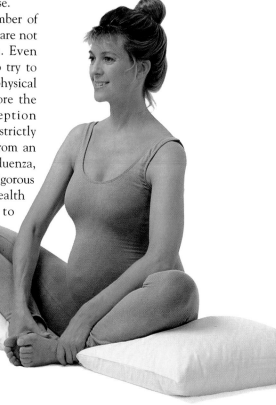

EXERCISE AND CHILDREN

Active children are much more likely to grow into active adults, so it is vital that a pattern for healthy living is set at an early age.

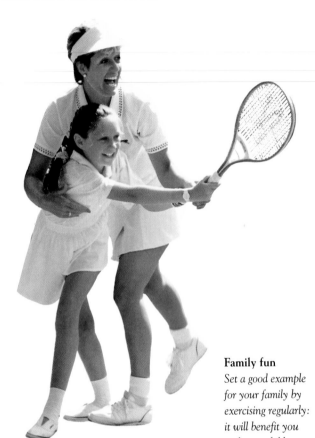

Family fun
Set a good example for your family by exercising regularly: it will benefit you and your children.

ALTHOUGH TODDLERS and young children nearly always seem to be rushing about, it does not take long for them to develop the habit of slumping in front of the television as soon as they get home from school. In addition, many schools are now devoting less time to sports due to a lack of staff with proper physical education training, especially in primary schools.

In some schools, there has been a tendency to concentrate on the minority who are good at sport, while neglecting the rest. In other schools, there have been moves to reduce the amount of competitive sport, because some educationalists believe that children who

Couch potatoes
A recent survey of 500 secondary school children showed that nearly two thirds of them got no vigorous exercise outside of school hours. If this way of life continues it is likely to cause serious health problems.

HOW TO GET CHILDREN TO EXERCISE

• Parents must take some of the responsibility for making sure their children get enough exercise.

• Children need to learn that exercise is fun, so try to find an activity that your child will enjoy, such as roller-skating or dancing.

• Encourage your child to join a local sports or youth club that organizes after-school activities.

• Tell your child that most sports will enable him or her to make new friends. Children are more likely to respond to this motive than to the distant threat of heart disease.

• Plan family outings that involve physical activity such as canoeing, hiking, or swimming.

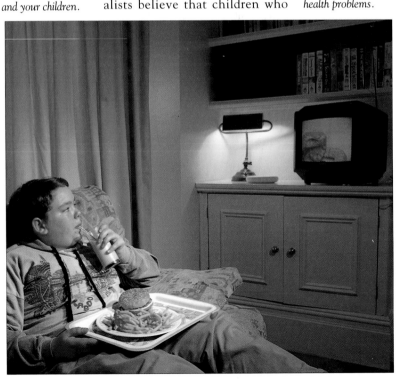

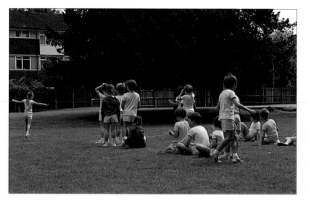

constantly lose may suffer long-term psychological harm.

The increased levels of violence in society have also led to many children not being allowed to play unsupervised in urban areas. The combined effect of all these various factors is that today's youngsters are involved in less day-to-day physical activity than previous generations.

All-around improvement

The inactive lifestyle of many of today's children is likely to produce unfit adults, whose health may suffer

Does your child exercise as much as you think?
Many playground and organized activities at school involve team games, which for many children simply mean standing around most of the time.

as a result. All children should get regular exercise because it reduces their risk of developing heart disease in later life. Activity produces many other benefits too. Fit children have strong muscles, which are very important for good posture and stable joints; they have better balance, coordination, and flexibility; and they are less likely to fracture bones, as exercise increases bone density.

Apart from the obvious physical benefits, regular exercise produces many more subtle skills. Children

who take part in physical activities learn how to interact and cooperate with other children. They also develop their own self-esteem by creating a strong sense of purpose.

The benefits of childhood exercise will last a lifetime

The U.S. has one of the highest rates of heart disease in the world. The root of this problem is thought to lie in childhood. Insufficient exercise increases the risk of becoming overweight, of having abnormally high cholesterol levels, and of suffering from high blood pressure – all of which can start to develop in your early teens, and significantly increase your chance of eventually developing serious heart problems.

It is essential that all children, and their parents, realize just how vital regular exercise is. If children discover the pleasures of exercise when they are young, they are likely to maintain this healthy habit for the rest of their lives.

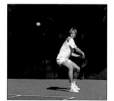

OVERTRAINING YOUNG ATHLETES

In contrast to the majority of children who need encouragement to do any exercise, there is a dedicated minority of young athletes who spend several hours each day training intensively.

This may be because of their own desire to excel. However, overenthusiastic parents or coaches can push too hard, so children must be allowed to slow down or change sports if they want to.

DO NOT OVERDO IT

Some children exercise too much. Stress caused by overtraining may cause a number of problems, which will end once the training schedule is reduced. These symptoms include loss of appetite, sleeping difficulties, constant exhaustion, recurrent sore throats or colds, and even the stopping of periods in young girls.

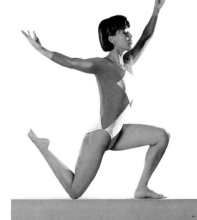

Injury prone
Many top athletes are still in their teens, especially in sports such as gymnastics, swimming, and tennis. Because their skeletons are not yet fully developed, they are vulnerable to more serious injuries than older competitors. The sort of trauma that might sprain a ligament in an adult, could cause a fracture or displacement of part of the bone in a growing child or adolescent.

EXERCISE AND PREGNANCY

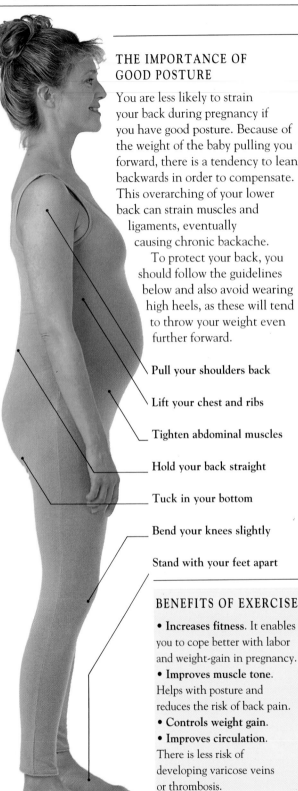

THE IMPORTANCE OF GOOD POSTURE

You are less likely to strain your back during pregnancy if you have good posture. Because of the weight of the baby pulling you forward, there is a tendency to lean backwards in order to compensate. This overarching of your lower back can strain muscles and ligaments, eventually causing chronic backache.

To protect your back, you should follow the guidelines below and also avoid wearing high heels, as these will tend to throw your weight even further forward.

Pull your shoulders back

Lift your chest and ribs

Tighten abdominal muscles

Hold your back straight

Tuck in your bottom

Bend your knees slightly

Stand with your feet apart

BENEFITS OF EXERCISE

- **Increases fitness**. It enables you to cope better with labor and weight-gain in pregnancy.
- **Improves muscle tone**. Helps with posture and reduces the risk of back pain.
- **Controls weight gain**.
- **Improves circulation**. There is less risk of developing varicose veins or thrombosis.
- **Decreases stress**.

Pregnancy places great physical demands on the body, but the fitter you are, the better you will cope.

WOMEN WHO ARE physically fit through getting regular exercise tend to develop fewer problems during pregnancy, labor, and childbirth. Being fit also helps women to regain their figures more rapidly once the baby is born.

Ideally you should try to get in shape before you become pregnant. However, it is never too late to take up exercise. You will still benefit from improving your fitness even well into your pregnancy.

Start by getting some form of gentle exercise each day, such as walking or swimming. Gradually increase the distance, building up to around 20 minutes at a time.

Exercising safely

If you are used to energetic exercise you can usually continue throughout pregnancy. But stop as soon as you feel tired, or out of breath.

Both stretching exercises and aerobics should be undertaken with extreme caution, especially during the last few months of pregnancy. Ligaments and tendons that support the joints and spine soften, increasing the risk of injury.

Avoid contact sports and those which risk a blow to the abdomen, such as skiing and horse-riding.

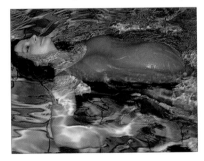

Swimming
Even late in pregnancy, swimming is an excellent form of exercise because the baby's weight is supported by the water. You should not, however, swim in extremely cold water, as this may induce abdominal cramps.

GENTLE YET EFFECTIVE EXERCISES

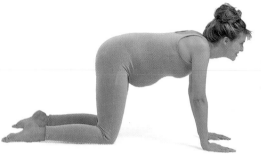

Pelvic tilts
Kneel on the floor with your back held flat. Tighten your buttock muscles, pull in your abdominal muscles, and gently tilt your pelvis forward, while breathing out. Hold for a few seconds. Pelvic tilting strengthens abdominal muscles and improves back and pelvis flexibility.

Pelvic floor exercises
Lie on your back, tighten your pelvic muscles, hold for a few seconds, and then slowly relax. Alternatively, while you are urinating, squeeze your muscles to stop the flow. Count to four and release. Repeat.

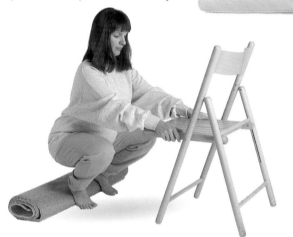

Squatting
Squatting prepares you for childbirth. It strengthens back and thigh muscles and increases the flexibility of the pelvis. Use a chair for support and a rolled-up rug under your heels to avoid overstretching your calf muscles.

Leg exercises
Begin by gently circling your feet and ankles, and then move your feet up and down to work your calf muscles. These exercises will improve the circulation in your legs, reducing aching and swelling.

EXERCISING AFTER CHILDBIRTH

Go slowly and avoid excessive stretching for the first few weeks, while your ligaments are still vulnerable to sprains. Be sure to continue your pelvic floor exercises (see above). After a caesarean section, ask your doctor when it will be safe to start your abdominal exercises.

Shoulder stretches
Clasp your hands behind your back and point one elbow up and the other down. Hold, and then repeat the other way round. Also, try putting your palms together and pulling your elbows back.

Pelvic thrusts
Lie on your back, bend your knees, and keep your feet flat on the floor. Breathe in, and then raise your hips off the floor as you breathe out. Hold this position for a few seconds, then slowly lower your hips as you breathe in again.

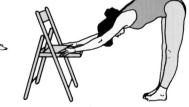

Forward bends
Bend from the hips and breathe deeply. As you exhale, pull in your abdominal muscles. Lean on a chair for support.

EXERCISE FOR THE OVERWEIGHT

Regular exercise will make you fitter and can help you lose weight.

BEING OVERWEIGHT should not be used as a general excuse for avoiding exercise, although it may influence the type and amount of exercise that can be undertaken. Unfortunately, many overweight people are too embarrassed to get involved in sports. Regular exercise, however, makes it much easier to lose weight. It will also make you fitter and improve your general health, no matter what your size.

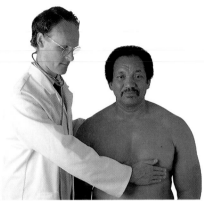

See your doctor first
Before you begin an exercise program, see your doctor to make sure your blood pressure is not abnormally high and that your heart, lungs, and joints are healthy.

CHOOSING AN EXERCISE

Pick an activity that you will enjoy, that your state of health will permit, and that will fit easily into your lifestyle. Otherwise you are unlikely to stick with it. Gentle walking and swimming are good choices, as they avoid putting too much strain on your spine and joints in the hips, knees, and ankles. Jogging is not a good choice; every time your heel strikes the ground the force through your foot is between three and eight times your body weight. Overweight people carry a greater load and therefore have a higher risk of developing an injury when they jog.

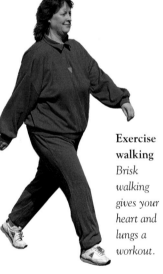

Exercise walking
Brisk walking gives your heart and lungs a workout.

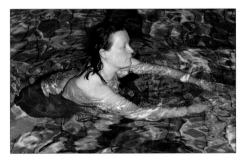

Swimming
If you are overweight, weight-bearing exercises like running can put a strain on your body. When you swim, however, your body is supported by the water, making it an ideal form of exercise.

Walk every day
Exercise does not always require special clothing or equipment. Walking whenever you can is an easy way to incorporate exercise into your daily life.

The right shoes
When walking, wear a cushioned insole and try to walk on soft ground: this will reduce the risk of suffering an injury from repeated, excessive jarring.

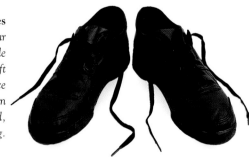

Why lose weight?

If you are overweight, you are putting extra stress on your heart, lungs, and joints. Being more than 20 percent over the maximum normal weight for your height and build (see p86) increases your risk of developing high blood pressure, diabetes, and a high cholesterol level, all of which make you more likely to suffer from angina, heart attacks, or strokes later in life.

Added stress on your joints means that osteoarthritis, caused by wear and tear on the cartilage surfaces, is more likely to occur with advancing years.

How does exercise help?

Regular exercise will help reduce your body's fat reserves by converting them into energy. Exercising at least three times a week makes you burn up more calories while you are exercising. It also raises your basal metabolic rate, which is the energy your tissues use up while your body is resting.

Exercise can help weight loss by taking your mind off food. Some people, however, find that exercise makes them hungrier. If this is the case, eat sensibly, choosing fruit, vegetables, and high-fiber foods that are low in calories. To lose weight you must control the amount, and more importantly, the types, of food that you eat.

Getting started

If you are excessively overweight, vigorous exercise is likely to make you extremely breathless almost immediately. You must therefore be prepared to start off your exercise program at a slow pace. Walking and swimming are probably all that should be attempted during those first few months, until you have begun to lose some weight, and there has been some improvement in your fitness level.

As you get fitter, try a variety of different activities to reduce the risk of injury and to keep up your interest. Proceed at your own pace and do not let others rush you.

Gradually increase the speed at which you exercise, walking or swimming faster over several weeks. Increase the time you spend exercising too. Be careful not to overexert yourself, as the resultant pain and exhaustion will only sap your motivation to continue.

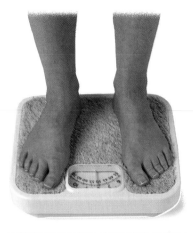

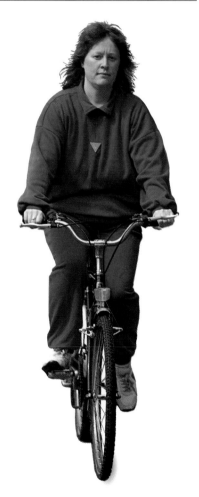

Cycling
Riding a bicycle is a particularly good form of gentle exercise if you are overweight because it does not put too much strain on any of your joints.

MONITORING YOUR PROGRESS
Getting Fitter

• Once you begin exercising regularly, your level of fitness will improve. You will soon be able to cope with a longer period of continuous exercise, or more vigorous exercise, before you have to stop because you feel tired or breathless.

• Being overweight and possibly out of shape to start with, you should expect to take longer to progress through the various stages of becoming fit and active.

• Do not be disheartened if you do not lose much weight at first. Regular exercise not only removes excess body fat, it also builds up muscles, so that initially your fat will be replaced by muscle. Muscle tissue, however, is much more efficient at burning calories than fat and so will aid weight loss.

• You will soon notice an improvement in your figure and posture. Within a few weeks the fat loss will greatly exceed any further muscle gain, leading to a steady reduction in your weight.

• Even if you do not change your diet, simply adding a brisk walk of 30 minutes a day to your routine will cause you to lose weight and help you become fitter as well.

EXERCISE FOR THE ELDERLY

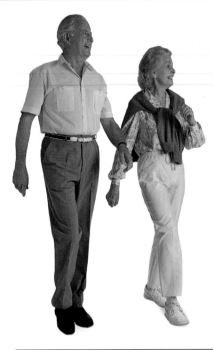

KEEPING YOUR BODY in good physical condition by getting some form of regular exercise helps maintain the normal functioning of joints, bones, muscles, tendons, and ligaments well into old age. There is convincing evidence that regular exercise is the best preventive medicine available.

Exercise reduces the risk of falls by keeping your joints mobile and maintaining your muscle strength, balance, and coordination. Falls are a common cause of serious injury,

Walking your way to fitness
If you have neglected to exercise for some time, you might find that walking is the best way to begin to improve your fitness.

Exercising slows down the natural stiffening associated with the aging of muscles and joints.

such as fractures of the wrist and hip, among the elderly.

In addition to helping to keep you mobile and independent, exercise slows down the development of osteoporosis. This condition is more common among women than men and causes the bones to become thinner and more fragile with advancing years. Elderly

INCREASING STRENGTH AND FLEXIBILITY

Loosening-up and stretching exercises can be done as a way of keeping fit or as a warm-up before going on to more strenuous exercise. They are especially important as you get older since you are more likely to suffer from stiff muscles and joints. These exercises can be done indoors, so even if you are unable to get out of your house, you can stay active and keep your muscles strong and your joints flexible.

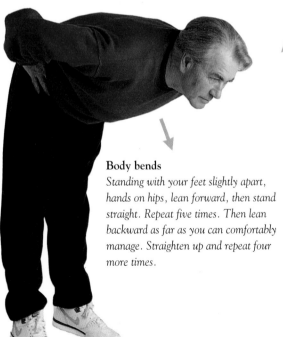

Body bends
Standing with your feet slightly apart, hands on hips, lean forward, then stand straight. Repeat five times. Then lean backward as far as you can comfortably manage. Straighten up and repeat four more times.

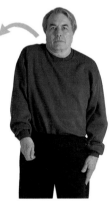

Shoulder rolls
Roll each shoulder forward then backward in turn. Repeat five times. These exercises can be done either sitting down or standing up.

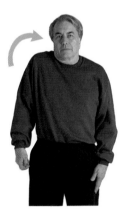

WHEN TO STOP

If you experience chest pain, pain in the neck or arms, feeling dizzy or faint, palpitations, or severe breathlessness during exercise, it may indicate that your heart is under excessive strain. If one of these symptoms does develop, rest at once and see your doctor.

people who have remained fit and active have stronger bones and so are much less vulnerable to fractures if they do fall.

Getting started

 Even when they are in their 70's, many people are capable of running a marathon or playing tennis. But it can be dangerous to overexert yourself if you have been inactive for many years. If you have not exercised for a long time, it is not too late to start a well-planned fitness program. You should, however, get a check-up from your doctor first.

Once your doctor has given you the all clear, you can begin to exercise cautiously. Now that you are older you will not be able to push yourself as hard as you once did. Walking or swimming are good gentle activities to start with. No matter what exercise you choose, it should make you a little breathless but not leave you gasping for air, tired but not totally exhausted.

Building up your fitness

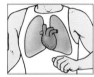 Working your body too hard when you are not sufficiently fit can be dangerous. The best approach is to increase your activity level gradually, for example by walking or swimming over a greater distance, or for a longer time, before resting. As your fitness level improves, you will soon be able to keep going longer. Your ultimate goal should be to manage 20 minutes of continuous exercise more than twice a week.

Remember that as you get older, it will take longer for your muscles to recover from exercise. If you are unused to exercise, you may feel a little stiff for a day or two afterward. If you injure yourself while exercising, your injuries will not heal as quickly as they once did.

Your exercise program

 The best way to make exercise a routine part of your lifestyle is to choose activities that fit easily into your daily routine. For example, rather than driving or taking the bus to the local shops, walk or cycle there. If you use public transport, get off the bus a couple of stops from your house and walk the rest of the way home. If you have a dog, increasing the length of your daily walks is a good way of providing more exercise for both of you.

Climbing the stairs, rather than taking the elevator, is an excellent exercise because it works your heart, lungs, and muscles. It may, however, put strain on arthritic hip and knee joints. If you have even a mild heart or lung disorder, it could cause chest pains or severe breathlessness. If you experience any of these symptoms, you should not climb stairs if you can help it.

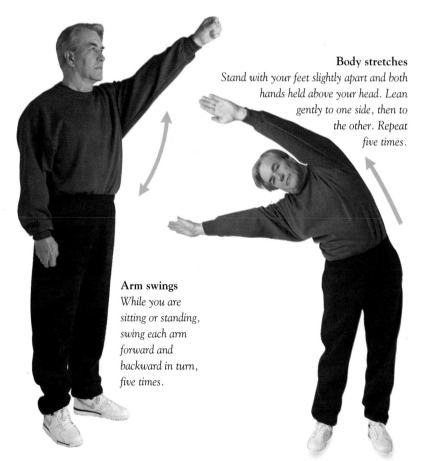

Body stretches
Stand with your feet slightly apart and both hands held above your head. Lean gently to one side, then to the other. Repeat five times.

Arm swings
While you are sitting or standing, swing each arm forward and backward in turn, five times.

COPING WITH ARTHRITIS

Older people should restrict or change their activities altogether if they find that a particular exercise aggravates the pain and stiffness in an arthritic joint.

EXERCISE AND ILL-HEALTH

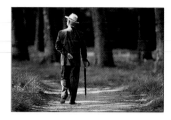

Enjoying life
Even serious illness need not keep you from exercising and continuing to remain fit and active.

Physical activity is not just for the healthy and the fit; regular exercise can actually ease or slow down the progression of many disorders.

ALTHOUGH THERE ARE a small number of medical disorders, such as anaemia or an infection, where exercise is not recommended, it is usually better to remain as active as possible. People who regards themselves as invalids, and therefore do not bother to get any exercise, are more likely to suffer a steady deterioration in general health, due to progressive loss of fitness.

Ask your doctor for advice

If you have any type of medical problem you should have a check-up before starting your exercise program. Discuss with your doctor the type of activities you might safely take part in.

Your doctor is likely to recommend that you take up some form of regular exercise as this can slow the progression of many disorders, reduce the risk of developing complications, and help you to remain independent and mobile. Even if physical activity does not directly help a particular condition, staying active is important for your overall health and morale.

World-class athletes with chronic disorders

As further proof that many medical disorders do not interfere with the ability to exercise vigorously, there are a number of successful athletes who compete at the highest levels, despite having conditions such as asthma and diabetes.

When taking up organized sports, the only limitation is that you must not take any medication for your illness which is prohibited in the sport you choose. However, in most cases, there are several alternative drugs that are acceptable to the sports authorities.

Take sensible precautions

If physical activity tends to bring on your asthma symptoms, such as coughing, wheezing, or tightness across the chest, it may be helpful to use your inhaler a few minutes before you begin to exercise. If this does not relieve your symptoms, talk to your doctor. You may need to change to a different drug.

Any diabetic involved in regular physical activity should check with his or her doctor on how best to adjust their diet. They may also need to change the timing and level of medication taken to control their blood sugar level. Most types of exercise reduce the amount of diabetic medication needed.

EXERCISE AND INFECTION

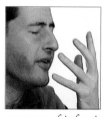

Exercise may make an infection worse. Exercise encourages the spread of an infection throughout the bloodstream to other organs. With some types of viral infection, this may lead to inflammation of vital organs, such as the heart (myocarditis), and liver (hepatitis). Do not exercise if you have any type of infection, including colds, influenza, bronchitis, cystitis, and even skin infections.

WHEN TO AVOID EXERCISE

Do not exercise when you have any of the following symptoms:

- Deep cough
- Sore throat
- Fever
- Swollen glands
- Cold sore
- Painful urination
- Genital discharge

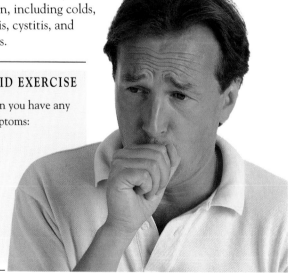

EXERCISE GUIDELINES FOR DIFFERENT MEDICAL CONDITIONS

CONDITION	SUITABLE EXERCISES	SPECIAL PRECAUTIONS
Anemia	None, until you are symptom-free and your blood tests are normal.	Vigorous exercise while you are anemic could put a dangerous strain on your heart, by depriving it of oxygen.
Arthritis	Swimming and cycling.	Ease up if your joints become stiffer, more painful, or more swollen. Wear warm socks and gloves when cycling to prevent stiffness.
Asthma	Swimming is the best possible sport.	When you go out in cold weather, wear a scarf across your nose and mouth.
Diabetes	Any sport should be perfectly safe, but always tell the people you exercise with that you are diabetic, in case you suffer a sudden "hypo" (a drop in blood sugar level).	You may need to increase your intake of carbohydrates before exercise. Carry a supply of sugar or sweets with you.
Epilepsy	Most forms of exercise, apart from boxing and wrestling. Always tell someone you exercise with that you are epileptic, in case you have a seizure. Only lift weights under supervision.	Wear protective headgear when you play any contact sport. Make sure you eat and drink enough before you exercise – hypoglycemia and dehydration may provoke a seizure.
High blood pressure	Any sport, apart from weight training and isometric strength exercises.	If you take beta-blockers which slow down your heart rate, you will not be able to gauge your condition from the speed of your pulse. Check with your doctor before starting.
Infection	None, until your fever resolves, and your other symptoms also improve.	Energetic exercise while suffering from an infection is likely to make the infection a lot worse and also delay your recovery.
Parkinson's disease	Any exercise that you are able to cope with will help to reduce muscle weakness and joint stiffness.	Warm up thoroughly before exercising in order to get the muscles working and the joints moving.
Peripheral vascular disease	Any sport will aid the circulation to your arms and legs. Try to exercise regularly.	If gangrene or ulcers develop as a result of your condition, rest the affected limb.
Stroke	Any exercise that you can cope with will help you regain the use of muscles and joints.	If you still have high blood pressure, avoid weight training and all types of isometric strength exercises.
Varicose veins	Any form of activity that exercises your legs will normally help to reduce discomfort and swelling.	Wear elastic support hose during vigorous exercise to minimize congestion in the veins and help reduce any pain.

EXERCISE AND HEART DISEASE

CONSULTING YOUR DOCTOR

If you have had a heart attack or suffer from heart disease, you will naturally be anxious about your state of health and may therefore restrict your overall level of activity. But exercise can dramatically improve your health. Physical inactivity is, in fact, one of the factors that puts you at risk of having another heart attack.

You should, however, consult your doctor before beginning even a gentle exercise program because exercise may, in some cases, cause pain or aggravate your condition.

Exercise can improve the quality of your life and health even when you have had a heart attack or suffer from heart disease.

Talk to your doctor
Discuss your plans for beginning to exercise to ensure that you do not endanger your health by overdoing things.

IN THE PAST, anyone with a heart condition was usually advised to rest because doctors thought that exercise would only make their condition worse. For example, after a heart attack, it was customary to be kept on strict bed rest for six weeks. For another six weeks, only restricted physical activities would be allowed.

Nowadays, doctors realize that controlled exercise, within sensible limits, is not only safe, but can also improve certain heart conditions. Prolonged rest after an uncomplicated heart attack ultimately does more harm than good. Most heart-attack patients are now encouraged to get out of bed within a few days and to start on a gentle program of rehabilitation exercises as soon as they possibly can.

The role of exercise

A program of aerobic exercise can improve the efficiency of the pumping action of the heart. Symptoms of heart failure such as breathlessness and swollen ankles can also be reduced by exercise.

Although exercise is now acknowledged to be the best medicine for most cases of heart disease, you must still be careful. Since everyone is different, it is essential to ask your doctor for some clear guidelines before you start your own exercise program.

EXERCISING SAFELY WITH A HEART CONDITION

• Get a check-up from your doctor before you start an exercise program.
• Start slowly, build up gradually.
• Stop exercising at once if you develop chest pain, pain in the neck and arms, severe breathlessness, palpitations, nausea, blurred vision, dizziness, or feel faint or light-headed.
• Do not exercise immediately after eating a large meal.
• Avoid exercising in very cold or very hot weather.
• Do not undertake strenuous activities, such as digging, heavy housework, or carrying or lifting heavy objects.

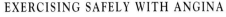

EXERCISING AFTER A HEART ATTACK

A heart attack occurs when one of the coronary arteries becomes blocked by a blood clot, resulting in damage to the area of heart muscle which that artery supplies with oxygen and nutrients.

It takes about six weeks for the scar in the heart muscle to heal completely after a heart attack, but gentle exercise can usually be started within days, if there are no complications, such as heart failure or an irregular heartbeat.

EXERCISING SAFELY WITH ANGINA

Angina is chest pain brought on by exertion or stress. It is eased by rest. Attacks of angina are caused by a lack of oxygen supply to the heart muscle, resulting from narrowing or spasm of the coronary arteries.

Gentle exercise is recommended for most people with angina. Stop if you have symptoms like chest pain or severe shortness of breath. As long as exercise does not provoke angina, it will enhance the efficiency of your heart, lungs, and muscles. Do not continue beyond the onset of chest pain.

Coronary arteries

Fatty plaque

Coronary heart disease
Deposits of fatty plaque on the walls of the coronary artery slow down the blood flow through the artery, causing angina.

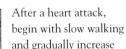

After a heart attack, begin with slow walking and gradually increase the pace and distance covered over a few weeks. Once you can cope with the exertion of climbing stairs without any difficulty, it should be safe to resume sexual relations with your partner.

After six weeks, when the damaged heart muscle has healed, you can usually return to normal physical activities. By doing some form of regular aerobic exercise, such as swimming or brisk walking and by building up to 20 minutes of exercise at a time, three times a week, you will significantly reduce your chances of having another heart attack.

EXERCISE AND HEART FAILURE

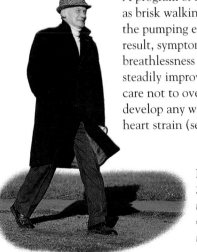

A program of regular aerobic exercise, such as brisk walking or swimming, can increase the pumping efficiency of the heart. As a result, symptoms of heart failure, such as breathlessness and swollen ankles, should steadily improve. However, you should take care not to overexert yourself. Rest if you develop any warning symptoms of excessive heart strain (see opposite page).

Regular physical activity
Swimming and walking improve the exercise tolerance of anyone who suffers from heart disease and therefore enhance their quality of life.

EXERCISE AND BACK PAIN

Regular exercise can help those who suffer from back pain to enjoy life to its fullest.

S TUDIES HAVE demonstrated that exercise can help people cope much better with back pain than they would if they had remained inactive. Before you start any exercise program, you should check with your doctor on the cause of your back pain. Some activities might make your condition worse.

Choosing an exercise

Swimming is an excellent exercise for anyone with chronic back pain, as it helps strengthen the back and abdominal muscles which support the spine. Water reduces the pull of gravity on your body, which means that you are unlikely to put an excessive strain on your back.

When doing the breast stroke, put your face in the water every few strokes. Keeping your head raised above the water all the time makes you arch your lower back, which could cause you to overstretch the spinal ligaments and aggravate your back pain.

Safety is paramount

If you go jogging when you have back pain, try to avoid running on hard surfaces. Wearing cushioned insoles will also reduce the jarring through your lower spine each time your feet strike the ground.

If you have had a previous back problem, such as a disk prolapse, it is essential that you take extra care while doing strength exercises, particularly if you are using weights. An exercise mat should always be used for floor exercises.

RECOVERING FROM BACK PAIN

Once an attack of back pain starts to ease off, you should be able to do a selection of gentle exercises to stretch and strengthen your back and abdominal muscles. They should not cause pain. If any of the exercises shown below does cause further pain or aggravates your existing pain, stop at once and continue with another exercise.

As soon as you can do all these exercises without discomfort, you will be ready to resume normal activities. By completing this exercise program and then persevering with at least some, if not all, of these back and abdominal muscle movements on a regular basis, you will reduce your risk of suffering from further episodes of back pain.

SPINAL STRETCHING EXERCISES

1 *Get down on your hands and knees. Bow your head. Lift one knee up toward your forehead. Stretch that leg straight out behind you, looking up at the same time. Repeat with the other leg.*

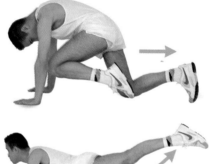
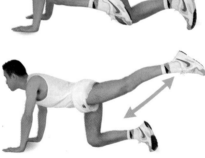

2 *Stand with your arms above your head, hands together. Gently lean backward, arching your back. Straighten up. Put your arms down by your sides. Bend slowly to one side, then to the other. Finally, hold your arms in front of you and turn to one side, then to the other.*

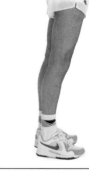

SPINAL MOBILITY EXERCISES

1 *Lie on your back with arms outstretched. Raise one leg straight up. Slowly swing it across the other leg toward the floor. Keep the shoulders still. Go only as far as is comfortable. Repeat with the other leg.*

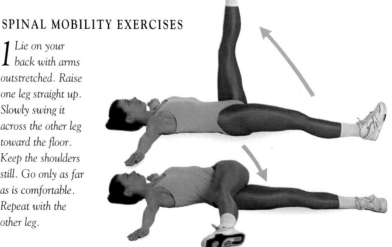

ABDOMINAL STRENGTHENING EXERCISES

Abdominal muscles support your spine. Gentle exercise that increases their strength will benefit your back.

1 Lie on your back. Slowly raise each leg about 4 in (10 cm) off the floor. Keep your knees straight.

SPINAL STRENGTHENING EXERCISES

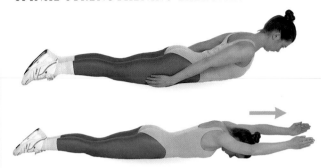

1 Lie flat on your stomach, arms down by your sides. Raise your head and shoulders up off the ground. Then repeat, first with your hands behind your head and elbows bent, second with your arms held straight out in front. There is no need to raise your head and shoulders any further than is comfortable. Hold each position for a few seconds.

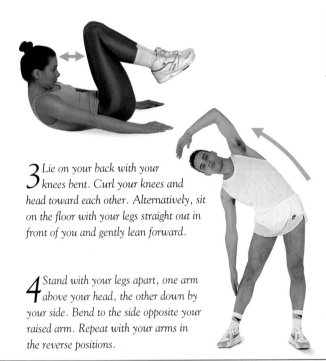

3 Lie on your back with your knees bent. Curl your knees and head toward each other. Alternatively, sit on the floor with your legs straight out in front of you and gently lean forward.

4 Stand with your legs apart, one arm above your head, the other down by your side. Bend to the side opposite your raised arm. Repeat with your arms in the reverse positions.

2 Lie flat on your stomach, arms by your sides. Raise each leg in turn and then both together, keeping your knees straight. Put your arms straight out in front of you. Raise your head and shoulders at the same time as you raise both legs.

2 Lie on your back with your arms out at right angles to your body. Move your right foot up so that it rests on the inside of your left knee. Then slowly turn your lower back to the left, so that your bent knee moves toward the ground. Only go as far as is comfortable, then repeat with the other leg.

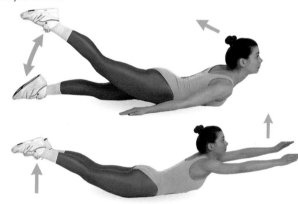

TESTING YOUR FITNESS

Most people do not know how fit they are – do you?

FITNESS TESTING enables you to determine your basic level of fitness so that you can safely embark on an exercise program. Testing also allows you to periodically assess and monitor your progress after you have been training for a few weeks.

The most accurate measurements of fitness are provided by tests carried out in an exercise physiology laboratory, using complex equipment and the services of specially trained staff. However, there are a several simple tests that you can do yourself to obtain a general idea of your level of fitness.

No single test can determine if you are fit or unfit. Instead, you need to assess the different components of your all-round fitness, which consist of strength, flexibility, and endurance. The following series of tests lets you evaluate your condition and then decide which type of fitness program would improve it.

HOW FIT ARE YOU REALLY?

Most people overestimate their fitness level. Even those who exercise very little and spend most of their time in sedentary activities often think that they are super-fit. Answer these questions to find out how fit you are.

Q *Do you walk each day, on average…*

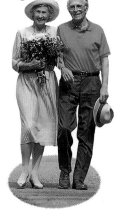

A
- More than 3 miles (5 km).
- Between 1 and 3 miles (1.5-5 km).
- Less than 1 mile (1.5 km).

Brisk walking, over a distance of at least 1.5 km (1 mile) a day, is an excellent form of aerobic exercise. It improves your endurance by enhancing the efficiency of your heart, lungs, and muscles.

Q *Do you get some form of vigorous physical exercise…*

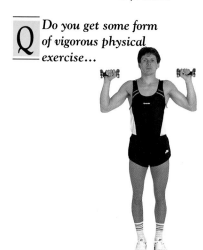

A
- At least four times a week.
- Two or three times a week.
- Once a week.
- Less than once a week.

In order to improve and maintain your overall level of fitness, you should take part in some form of physical activity for around 20 minutes, without a break, at least two or three times a week.

WARNING SIGNS

It is perfectly normal to become tired and a little breathless and for your heart to beat much faster during a test of your endurance. But you should rest immediately if you develop any of the following warning symptoms of excessive strain on the heart: chest pain (angina) or pain in the neck and arms; palpitations or skipped heart beats; nausea, dizziness, light-headedness, or feeling faint; severe breathlessness; or extreme fatigue.

TESTING STRENGTH

Strength is the ability to carry, lift, push, or pull a heavy load. To measure your muscle strength, count how many sit-ups you can do in 60 seconds. Around 20 to 25 sit-ups in a minute is average for anyone under 50 – less than this, and you need to do some abdominal strengthening exercises.

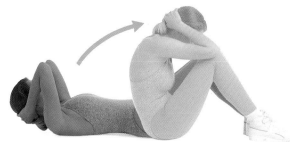

- *Lie on your back with your knees bent and your ankles secured under a solid object or being held by someone. Clasp your hands behind your head. Pull yourself up to a sitting position using your stomach muscles. Keep your knees bent to avoid lower back strain.*

Q *Faced with climbing three flights of stairs would you...*

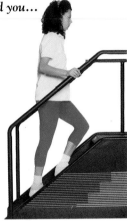

 Q *When you travel to work or to shops would you...*

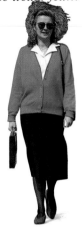

Q *At weekends and in the evenings do you spend most of your free time...*

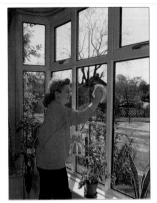

A • Be able to reach the top in one go, without any difficulty whatsoever?
• Struggle to the top and end up gasping for breath.
• Have to stop several times to catch your breath.
• Look for the elevator or escalator.

Stair-climbing is a good test of the fitness of your heart, lungs, muscles, and circulation. If you avoid climbing stairs, you are missing an opportunity to keep fit.

A • Be capable of running for a bus or train.
• Consider walking part of the way.
• Use public transport, or your car, to get as close to your destination as possible.

Many people could increase their fitness, without disrupting their lifestyle, by adding a little more exercise to their daily routine. Regularly choosing to walk or cycle to local shops, for instance, will help to keep you fit and healthy.

A • Involved in sporting activities.
• Taking care of manual jobs around the house and in the garden.
• Sitting in front of the TV or reading.

Sitting passively in front of the TV does not help to build up your strength, flexibility, or endurance. Use your spare time sensibly; take up a new and more energetic pastime and create a healthier future for yourself.

TESTING FLEXIBILITY

Flexibility is the ability to bend, stretch, and twist. You can assess your flexibility by performing a simple sit-and-reach test. Anyone whose flexibility is limited due to tight back or hamstring muscles should do regular stretching exercises.

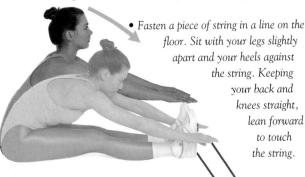

Fasten a piece of string in a line on the floor. Sit with your legs slightly apart and your heels against the string. Keeping your back and knees straight, lean forward to touch the string.

TESTING ENDURANCE

Endurance is the ability to keep on exercising. It reveals your general fitness level by showing how efficient your heart, lungs, muscles, and circulation are. You can test your own endurance level by seeing how well you cope with everyday physical activities.

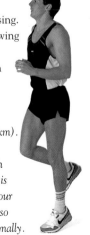

• *Walk briskly or jog slowly for 1 mile (1.5 km). You should not become breathless or tired.*
• *Walk steadily up three flights of stairs, each consisting of 15 to 20 steps. Your endurance is below normal if you have to pause to catch your breath or ease your aching legs, or if you are so breathless at the top that you cannot talk normally.*

HOW FIT IS YOUR HEART?

If climbing stairs leaves you breathless, your heart and lungs are probably out of shape – but do you really know how fit they are?

THE CONDITION OF your heart at rest and the way it responds during and after physical exercise are reliable indications of your overall fitness level. By performing a few simple tests, such as taking your resting pulse and measuring your pulse recovery 30 seconds after intense activity, you can easily assess the fitness of your heart.

Heart rates vary greatly. The resting pulse of a very fit person can be as low as 40. The average, however, is about 80. After exercise, the pulse of a trained athlete will recover in under a minute. For most people, however, it will take between four and five minutes, depending on the person's age.

Your target heart rate

You can gauge how hard you need to exercise to improve the functional efficiency of your heart by calculating your so-called "target heart rate." The target for each individual can be worked out using a simple mathematical formula based on their age and resting pulse (see opposite page).

If you regularly exercise hard enough to achieve your target pulse, you can monitor the improvement in the fitness of your heart. Take the measurements of your resting and recovery pulse rate every few weeks, or months, and compare it with your previous pulse rates.

WHAT IS YOUR RESTING PULSE?

Your resting pulse is the pulse you take when you first wake up in the morning. In general, as the fitness of your heart improves, your resting pulse becomes slower, stronger, and more regular. Women tend to have a slightly higher resting pulse than men. The resting pulse also increases a little with advancing years.

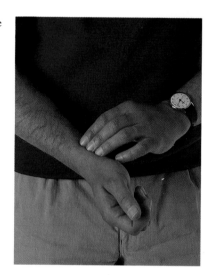

Taking your pulse
The easiest place to locate and record your pulse is on the front of your wrist, at the base of your thumb. Use your fingertips to press firmly over the pulsating artery. Count the beats for 15 seconds – then multiply by four to get a heart rate per minute.

Interpreting your pulse rate
The table below shows the relationship between your age, sex, resting pulse, and level of fitness. A resting pulse over 100 beats per minute could indicate a problem. You should therefore consult your doctor.

FITNESS LEVEL	BEATS PER MINUTE AT REST			
AGE	20 – 29 yrs	30 – 39 yrs	40 – 49 yrs	50+ yrs
MEN				
Excellent	under 60	under 64	under 66	under 68
Good	60 – 69	64 – 71	66 – 73	68 – 75
Fair	70 – 85	72 – 87	74 – 89	76 – 91
Poor	over 85	over 87	over 89	over 91
WOMEN				
Excellent	under 70	under 72	under 74	under 76
Good	70 – 77	72 – 79	74 – 81	76 – 83
Fair	78 – 94	80 – 96	82 – 98	84 – 100
Poor	over 94	over 96	over 98	over 100

WHAT IS YOUR PULSE RECOVERY TIME?

Another indicator of the fitness of your heart is how quickly your pulse returns to normal after it has speeded up during a period of vigorous exercise. If you exercise regularly, your pulse recovery time will gradually speed up, so that after 30 seconds of rest, your pulse rate comes down closer to your normal resting value.

WARNING

Do not attempt this test if your resting pulse is over 100 or if you feel unwell. Stop if you feel faint or develop chest pain, pain in the neck or arms, severe breathlessness, palpitations, or dizziness.

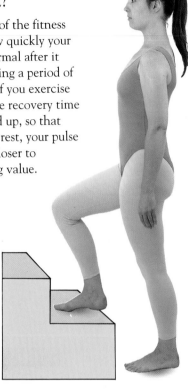

How to measure it
Using the step-up routine, strenuous exercise is possible even indoors. It does not require any specialized equipment. Find a stair, about 8 in (20 cm) high, and step up and down off it, moving one foot after another. Aim for about 24 step-ups a minute for three minutes. After 30 seconds rest, take your pulse at the wrist: count over a 15 second period and then multiply by four to get a heart rate per minute.

How to interpret it
The table below shows the relationship between your age, sex, pulse recovery at 30 seconds, and level of fitness.

FITNESS LEVEL	BEATS PER MINUTE AFTER EXERCISE			
AGE	20 – 29 yrs	30 – 39 yrs	40 – 49 yrs	50+ yrs
MEN				
Excellent	under 76	under 80	under 82	under 84
Good	76 – 85	80 – 87	82 – 89	84 – 91
Fair	86 – 101	88 – 103	90 – 105	92 – 107
Poor	over 101	over 103	over 105	over 107
WOMEN				
Excellent	under 86	under 88	under 90	under 92
Good	86 – 93	88 – 95	90 – 97	92 – 99
Fair	94 – 110	96 – 112	98 – 114	100 – 116
Poor	over 110	over 112	over 114	over 116

TARGET HEART RATES

To make your heart fitter, you must raise your pulse as near as possible to your target heart rate while exercising. Calculate your target heart rate as shown below. At first, it may be hard to meet your target; as you get fitter, it will become easier.

220 minus your age
= **Theoretical maximum pulse**

Theoretical maximum pulse minus resting pulse
= **Pulse range**

Pulse range divided by two plus resting pulse
= **Target heart rate during exercise**

For example, a woman of 50 years of age who has a resting pulse of 80, will have a theoretical maximum pulse of 220 minus 50, which equals 170. Her pulse range is therefore between the resting value of 80 and this maximum of 170, a difference of 90. Half of this difference (which equals 45), added to her resting pulse (80), produces a target heart rate of 125 beats per minute.

Monitoring your exercise pulse
Take your pulse after exercising hard for a few minutes. Count your pulse rate for 15 seconds; any longer and your pulse will start slowing down. Multiply by four to get a heart rate per minute.

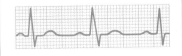

SETTING YOUR FITNESS GOALS

Set targets that are right for your level of fitness and choose a type of exercise you will enjoy.

KEEP AN EXERCISE DIARY

A daily record of the type and amount of exercise you have taken will allow you to monitor your progress. As your fitness improves you can increase the time or distance you walk, jog, cycle, swim, or row, by about 10 percent a week. If you find the next level of exercise uncomfortable, ease off a little. A week in your diary might look something like this:

Ted Robinson *is a 63-year-old retired surveyor whose hobbies are bowling, bridge, and bird-watching. His only health problem is some stiffness in his back. Ted does not smoke and is reasonably fit. He would, however, like to become fitter in order to improve his bowling game and to get ready for a walking holiday in France during the spring bird migration.*

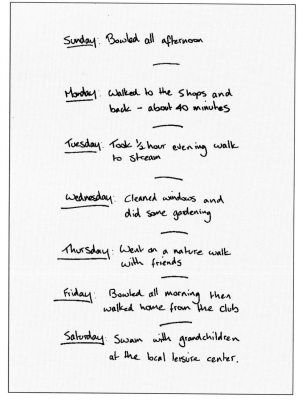

Sunday: Bowled all afternoon

Monday: Walked to the shops and back – about 40 minutes

Tuesday: Took ½ hour evening walk to stream

Wednesday: Cleaned windows and did some gardening

Thursday: Went on a nature walk with friends

Friday: Bowled all morning then walked home from the club

Saturday: Swam with grandchildren at the local leisure center.

Exercise is easy
Ted's diary reveals that he already leads a reasonably active life. But he still wants to improve his fitness. He decides to swim twice a week to reduce stiffness in his back and to go for more evening walks. He also joins a local hiking group on their nature hikes twice a month.

CHOOSING THE RIGHT balance of activities to suit your personal objectives and putting in the appropriate amount of time and effort to suit your current level of fitness is the key to creating a successful exercise program. The routine you eventually decide on should include a combination of aerobic, muscle-strengthening, and flexibility exercises.

Defining your objectives
Decide why you want to improve your fitness and make a note of your objectives. It will be much easier to keep yourself motivated once you are clear about your reasons for wanting to exercise more. Setting yourself realistic targets and working your way gradually toward them will help you achieve your exercise goals.

Whatever your objectives, you should devote at least 20 minutes of your time, three times a week, to physical activity.

A balanced routine
Aerobic activities, such as brisk walking or swimming, will improve your endurance, enabling you to exert yourself for longer periods without getting tired.

Muscle-strengthening exercises will tone up your muscles and improve your figure and posture.

Stretching exercises will help to keep your body supple and counteract the aches, pains, and stiffness that are the result of a sedentary, inactive lifestyle.

To reduce tension and relieve anxiety, try doing relaxation exercises. They will also help you sleep. In addition to specific relaxation routines, many sports aid relaxation as long as they are not played in a fiercely competitive way.

PERSONAL FITNESS PLANS

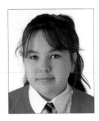

SAMANTHA WALKER is 13 years old, eats only junk food, and watches TV for three hours a day. She weighs 30 lb (14 kg) more than she should and is teased at school. She gets breathless when running up stairs and cannot touch her toes.

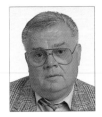

GEORGE GRESTY is a 54-year-old salesman. He smokes heavily and has not exercised properly for many years. He is 20 percent overweight. George's doctor has advised him to stop smoking and to lose weight to help reduce his blood pressure.

Discussion

You cannot force children to exercise, but you can make it fun and then they will want to take part. Children also need encouragement from their friends. Samantha's weight problem, however, requires more than just exercise. She needs advice on her dietary habits to help her see how harmful junk food is.

Fitness goals

- *lose 20 lb (9 kg) in 12 weeks.*
- *tone muscles and reduce fat.*
- *enhance flexibility.*

Exercise plan

- Walk 1 mile (2 km) to school every day.
- Go swimming with her family one evening a week.
- Go with friends either to the tennis club or roller skating once a week.

Discussion

George should start slowly and build up his exercise routine gradually because he is out of shape. Although George's blood pressure is not dangerous (it was only slightly raised), he should be aware of the warning symptoms of overstraining his heart, such as chest pain and palpitations.

Fitness goals

- *start taking exercise.*
- *lose 30 lb (14 kg) over the next 4–6 months.*
- *stop smoking.*

Exercise plan

- Daily walk, gradually increasing speed and distance.
- A supervised session in the multigym with two colleagues twice a week.
- Swim with his wife and children on the weekend.

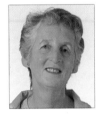

ELSIE TAYLOR, 68, has mild heart failure and osteoarthritis. Joint pain and stiffness have made it impossible for her to go outdoors unaided. Although cooking and housework are hard to manage, Elsie wants to stay independent.

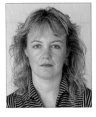

JOANNE BESFORD is a 29-year-old shop assistant who works six days a week. She suffers from aching legs and swollen ankles in the evening. Although Joanne does not play any sport, she would like to go on a skiing holiday in two months time.

Discussion

Elsie asks her doctor if exercise would help. The doctor advises her to do gentle loosening-up, stretching, and strengthening movements. They should also help her heart condition, but she should ease up if she starts to get very tired or out of breath. Special gadgets can make housework and cooking easier.

Fitness goals

- *improve her joint mobility and muscle strength.*
- *maintain her balance and coordination.*

Exercise plan

- Exercise at home, doing arm swings, shoulder rolls, body stretches, and ankle rotations.
- Attend a day center once a week for an "exercise for the elderly" session.

Discussion

Lack of fitness can cause skiing injuries. Unfit people fatigue quickly, making injury far more likely. To get fitter, Joanne should take a walk in her lunch break and use the stairs not the elevator. In addition to exercise, Joanne's leg symptoms would be helped by wearing support hose while at work.

Fitness goals

- *get fit for her skiing holiday.*
- *prevent some of her unpleasant leg and ankle symptoms.*

Exercise plan

- Join a health club. Attend three sessions a week.
- Leg exercise program morning and evening.
- When standing for long periods, Joanne should alternately push her toes, then heels, up off the floor.

PREPARING YOUR BODY FOR EXERCISE

Warming up before exercising and cooling down afterward is an essential part of any strenuous activity.

THE BODY has been compared with a finely-tuned machine. Like most machines it cannot work at full efficiency or at its maximum capacity as soon as it is activated. The muscles must be sufficiently warmed up if they are to function properly and without risk of injury.

The body needs to be correctly prepared for strenuous exercise if you are to achieve the maximum benefit with the minimum risk of injury. If you do not warm up, you will expose your body to the danger of developing a variety of aches and pains, or even an injury.

Perils of improper preparation

Even people who are in generally good condition risk suffering an injury if they suddenly force their muscles to stretch and contract. Stopping abruptly after exertion, without easing the muscles back into a resting condition, is likely to cause as much soreness and stiffness as suffered by the unfit beginner who has pushed too hard and too fast. Pulled muscles and muscle strains may result from exercising without warming up fully and carefully first.

WARM UP FOR SAFETY

Although liniments and lotions may feel good and relieve some pain and stiffness, they should never be used instead of a warm-up routine; they do not help prevent injuries.

HOW TO WARM UP

The best way to make sure that you warm up properly each time you exercise is to establish a set routine of loosening up, stretching, and gentle aerobic activities. A complete warm-up should last at least 10 minutes and should be done not more than 10 minutes before you begin exercising vigorously. A massage is also a good way of warming up as it increases blood flow through the muscles. However, the massage should always be followed up with a series of muscle stretches.

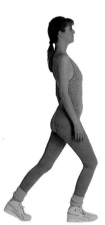

Calf stretches
Stand with one leg in front of the other. Gradually lean your weight onto your front leg, bending the knee. This stretches the calf muscles of the leg extended behind you. Hold for a count of five.

Speeding up
Gentle aerobic activity, like a brisk walk or slow jog, speeds up your heart rate and increases blood flow to your muscles and tissues.

Shoulder and chest stretches
Clasp your hands behind you. Slowly move your arms up. Hold the pull for a count of five.

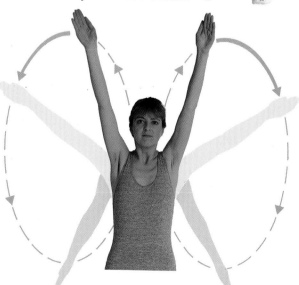

Loosening up
To loosen up your shoulder joints and warm up your upper arm muscles, make large circling movements with your arms held straight. Rotate your arms forwards five times, then back five times.

HOW TO COOL DOWN AFTER EXERCISE

You should always "cool down" for a few minutes after exercising by walking around and by repeating the same routine of loosening-up and stretching exercises you did to warm up. A proper cooling-down period keeps the blood flowing through your muscles. Any lactic acid that has built up inside the muscle cells can then be dispersed in the circulation to the liver where it is broken down. If you stop exercising suddenly, the lactic acid left behind in your muscles may cause cramps. It also tends to increase the amount of muscle soreness and stiffness you may suffer over the following two days.

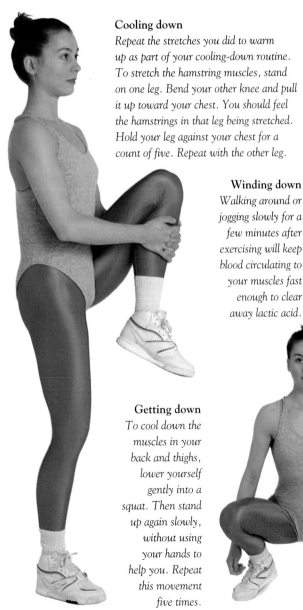

Cooling down
Repeat the stretches you did to warm up as part of your cooling-down routine. To stretch the hamstring muscles, stand on one leg. Bend your other knee and pull it up toward your chest. You should feel the hamstrings in that leg being stretched. Hold your leg against your chest for a count of five. Repeat with the other leg.

Winding down
Walking around or jogging slowly for a few minutes after exercising will keep blood circulating to your muscles fast enough to clear away lactic acid.

Getting down
To cool down the muscles in your back and thighs, lower yourself gently into a squat. Then stand up again slowly, without using your hands to help you. Repeat this movement five times.

The benefits of warming up

The main reason for warming up is to protect muscles, tendons, and ligaments from tearing during any violent stretching movement. This is especially important for activities such as throwing or kicking a ball that require a variety of movements of considerable force.

Warm-up exercises increase blood flow through soft tissues by widening the blood vessels in and around them. As a result their temperature goes up and they become more elastic and supple.

Do not begin warming up too soon. If more than 10 minutes elapse after you finish your warm-up routine and before you begin to exercise, your body will cool down and you will lose all the benefits.

In addition to protection against injury, your body will often simply feel better prepared for exercise. Warming up can certainly help in the psychological preparation for sporting activities, particularly in competitive events.

Cooling down

It is almost as dangerous to stop abruptly after an exercise session as it is to begin suddenly. Taking the time to cool your muscles down properly, will protect you from cramps and reduce muscle stiffness. Cooling down causes muscle capillaries to shut down and stops blood "pooling." which could lead to a sudden decrease in blood pressure.

After exercising vigorously, you should gradually reduce the level of exertion by jogging slowly or walking briskly. Then repeat the muscle stretching and loosening exercises you did in your warm-up routine. Now you are ready to stop, confident that you have done all you can to protect yourself from injury.

GETTING STARTED

Fitness cannot be achieved overnight, but with the right start you can be well on your way in a month.

DO YOU NEED A CHECKUP?

It is usually possible to exercise even if you have a serious medical disorder, but you must take appropriate precautions. Your doctor will be able to diagnose any complaint that could make strenuous physical activity dangerous. You should visit your doctor for a routine check-up before you begin any exercise program if any of the following circumstances apply to you:

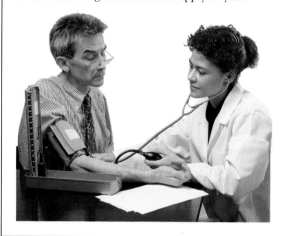

- Aged over 60.
- Over 35 and very unfit.
- Obese.
- Smoker.
- History of high blood pressure, heart disease, diabetes, or other health problems.
- Family history of heart disease before 50.

THE BEST FORM of exercise to choose is one that you enjoy and that fits easily into your everyday life. Cycling rather than driving to shops and climbing the stairs rather than taking the lift are two simple ways of becoming fitter.

It is important not to build up your fitness too quickly. You need to begin at a level of activity that will benefit rather than punish your body. Then, gradually increase the length of time and the amount of effort you put in as your fitness level improves.

Easy does it

There is no need to push yourself flat out in order to boost the efficiency of your heart, lungs, and muscles. You should, however, exert yourself enough to get sweaty and breathless and to

INCREASING YOUR OPTIONS

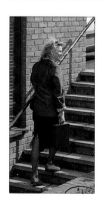

Becoming fit opens a whole range of exercise options to you. When you first begin, climbing stairs may leave you breathless. As you become fitter, however, you can begin to experiment with different types of exercise.

The first step
Take advantage of everyday opportunities to improve your fitness. Climbing the stairs rather than taking the elevator, walking to shops, and cycling to work will soon improve your overall level of fitness.

Adding variety
Exercise machines can add variety to your fitness routine. Rowing machines, exercise bicycles, treadmills, or stair-climbing machines all strengthen your cardiovascular system.

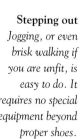
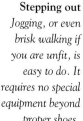

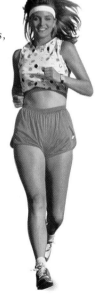

Stepping out
Jogging, or even brisk walking if you are unfit, is easy to do. It requires no special equipment beyond proper shoes.

KNOW YOUR LIMITATIONS

An essential part of exercising safely is to be aware of the warning symptoms that suggest you may be overstraining or damaging part of your body.

Some people can injure themselves by straining too hard in an effort to get fit. Others develop injuries by competing too hard against an opponent. When playing a competitive game like squash, it is safer to compete against your previous performance rather than your opponent. Even serious athletes risk injury if they overtrain.

BODY TISSUE	WARNING SYMPTOMS	WHAT TO DO
Heart	Chest pain; pain in the neck, jaw or arms; palpitations; severe breathlessness; dizziness, light-headedness, and feeling faint.	Stop at once. See your doctor for a check-up as soon as possible.
Joints	Pain, stiffness, and swelling.	Ease up your training routine and put cushioned insoles in your exercise shoes.
Muscles	Pain, soreness, and stiffness after an exercise session that do not go away before your next session.	Allow longer between exercise sessions for muscles to recover. Warm up and cool down properly. Ease up on strengthening exercises.
Kidneys	Blood in urine.	See your doctor, who may advise you to cut down distance running. If urine does not return to normal or other symptoms develop, further investigation is needed.
Bowels	Diarrhea or blood and mucus in stools.	Consult your doctor. Cut down on your training if you run long distances.

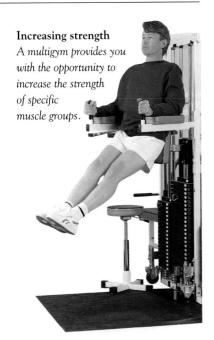

Increasing strength
A multigym provides you with the opportunity to increase the strength of specific muscle groups.

feel your heart beating faster. If you are jogging or walking, go at a pace that allows you to talk when you want to, not at an all out sprint.

People who are badly out of shape may have to stop often to avoid breathlessness or regain their strength. Slowly, over a period of several weeks, even the most unfit will find that they can keep going for longer periods without a break.

When to take a break

Although the ultimate goal is to exercise continuously for at least 20 minutes, you should not force yourself to continue if you do not feel well. If you work your body too hard you will only become injured or feel so stiff or sore for the next few days that you will not want to exercise again for a while. If you have an infection, you should not exercise at all (see p136).

A regular habit

For exercise to improve your over-all fitness, you should aim to work out vigorously three times a week. Each session should last between 20 and 30 minutes.

Once you have achieved your desired level of fitness, continue exercising to ensure that you stay in shape. The benefits of exercise soon wane if you do not keep it up. A day or two off will not effect your endurance, but two or three months of inactivity will cause a dramatic decline in your fitness.

HOME EXERCISE PROGRAM

Exercising at home can be fun and effective; it also builds up your confidence to take part in other sports.

ONE GOOD WAY of making sure that you find the time to work out regularly, without disrupting other commitments, is to exercise at home. Home exercise programs can be just as effective as any other form of physical activity. Many people actually prefer to exercise in the privacy of their own home, until they feel more confident and are in better shape.

Push-ups
Push-ups strengthen the triceps muscle at the back of each upper arm and the pectorals across the front of your chest. If you find this exercise too difficult, try it with your knees touching the floor.

The simple route to fitness

There are many types of exercise that can be performed in your home, with no need for any special equipment. For some activities you can make use of a piece of furniture or a door frame to provide support.

By performing a series of simple exercises, which work different muscles and joints, you can improve your strength and flexibility. Spend 30 seconds on each exercise, and then change to the next. Perform each exercise in your routine three times in all. Once you are fit enough to keep going for more than 12 minutes, without stopping for more than a few seconds between the different activities, you will be enhancing the efficiency of both your heart and your lungs.

Sideways bends
Stand up straight with your arms above your head. Tilt your spine first to the left and then to the right. This will strengthen your spinal muscles and improve their flexibility.

Jumping rope
Use a rope that is long enough to reach your armpits when you stand on its center. When you jump, bend your knees, do not jump higher than 4 in (10 cm), and always land firmly on the balls of your feet.

HOME EXERCISE EQUIPMENT

A wide variety of exercise machines are now available for use in your own home, ranging from fairly simple devices to expensive, highly sophisticated ones that use a computer to monitor your level of progress. Apparatus such as exercise bicycles, treadmills, and rowing, stair-climbing, and skiing machines are now available that can effectively simulate many different physical activities. Although, in theory, these machines offer you an enjoyable

Exercise bicycle

Motivating yourself

Although it does not matter when you exercise, if you set aside the same time of day each day for your workout, you are more likely to get into the habit. Put some music on in the background to liven up your routine, but choose a tempo that helps you pace yourself and stay comfortable. Exercise videos have become extremely popular; not only do they show how each movement should be done, but they also provide extra motivation and a feeling of actually belonging to a health club.

Exercise safely

Always wear suitable exercise shoes and loose-fitting, comfortable clothing. Move furniture you might knock into or fall over, and make sure that anything you are going to use for support is secure. Buy a cushioned exercise mat to protect your feet and ankles if you plan to include any high-impact aerobics in your exercise program.

Before you begin exercising warm up properly with a range of loosening-up and stretching exercises. This will reduce the risk of suffering from strains and sprains.

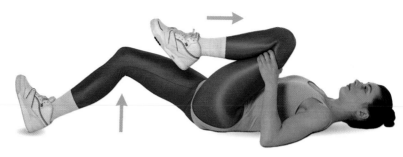
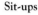

Leg raises
Lie on your back on the floor. Bend your legs and draw your knees one at a time toward your chin. This exercise will help develop your abdominal muscles.

Sit-ups
Sit-ups improve your figure and protect your back from injury by strengthening your abdominal muscles. Never perform a sit-up with your knees straight – this will overstretch the ligaments that support your spine.

BEWARE OF COSTLY MISTAKES

During the initial surge of enthusiasm many people rush out and buy home exercise equipment which is then rarely used. It is better to start with simple exercises and, when you have managed to keep to your routine for a few weeks, select equipment which you have already tried in a gym.

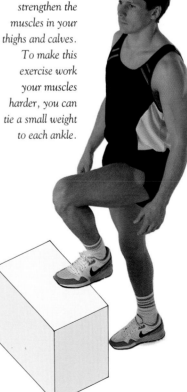

Step-ups
Step-ups strengthen the muscles in your thighs and calves. To make this exercise work your muscles harder, you can tie a small weight to each ankle.

form of exercise, which is readily accessible and convenient to use, in practice they are often expensive dust-gatherers. It takes a lot of willpower to exercise regularly on your own machine at home. Before you go out and buy one, ask yourself whether this is really the sort of activity you will enjoy. More importantly still, would you really use this machine two or three times a week? No-one's health has ever been improved by simply owning exercise equipment.

Rowing machine

EXERCISE IN THE GYM

ALTHOUGH HEALTH clubs and gyms have many different types of exercise machines that can be used for aerobic training, most people go specifically to exercise on the multigym apparatus.

These weightlifting machines allow you to push or pull against a variable load so that each muscle group can be strengthened in turn. Because they eliminate the risk of dropping a heavy weight, they are safer to use than free weights.

Designed to avoid injury

On mechanical weightlifting equipment, a system of pulleys moves fixed weights. Because the person using the machine does not hold the weights, there is no risk of being trapped beneath a weight. These machines also reduce the strain on your muscles when they reach the limit of their strength and heighten the tension during the muscle-relaxation phase.

The use of today's sophisticated gym apparatus rather than free weights has reduced the incidence of muscle and tendon injuries that once plagued weightlifters.

Aerobic apparatus

In addition to normal multigym equipment, most gyms and health clubs provide a range of exercise machines for aerobic activity. The most popular types of aerobic apparatus are the exercise bike, the treadmill, and stair-climbing and rowing machines.

Although a treadmill is no more effective than a brisk walk, it is safer than walking at night. As it is used indoors, you can exercise even when the weather is bad. The level surface of the treadmill is also less likely to cause stress injuries than walking along uneven pavements.

Sophisticated gym apparatus puts each muscle group safely through their full range of movement.

Stair-climbing machines are good for people who do not have easy access to a flight of stairs. These machines are becoming very popular and are an entertaining and different way to keep fit.

All these types of exercise are ideal as part of a warm-up routine before starting any muscle-strengthening exercise. A session of just 12 minutes on one of these machines can improve heart and lung fitness.

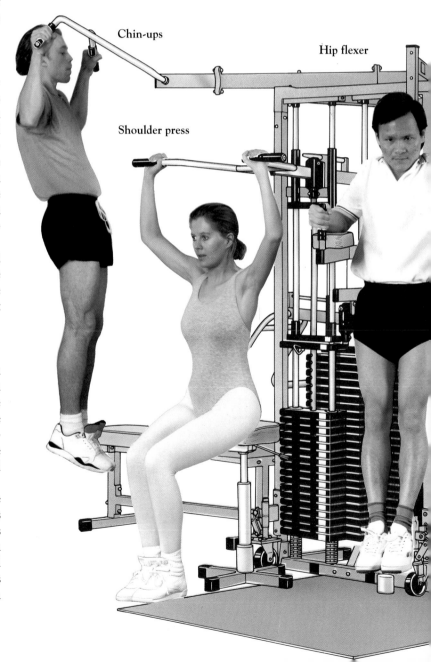

Chin-ups

Hip flexer

Shoulder press

BE SAFE, NOT SORRY

A multigym apparatus can be dangerous if it is used incorrectly. It is essential that all beginners are supervised and receive proper instruction from a qualified trainer. Following this sensible precaution will stop you from doing anything that could injure you.

TYPES OF EXERCISE

Chin-ups strengthen arms, shoulders, and also the upper back muscles.

Shoulder press strengthens both the upper arm muscles and the shoulders.

High pulley strengthens the shoulders and upper back muscles.

Chest press strengthens the muscles in the chest, upper arm, and back.

Hip flexor strengthens both the abdominal and the hip muscles.

Abdominal conditioner strengthens the abdominal muscles.

Leg press strengthens thigh and hip muscles.

Low pulley strengthens upper arm muscles.

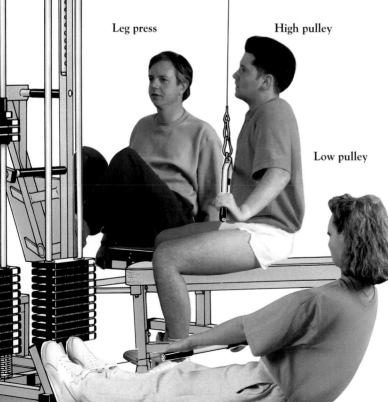

Leg press   High pulley

Low pulley

GETTING THE MOST OUT OF THE MULTIGYM

• Multiple repetitions with small loads are safer than using large weights to improve your muscle strength and tone.
• Build up your workload gradually and keep a record of your progress. If you push too hard you risk straining a muscle or tendon.
• Leave at least one day between gym sessions. This will give your muscles time to recover.
• Warm up with loosening-up and stretching exercises before you start.
• If you exercise with heavier loads to develop your muscle bulk, proceed carefully to avoid injury.
• Ideally, an instructor should always be present when you work out.

ARE YOU EXERCISING SAFELY?

If you take sensible precautions when you exercise you will avoid many injuries.

WHILE SOME SPORTS injuries are clearly unavoidable accidents, many could be prevented by taking special precautions before beginning to exercise or by paying better attention to safety guidelines.

The following questions highlight the many different aspects of injury prevention. Learning from your answers will help you safely enjoy all the benefits of physical activity.

Q *Do your muscles feel stiff or sore before you exercise?*

A
- Never.
- Occasionally.
- Yes, always.

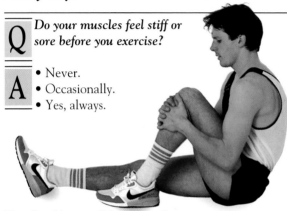

You should not still be aching from your previous exercise session when you start to exercise again. This is a symptom of overtraining – allow yourself a little longer to recover.

Q *Does exertion give you any of the warning symptoms of heart strain, such as chest pain or pressure; pain in the neck, jaw, or arms; palpitations; nausea; severe breathlessness, dizziness, light-headedness, or feeling faint?*

A
- Very rarely.
- Sometimes.
- Always.

One essential aspect of exercising safely is to be able to recognize the danger signals that could indicate that you are overtaxing your heart. If you develop any of the above symptoms during exercise, rest immediately. Do not begin to exercise again until you have been examined by a doctor. By listening to your body you will reduce the risk of aggravating any underlying heart problems.

Q *Are you over 35 years of age, a smoker, or overweight? Has a close relative died at an early age from heart disease?*

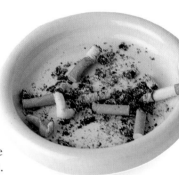

A
- No.
- Yes, to only one of these questions.
- Yes to two or more of these questions.

If you answer yes to two or more of these questions have a check-up, either at the gym or with your doctor, before you start an exercise program. Although very few people die during exercise, you could put your health at serious risk if you exercise too strenuously when you have a condition such as high blood pressure or heart disease.

Q *Have you suffered an injury recently?*

A
- No.
- Yes, but it is no longer swollen or painful.
- Yes.

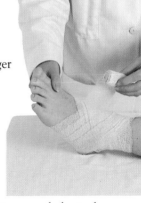

If you have been injured and it is still painful, tender, stiff, or swollen, you need to have further treatment before you can safely return to normal physical activities. If you exercise too soon you run the risk of making the injury worse, or even inflicting permanent damage on yourself. Also, when you are suffering from an injury you will naturally try to protect the painful area. This will cause you to use a bad technique and increase your risk of suffering from a second injury.

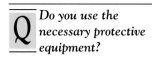

 Q *Do you use the necessary protective equipment?*

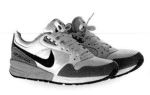

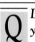 **A**
- Always.
- Only occasionally.
- Never.

Always wear the right protective equipment for the sport you are playing. Find out what you might need and buy the design or model that best suits your needs. Always use equipment that is the correct size. This applies to rackets, bats, and gloves, not just protective equipment like helmets and pads.

 Q *Do you warm up before you exercise?*

A
- Always.
- Only briefly.
- No.

Always warm up for 10 minutes before any strenuous activity. A routine of loosening and stretching exercises is best as it increases blood flow through tissues, making them more elastic and less likely to be damaged.

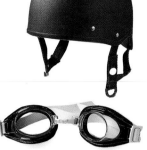

Q *Do you think your technique could do with some improvement?*

 A
- No, it is correct.
- Yes, a little.
- Definitely.

Since many injuries are caused by faulty technique, be sure yours is correct. For example, tennis elbow may result from failing to hit the ball in the center of the racket or from turning your wrist awkwardly when serving. Golf, rowing, and baseball are other sports where bad technique leads to injury.

Q *Before exercise do you drink alcohol or take any drug that could make you feel dizzy or drowsy?*

A
- Never.
- Sometimes.
- Often.

Do not drink before exercising. Even a small amount of alcohol reduces reaction times and impairs coordination, increasing your risk of injury. Many drugs can also do this, including antihistamines and sleeping tablets taken the night before. Do not exercise until the effects have worn off.

Q *Do you exercise when suffering from the symptoms of an infection, such as a sore throat, swollen glands, fever, or a deep cough?*

 A
- No.
- Sometimes.
- Frequently.

If you exercise when you have an infection not only will your performance be impaired but you are likely to make the infection considerably worse. With some viral infections, strenuous exertion can result in dangerous complications, such as inflammation of the heart muscle (myocarditis) or of the liver (hepatitis). Rest until your infection has cleared up.

Q *Do you ever wear exercise shoes that are excessively worn or do not fit properly?*

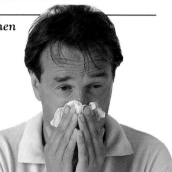

 A
- Never.
- Occasionally.
- All the time.

To prevent foot and leg injuries it is important not to wear shoes that are uncomfortable, poorly fitting, or starting to wear out. Choose a pair that provides adequate cushioning and is designed for the sport you intend to take part in.

FOODS, FLUIDS, AND EXERCISE

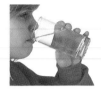

The foods you eat and the fluids you drink determine not only how healthy your body is but also how well you cope with energetic exercise.

Drinking water
Fluid lost due to perspiration during vigorous exercise must be replaced if the body is to work efficiently. Water is the best choice.

CARBOHYDRATES ARE the best type of food to eat if you plan to get some vigorous exercise within the next few hours. They are rapidly digested and absorbed to provide an immediate and readily available energy supply.

While you are exercising your digestive processes slow down. Blood is diverted away from your stomach and intestines to supply your muscles. Eating less than an hour before exercising may make you feel nauseous, due to food remaining in your stomach. Avoid any strenuous activity if you feel

hungry, or if you have not eaten for more than five hours, because you are likely to suffer hunger pains. The best time to eat is about three hours before you exercise. Never chew gum while exercising – if you accidentally inhale the gum it could block your windpipe.

Drink enough fluids
An adequate fluid intake is needed to replace water lost in sweat. You may need to drink liquid during exercise if you continue for longer than 45 minutes, especially in hot weather when you perspire more.

Food for thought
Food provides the energy for activity, so dietary decisions inevitably affect your sporting performance. For example, foods such as potatoes and pasta are rich in carbohydrates and supply energy more rapidly than those which are high in either protein or fat.

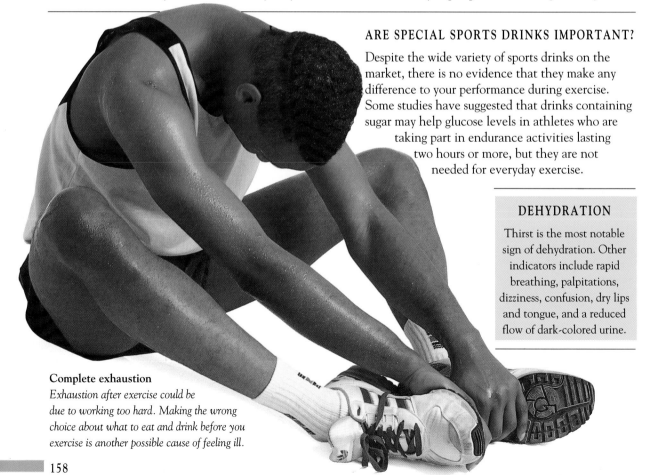

ARE SPECIAL SPORTS DRINKS IMPORTANT?

Despite the wide variety of sports drinks on the market, there is no evidence that they make any difference to your performance during exercise. Some studies have suggested that drinks containing sugar may help glucose levels in athletes who are taking part in endurance activities lasting two hours or more, but they are not needed for everyday exercise.

DEHYDRATION

Thirst is the most notable sign of dehydration. Other indicators include rapid breathing, palpitations, dizziness, confusion, dry lips and tongue, and a reduced flow of dark-colored urine.

Complete exhaustion
Exhaustion after exercise could be due to working too hard. Making the wrong choice about what to eat and drink before you exercise is another possible cause of feeling ill.

CARBOHYDRATE LOADING

Glycogen (also known as starch) is stored in muscles and converted into glucose during exercise to give energy. Many professional athletes boost their glycogen stores, and hence their energy stores, by a procedure known as carbohydrate loading. First of all they deplete their glycogen stores by training intensively. Then for three days before the competition they eat large amounts of carbohydrates that are rich in starch.

Foods that pack a powerful punch
Potatoes, pasta, legumes, grains, and cereals all contain large quantities of carbohydrates and are therefore ideal for boosting the body's stores of glycogen.

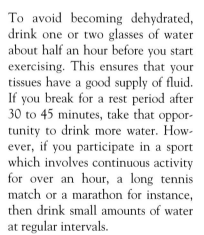

To avoid becoming dehydrated, drink one or two glasses of water about half an hour before you start exercising. This ensures that your tissues have a good supply of fluid. If you break for a rest period after 30 to 45 minutes, take that opportunity to drink more water. However, if you participate in a sport which involves continuous activity for over an hour, a long tennis match or a marathon for instance, then drink small amounts of water at regular intervals.

Feeling thirsty is not a reliable guide to how much fluid you have lost, so get into the habit of drinking liquids during any prolonged exercise session, even when you do not feel thirsty.

As soon as you finish exercising drink some more fluid, particularly if you have been perspiring heavily.

Benefits of a balanced diet
The more active you are, the higher your calorie intake should be. A balanced diet should satisfy all your body's needs for vitamins, minerals, and other nutrients. Many people mistakenly believe that if you play sport or exercise regularly you need to take food supplements to satisfy these increased energy requirements. However, supplements do not speed up your recovery from an injury and will not normally make any difference at all to your overall level of fitness.

CAFFEINE

Water remains the best source of fluid to prevent dehydration during exercise. Tea, coffee, and cola contain caffeine, a diuretic drug that increases the amount of urine produced and can thus lead to dehydration.

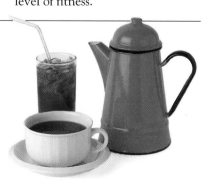

SALT-LOSS AND EXERCISE

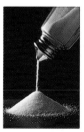

Salt tablets are rarely needed, even by people who exercise vigorously for long periods of time in very hot, humid environments. Although everyone loses salt as well as water when they sweat, in the vast majority of cases the body can compensate for this loss by reducing the level of salt in the urine. Taking salt tablets when you do not need them is not recommended as they may cause cramps.

CLOTHING AND EQUIPMENT

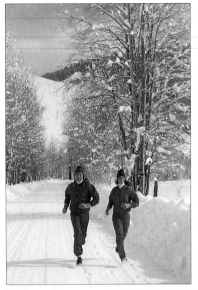

One easy way to avoid injury during exercise is to make sure that your clothing is suitable and that you use the recommended equipment.

WHEN YOU TAKE part in any form of exercise every piece of clothing and equipment plays a part in determining how safe you are. Clothes should be comfortable, fit properly, and offer adequate protection against the weather. For example, tight underclothing can soon rub skin raw or restrict your circulation, and socks that are too big will bunch up inside your shoes to cause painful blisters.

Protective equipment can shield all the different parts of your body from collisions with moving objects, other players, and the ground. Women may find that sporting bras are an asset and some sports require men to wear jock straps and cups for safety. To get the best advice on what equipment is appropriate for your chosen activity, consult an expert, such as the coach at your local club.

Cold weather
Several layers of thin clothing provide better insulation than one layer of thick material. Wear a hat to prevent loss of body heat through your head. After exercising be careful not to get chilled – change out of clothes that have become drenched with perspiration.

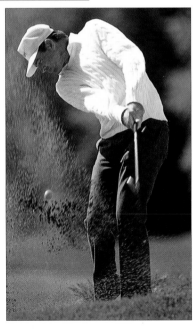

Hot weather
Cotton clothes are preferable to synthetic fibers in hot weather. They encourage efficient loss of body heat by speeding up the absorption and therefore the evaporation of sweat. Choose loose-fitting clothes which are light-colored to reflect the sun's rays. Wear a hat or sun visor to prevent heat stroke.

Essential equipment
Skiers, like participants in all potentially dangerous sports, need special clothes and equipment for safety.

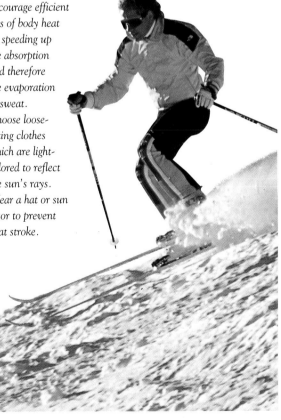

SENSIBLE PRECAUTIONS

Many minor accidents and even some serious eye injuries are caused by jewelry. Remember to take off your watch and any other items of jewelry before you participate in any sport, particularly contact sports. Tape over your rings if you do not wish to remove them. If you need to wear glasses buy a pair that have plastic lenses and make sure that they are fastened securely.

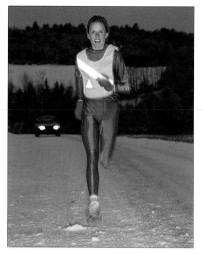

Safety at night

If you go out walking, jogging, or cycling after dark, wear white or light-colored clothing and fluorescent reflecting bands so that drivers can see you clearly.

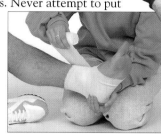

STRAPPING FOR SAFETY

Your doctor may suggest strapping a joint with adhesive tape or an elastic bandage after a ligament injury. Although strapping gives support and reduces the risk of a subsequent injury, do not start exercising again until the original injury has healed. Strapping can also be used as a preventative measure: it protects ligaments during fast twisting movements. Never attempt to put on strapping if you have not been shown the correct technique – too loose and it will be useless, too tight and it may actually provoke an injury.

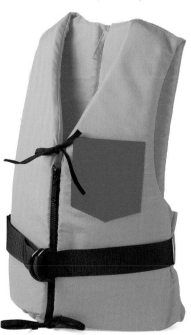

Life jackets

Every activity on water is potentially dangerous. A blow to the head can knock you unconscious and put you at risk of drowning. Therefore, even good swimmers should wear a life jacket while canoeing, sailing, or water-skiing. Children must wear a life jacket when they take part in any form of water sport.

Cycle helmet

Padded football helmet

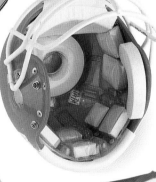

Helmets

Although helmets are routinely worn in cycling and horse riding, protective headgear is advisable in all sports where there is a risk of receiving a blow to the head. Good helmets carry an authorized safety standard mark of approval.

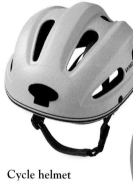

Gum shields

Gum shields are recommended for most contact sports. They protect your teeth, lips, and tongue. They also reduce the risk of concussion or a broken jaw. Ask your dentist for a made-to-measure shield.

Goggles

A pair of goggles, made of shatter-proof plastic, is essential in sports such as squash and handball to prevent serious eye injuries. Swimming goggles prevent chlorinated water from irritating the eyes.

SENSIBLE FOOTWEAR

Wearing the right shoes could stop you from developing a wide variety of problems.

SHOES THAT DO not fit properly or that do not provide adequate support or protection can cause injuries to your feet, the muscles and tendons in your legs, or even your back. Poorly fitting shoes can cause blisters and bruised nails, while shoes that do not provide enough support increase the risk of a sprained ankle. Lack of proper cushioning can result in back pain, joint injuries, and stress fractures.

Choosing the correct shoe

Different patterns of movement make different demands on your feet. Jogging shoes, for instance, need rigid heel support, flexible fronts, elevated soles at the heel, shock-absorbing heel cushions, and rough tread for outdoor running. Flared heels are to be avoided as they may encourage your foot to turn over on its side.

Footwear for racket sports needs good support at the front of the foot and shock-absorbent material under the ball of the foot. Avoid those that have elevated heels. Aerobics shoes need cushioning and ankle support. The tops should be cut low at the back to avoid pressure on the Achilles tendon.

Throw away well-worn shoes

Replace your shoes once they start to show signs of wear and tear. Abnormal wear may interfere with your foot posture when you walk or run, putting additional stress on the ligaments and tendons in your legs and lower back.

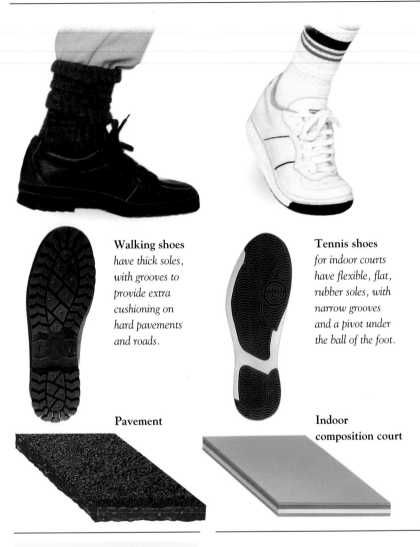

Walking shoes
have thick soles, with grooves to provide extra cushioning on hard pavements and roads.

Pavement

Tennis shoes
for indoor courts have flexible, flat, rubber soles, with narrow grooves and a pivot under the ball of the foot.

Indoor composition court

HOW TO CARE FOR YOUR SPORTS SHOES

• **Always break in a new pair**. To help prevent blisters, try one or two short exercise sessions when you first get your shoes.

• **Dry shoes naturally**. Never dry shoes on a radiator. The uppers will harden and lose their flexibility.

• **Replace old shoes**. No matter how comfortable your shoes are, abnormal or excessive wear of either the outer sole or the cushioned insole could cause you to develop an injury.

THE WELL-DESIGNED SPORTS SHOE

Heel counter

A stiff heel counter should keep your foot stable, but still allow movement in aerobics. It protects the Achilles tendon by supporting the back of the ankle.

Outer sole

The sole must be able to withstand rough treatment, be waterproof, and provide insulation from the cold. It should not be too rigid. Grip is enhanced by varying the thickness of the tread. Sole height should be slightly greater at the heel.

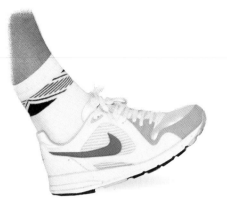

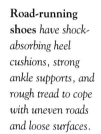

SOLES FOR DIFFERENT SURFACES

There are hundreds of different sports shoes on the market, but many of them are more for fashion than sport. All have some characteristics in common – they are comfortable and help absorb shock. Cross-training shoes are specifically designed to enable you to use just one pair of shoes for several different sports. They are expensive and not ideal for any type of physical activity. Their soles are thicker than tennis shoes, heavier than aerobics shoes, and less able to absorb shock than running shoes.

Road-running shoes *have shock-absorbing heel cushions, strong ankle supports, and rough tread to cope with uneven roads and loose surfaces.*

Aerobics shoes *have light, flexible soles with a smooth tread, they are designed to be used on polished wooden gymnasium and dance floors.*

DO YOUR SHOES WEAR OUT UNEVENLY?

If your shoes always wear out in one particular area of the sole you probably have an abnormal foot posture, for example a collapsing arch or excessive pronation (where the sole of the foot turns inward). A specially made orthotic appliance fitted inside your shoe will quickly and effectively solve this problem.

Gravel

Wood

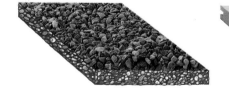

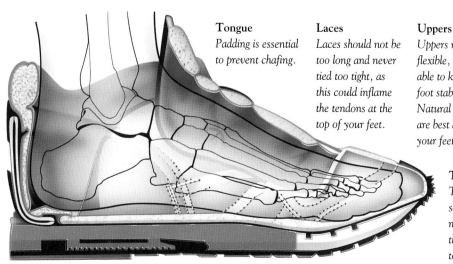

Tongue
Padding is essential to prevent chafing.

Laces
Laces should not be too long and never tied too tight, as this could inflame the tendons at the top of your feet.

Uppers
Uppers need to be flexible, firm, and able to keep your foot stable. Natural materials are best as they let your feet breathe.

Cushioned insole
Each time you take the weight off either of your feet, the insole should spring back to its original shape. Ordinary foam is not adequate.

Toe wrap
This area of the shoe is easily scuffed and therefore needs to be made of a strong material to reduce the rate of wear and tear and also to protect your toes.

Overtraining

Exercising can do more harm than good if you do not rest and recover between sessions.

THERE IS NO need to push yourself to the limit each time you exercise. A moderate amount of physical activity is enough to keep most people fit. Others, however, enjoy exercise and sport so much that they train more often. A few train to excess and damage their bodies in the process.

What is overtraining?

You are overtraining if you do not allow your body time to recover between exercise sessions, but carry on exercising despite feeling stiff and sore from your last workout. Some people become obsessed with exercise and push themselves too hard. Warning signs such as sickness, injury, exhaustion, or physical performance that is well below normal soon show up.

Even professional athletes do not exercise at their maximum level every day. They generally rest or exercise less on alternate days.

How much recovery time does your body need?

If you exercise strenuously, for example swimming 50 lengths of the pool or completing three long circuits in the gym, it is important to allow your body time to recover between sessions. The usual recovery time for muscles that have been worked to their maximum capacity is about 48 hours. This is true for everyone, no matter how fit.

After a vigorous workout, your muscles are likely to feel a little stiff and sore, particularly if you

ILLNESS DUE TO EXERCISE

Exercising too hard can give you more than just sore muscles. It can cause a variety of different medical disorders. Other parts of your body, from your digestive tract to your urinary system, can also be affected.

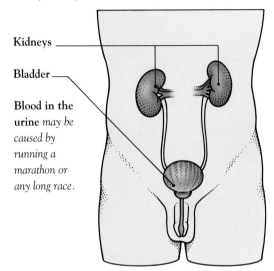

Kidneys

Bladder

Blood in the urine *may be caused by running a marathon or any long race.*

Runner's hematuria

After running a long distance, you may notice that your urine is cloudy or has blood in it. This condition, known as runner's hematuria, usually clears up in a couple of days. If it does not, or if you have any other symptoms, see your doctor.

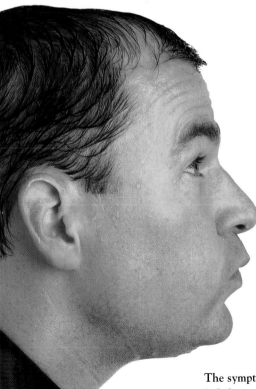

Heat exhaustion

Training too hard in hot weather can cause heat exhaustion (or even heat stroke, which can be fatal). Heat exhaustion is due to failure of the body's heat-regulating systems. Wear a hat and light-colored clothing to avoid overheating. If symptoms are not helped by drinking plenty of water and lying in the shade, consult a doctor.

The symptoms of overheating *include nausea, dizziness, fatigue, and muscle cramps.*

If you develop any unusual symptoms while you are following a training schedule, report them to your doctor. Most symptoms caused by vigorous exercise cease as soon as you start exercising less.

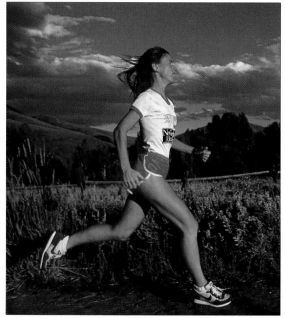

Menstrual changes *due to excessive exercise can involve irregular bleeding but in extreme cases menstruation can stop altogether; this is known as amenorrhea.*

Amenorrhea

Exercise reduces the production of hormones by the pituitary gland. These hormones help to control the menstrual cycle. Periods may stop altogether but they usually return if you stop pushing yourself so hard. Always consult your doctor if you notice any change in your menstrual cycle.

have just started on an exercise program. These symptoms are partly the result of minor damage to individual muscle fibers and partly due to an excessive build-up in the muscle cells of lactic acid, which is produced by anaerobic metabolism in the cells.

Normally the discomfort and stiffness eases within the first two days after the exercise. The muscle fibers heal and the lactic acid is absorbed into the bloodstream to be carried to the liver where it is broken down. Typically the symptoms get worse on the second day, before they disappear.

How to avoid overtraining

By following just one simple rule you can avoid the various problems associated with training too much. Never attempt any strenuous activity while your muscles are still stiff and sore from your last workout.

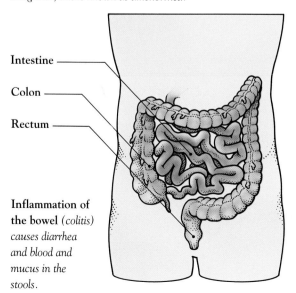

Intestine ———

Colon ———

Rectum ———

Inflammation of the bowel (*colitis*) *causes diarrhea and blood and mucus in the stools.*

Runner's diarrhea

This condition is a form of colitis caused when blood is diverted from the digestive tract to your muscles during an excessively long period of exercise. Easing up on your training should relieve the symptoms.

SYMPTOMS OF OVERTRAINING

You are exercising too much and need to reduce your level of training if you develop any of the following list of symptoms:

• Reduced appetite.
• Difficulty sleeping.
• Constant feeling of exhaustion.
• Waking up tired and listless.
• Unplanned loss of weight.
• Loss of desire to keep fit.
• Recurrent infections or minor injuries.

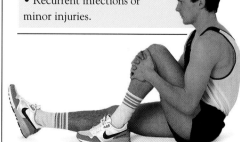

SPORTS INJURIES

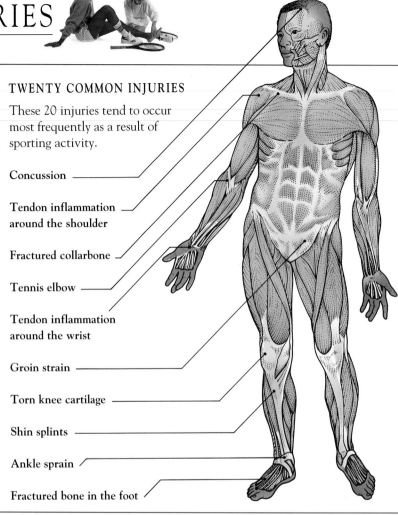

Recovery from most injuries does not require professional help.

ANY PART OF YOUR body may be injured during sport or physical exercise. The injury may be caused by a direct blow, by overstretching, or by repetitive movements of one particular body part.

Around 80 percent of all sports injuries involve soft tissues, such as muscles, tendons, ligaments, and joint linings. Only about 20 percent involve a bone being broken or damage to an internal organ.

Although some of these injuries have been given a name that includes a sports prefix, for example tennis elbow or baseball finger, they are not specific to those sports. They can just as easily occur as a result of many other activities. In fact tennis elbow happens more often as a result of painting a ceiling or sawing wood, than after a hard game of tennis.

TWENTY COMMON INJURIES

These 20 injuries tend to occur most frequently as a result of sporting activity.

Concussion

Tendon inflammation around the shoulder

Fractured collarbone

Tennis elbow

Tendon inflammation around the wrist

Groin strain

Torn knee cartilage

Shin splints

Ankle sprain

Fractured bone in the foot

SOFT TISSUE INJURY

Many sporting accidents lead to the appearance of a bump or a bruise over the following few days. Soft tissue injuries (in the muscles, ligaments, tendons, or joint linings) cause inflammation with redness, warmth, tenderness, and swelling at the site of the injury.

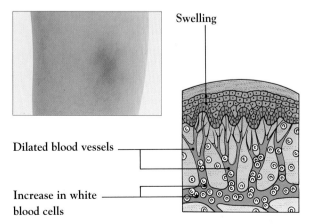

Swelling

Dilated blood vessels

Increase in white blood cells

Bruising
Blood vessels damaged by the injury dilate and cause internal bleeding. Fluid then leaks into the tissue, resulting in inflammation and an associated increase in the number of white blood cells.

FIRST AID FOR SOFT TISSUE INJURIES

"RICE" stands for Rest, Ice, Compression, and Elevation.

Following any soft tissue injury, you should use the RICE first-aid routine for the initial 48 hours. If you do, the symptoms will be reduced and recovery from the injury will be much quicker.

If the symptoms do not improve or if pain persists after 48 hours you should always consult your doctor so that he or she can rule out the possibility of a fracture or other serious injury.

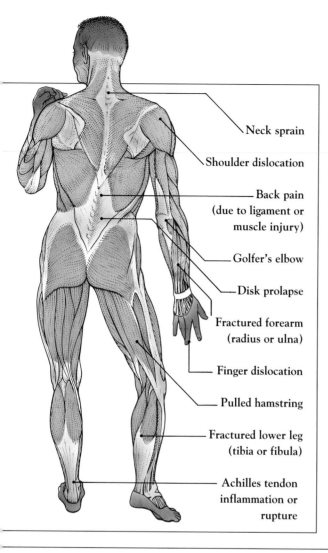

Neck sprain

Shoulder dislocation

Back pain
(due to ligament or
muscle injury)

Golfer's elbow

Disk prolapse

Fractured forearm
(radius or ulna)

Finger dislocation

Pulled hamstring

Fractured lower leg
(tibia or fibula)

Achilles tendon
inflammation or
rupture

EXERCISE FOR RECOVERY

As soon as the pain and swelling subside and you are able to move the injured area without making the pain worse, you can safely start some gentle exercises. As your injury continues to heal, build up the range of each movement, the number of repetitions you perform, and the time you spend on them.
Your doctor or physiotherapist can recommend a program of rehabilitation exercises. These will normally include:

- Stretching exercises to restore mobility and flexibility.
- Strengthening exercises to build up muscles and correct weakness or wasting caused by inactivity.
- Exercises to restore balance and coordination.
- Aerobic exercises to build up fitness.

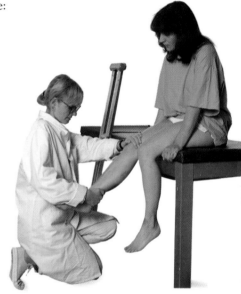

 1 **Rest** – *Resting the injured part and avoiding unnecessary movement allows the damaged tissues to begin healing and reduces the amount of further bleeding and swelling.*

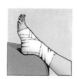 *2* **Ice** – *Apply an ice pack to the injured area for a period of 10 minutes every three hours. The cold relieves pain and limits swelling and bruising by narrowing the damaged blood vessels.*

 3 **Compression** – *A compression bandage helps reduce bleeding and swelling. You may need help to put the bandage on. It should extend well above and below the injury, but should not be so tight that it cuts off the circulation across the injured area. Use crepe or elastic bandages.*

 4 **Elevation** – *Raising the injured area (above the heart when possible) reduces bleeding and swelling. It also helps drain away any fluid that has accumulated due to inflammation of the tissues caused by the injury.*

MONITORING YOUR RECOVERY
Resuming your usual activities

You should be ready to go back to your usual activities once you can pass the following fitness tests:
- The injured part can be moved freely without pain or stiffness.
- Stretching of the surrounding muscles is not painful.
- Balance and coordination are back to normal.
- Resisted movement is not painful.
- There is no pain, stiffness, or swelling during or after exercise.
- The cause of the original injury has been identified, so that the chances of it occurring again can be reduced.

TREATING INJURIES

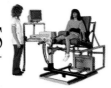

There are several simple and effective treatments for every different kind of soft tissue injury.

COMPLETE RECOVERY from a sports injury may take several weeks, even if you have followed the correct first-aid measures. If you are not getting any better and have persistent pain, tenderness, stiffness, or swelling, then consult a specialist in sports medicine. You may have an injury that requires extra treatment, such as physiotherapy, a corticosteroid injection, or even surgery.

FIRST AID

Proper first-aid treatment (see p166) in the first 48 hours after an injury will reduce the pain, relieve symptoms, and speed your recovery time.

MASSAGE

Physiotherapy often includes massage, a technique which can help relax muscle spasm and improve the flow of blood through an injured tissue.

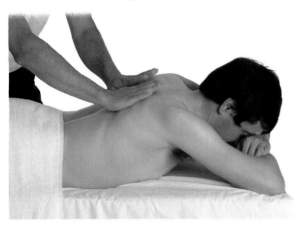

Physiotherapy

A wide range of physical treatments are available to relieve pain, heal damaged or inflamed tissues, and speed up recovery. For many sports injuries, rest alone is not the solution. A physiotherapist, using a combination of exercise and specialist healing treatments, such as applying heat sources or using ultrasound or laser treatment, can make your recovery more rapid.

EXERCISES

During the early stages of recovery, exercises may be carried out in water. Known as hydrotherapy, this form of treatment is highly successful because the water reduces the pull of gravity on the injured part, making movements easier and therefore less painful.

Other exercises to aid recovery include passive exercises, where a physiotherapist manipulates the affected limb, or assisted-active exercises in which part of the body is supported during movement.

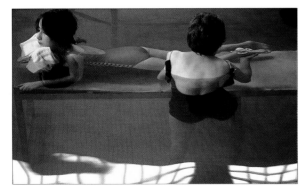

LASER THERAPY

A low-intensity laser beam can reduce pain, inflammation, and swelling at the site of an injury, thereby assisting the healing of the

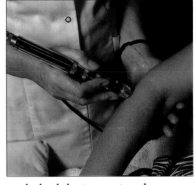

damaged tissues. It works both by improving the flow of blood and by reducing the production of prostaglandins – chemicals which cause pain and inflammation that are released after an injury.

The skin is first cleaned with an antiseptic swab to remove natural oils which might reduce the efficiency of transmission. The laser is then focussed onto the injured part from a hand-held treatment probe which rests lightly against the skin or is positioned just above it. Protective glasses are worn to prevent the remote possibility of the laser causing eye damage.

HEAT TREATMENT

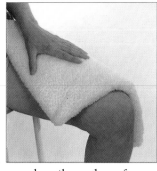

A heating pad, infrared lamp, short-wave diathermy machine, or any other type of heat source may be used to relax muscle spasm, relieve pain, and improve blood flow through damaged tissues. Treatment should not be started until two days after the injury occurred, to give blood vessels time to heal and thus avoid aggravating any bleeding or swelling.

ULTRASOUND TREATMENT

High-frequency sound waves, produced by passing an electric current through a crystal, may be used to treat many types of sports injury. Ultrasound waves relieve pain and swelling and enhance healing by reducing inflammation and improving blood flow.

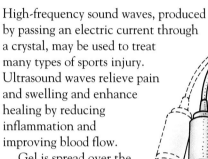

Gel is spread over the injury site to improve transmission and the device is moved continuously to stop the skin from becoming too hot.

NON-STEROIDAL DRUGS

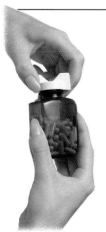

A non-steroidal anti-inflammatory drug (NSAID) is often prescribed to promote recovery from an injury. Clinical studies have shown that these drugs are more effective than other painkillers at relieving pain and tenderness. The best known examples of NSAIDs are aspirin and ibuprofen.

NSAIDs block the release of prostaglandins, chemicals which cause pain and inflammation. Prostaglandin release starts soon after suffering an injury, so NSAIDs should be taken as soon as possible for maximum benefit.

MANIPULATION

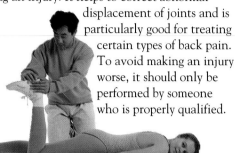

Manipulation is an effective physical method of treating an injury. It helps to correct abnormal displacement of joints and is particularly good for treating certain types of back pain. To avoid making an injury worse, it should only be performed by someone who is properly qualified.

INTERFERENTIAL TREATMENT

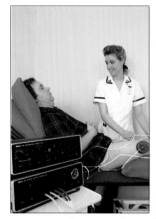

This electrical treatment involves passing two sources of alternating current through the injured tissues, from either two or four electrodes that are held onto the skin surface by suction pads. The interference waves produced by an interaction between these electric currents temporarily relieve pain and relax muscle spasm. A course of this treatment can help reduce swelling and inflammation, and speed up healing by improving blood flow.

STEROID INJECTIONS

A corticosteroid drug may be required if the injury has remained tender due to persistent inflammation. Prior to the injection the skin overlying the injury is cleaned with antiseptic and a local anesthetic may be given. Often the anesthetic and steroid are mixed together in the same sterile syringe and then injected.

Following a steroid injection, you should rest the injury for at least two days. As the anesthetic wears off be prepared for a slight increase in pain. It normally takes around five days to gain the full benefit from the steroid. Occasionally a second injection is required.

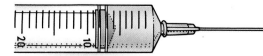

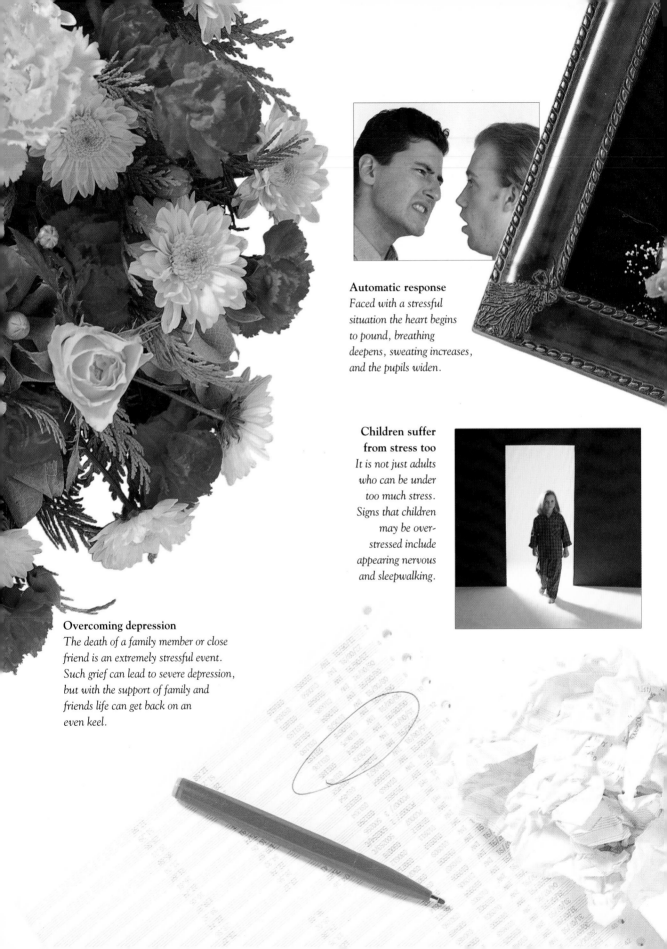

Automatic response
Faced with a stressful situation the heart begins to pound, breathing deepens, sweating increases, and the pupils widen.

Children suffer from stress too
It is not just adults who can be under too much stress. Signs that children may be over-stressed include appearing nervous and sleepwalking.

Overcoming depression
The death of a family member or close friend is an extremely stressful event. Such grief can lead to severe depression, but with the support of family and friends life can get back on an even keel.

CHAPTER SIX

MANAGING STRESS

EVERYONE NEEDS A CHALLENGE, but if the challenge becomes impossible to meet, it can produce intolerable levels of stress.

Stress stimulates and motivates people. Usually, minor daily stresses are accepted as just part of the day, something that makes life interesting and challenging. But if a great many demands are made on you these minor difficulties can lead to too much stress and damage your health, causing insomnia, tension, back and neck pain, and other stress-related illnesses.

Some people seem to thrive on stress, while others cannot tolerate it. By analyzing your emotional habits and behavior you can find out how stress affects you and learn to recognize the warning signs of excessive stress. With this knowledge you will be able to combat the cause of the stress before it becomes a major problem. There are many different ways of easing this tension. Relaxation exercises, meditation, yoga, or physical exercise can all help.

In the US, it is estimated that seven million people consult their family doctors each year because they feel depressed or anxious. Surveys have shown that almost the same number suffer symptoms of these stress-related illnesses but do not seek medical advice.

If you are having emotional difficulties that are interfering with your health or wellbeing, it is best to discuss them with your doctor. Seeking help is the most important step toward finding a solution to your problems. Counseling, behavior therapy, a short course of medication, or psychoanalysis can all be beneficial.

Marriage troubles
Relationships can be one of the main causes of high levels of stress.

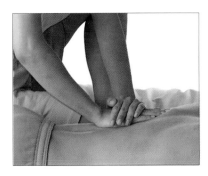

Massage the cares away
A soothing massage can reduce pain, relax muscles, and make the skin more supple. As you become more relaxed your level of stress will fall.

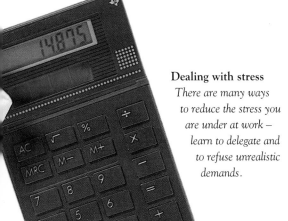

Dealing with stress
There are many ways to reduce the stress you are under at work – learn to delegate and to refuse unrealistic demands.

ARE YOU UNDER STRESS?

All sorts of different events and situations can put you under too much stress.

STRESS IS A COMMON problem that can build up gradually. You may not be aware of just how much stress you are under until it has reached a critical level. Therefore it is important that you learn to recognize the types of symptoms that may indicate that your level of stress is too high.

Find out how vulnerable your personality is to the harmful affects of stress; assess the current level of stress in your life; and learn whether you are suffering from any stress-related symptoms by answering the following questions:

 Q *Are you competitive and aggressive in everything you do?*

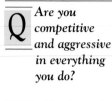

A
• No, I avoid unnecessary confrontation.
• Yes, I strive to be successful at play as well as at work.

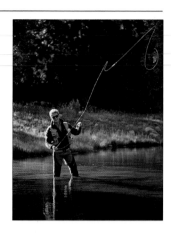

There is nothing wrong with wanting to be successful. It is a good idea, however, to take part in at least one noncompetitive activity in order to reduce tension.

 Q *Do you go over and over the events of the day and worry about them?*

A
• No.
• Sometimes.
• Yes.

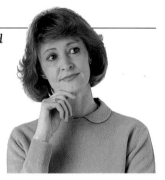

Constantly brooding about the past or worrying about future events increases the amount of stress in your life. Try not to worry so much; it is pointless fretting about events over which you have no control.

 Q *Do you find it hard to express your feelings and anxieties out loud?*

A
• No.
• Yes.

People who constantly bottle up their emotions are more likely to develop a harmful build-up of stress. Being able to cry or shout out loud occasionally is a good way to release pressure.

 Q *Do you lack ambition and always rely on other people to spur you into action?*

A
• No.
• Sometimes.
• Yes.

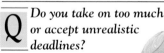

If you just allow events to happen to you and never take control of your life you are increasing your risk of suffering from stress. Be positive: you can beat your apathy, boost your confidence, and eliminate stress.

Q *Do you take on too much or accept unrealistic deadlines?*

A
• No.
• Yes, but this is the nature of my work.
• Yes, but I like to push myself hard.

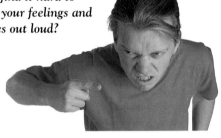
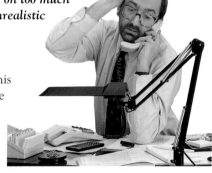

The ability to say "no" to excessive demands is a skill. If you create your own stress by pushing yourself too hard, try to manage your time better, increase the amount of work you delegate, and find time to relax.

Q *Do you find it hard to relate to people?*

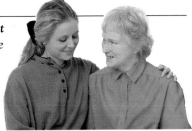

A
• No.
• Yes.

If you do suffer from too much stress you are likely to recover more quickly if you have close friends or relatives that you can confide in. Friendly advice or a shoulder to cry on can make all the difference and enable you to cope until the crisis is over.

Q *Are you suffering from any symptoms of stress?*

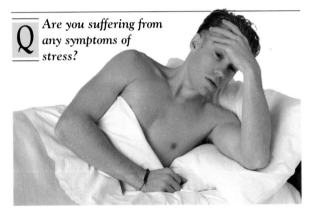

A • If you are suffering from more than four of the symptoms listed in the table to the right you are likely to be overstressed. To maintain your health you need to identify the sources of stress in your life and try to alleviate them.

Q *Has your life changed much in the last six months?*

A • Some areas of my life have changed but others are exactly the same.
• No, everything is the same as it was.
• Yes, many aspects of my life have changed.

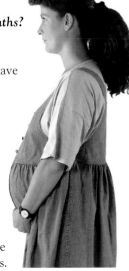

New activities and events add variety to life, reduce stress, and help to keep you healthy. However, too much or too little change can actually cause stress.

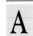
Q *How many interests and activities do you have outside of work?*

A
• Many.
• Only a few.
• None.

Working for excessively long hours, without allowing yourself time to wind down, increases your risk of becoming over-stressed. Any activity that you enjoy will help to relieve tension and keep you happy and relaxed.

SYMPTOMS OF STRESS

• Regularly having difficulty falling asleep.
• Often wanting to cry.
• Constantly feeling tired and lethargic.
• Rarely laughing or smiling.
• Difficulty concentrating or making decisions.
• Suffering from nervous tics.
• Having recurrent headaches or muscle pains.
• Being unable to talk to other people.
• Becoming increasingly short-tempered.
• Feeling unable to cope.
• Starting to drink or smoke more.
• Developing explosive rages.
• Losing interest in sex.
• Constantly having gloomy, pessimistic thoughts.
• Eating when not hungry.
• Lacking in enthusiasm.
• Driving fast and dangerously.

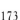

THE STRESS BALANCE

Finding the right stress balance is difficult since one person's challenge is another person's stress.

STRESS RATING SCALE

Psychologists have calculated the stress value of different events and have provided a rating for each one. Everyone deals with stress differently, so these values are only approximate. They can help you predict your chances of experiencing significant mental or physical ill-health due to the effects of stress.

Add up the points given for any of the events below that have happened to you in the last six months. If your total is over 40, you have a high risk of developing a stress-related illness or exhaustion.

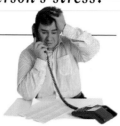

DEALING WITH STRESS

Some people thrive on stress and seek it out; others find it too much to take and avoid it. The way in which each individual is able to handle stress is determined partly by personality and partly by ability to cope under different types of pressure.

STRESS IS A FACT of life that has both positive and negative aspects. Stress adds spice to your life, challenges you, and drives you on. Too much or too little stress can harm your emotional wellbeing.

The risks and benefits of stress
Problems occur when stress is constant, rather than temporary. Ideally, stress should arise as you meet a particular challenge, and subside once those demands or difficulties have been resolved.

Short bursts of stress – whether enjoyable or upsetting at the time – are followed by a return to a resting state. But if stress and tension are unrelenting, rest is impossible and symptoms of either physical or mental illness can result.

2 points	3 points	5 points	6 points	7 points
Minor violations of the law	*Change in sleeping habits*	*Moving home*	*Child leaving home*	*New job*
	Going on vacation	*Changing school*	*Starting or leaving school*	*Foreclosure of mortgage or loan*
	Christmas	*Building an extension or making extensive home improvements*	*Arguments at work or at home*	*Change to different type of work*
	Change in eating habits	*Job under threat*	*Rapid promotion*	
	Change in social activities	*Change in work habits or conditions*	*Jet lag (twice or more)*	
	Change in church activities	*Spouse begins or stops work*	*Minor illness or injury*	
	Change in recreation		*Large mortgage*	
			Debt problems	

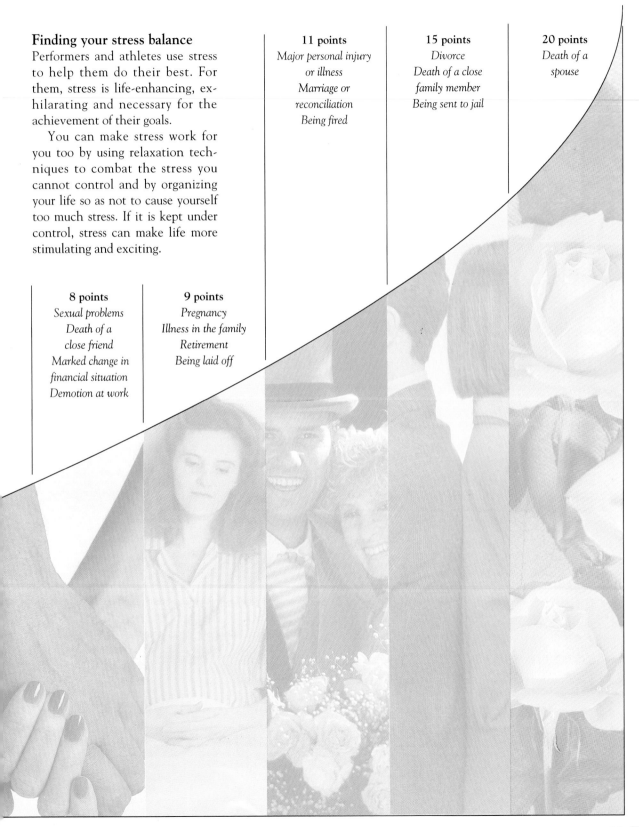

Finding your stress balance

Performers and athletes use stress to help them do their best. For them, stress is life-enhancing, exhilarating and necessary for the achievement of their goals.

You can make stress work for you too by using relaxation techniques to combat the stress you cannot control and by organizing your life so as not to cause yourself too much stress. If it is kept under control, stress can make life more stimulating and exciting.

11 points
*Major personal injury
or illness
Marriage or
reconciliation
Being fired*

15 points
*Divorce
Death of a close
family member
Being sent to jail*

20 points
*Death of a
spouse*

8 points
*Sexual problems
Death of a
close friend
Marked change in
financial situation
Demotion at work*

9 points
*Pregnancy
Illness in the family
Retirement
Being laid off*

STRESS WARNING SIGNS

KEY STRESS SYMPTOMS

If you experience any of the following symptoms you may be under too much stress:

 • Constantly feeling tense or on edge.

 • Finding it difficult to fall asleep or relax.

 • Being indecisive or lacking concentration.

 • Becoming irritable and impatient.

 • Aching limbs or recurrent headaches.

 • Smoking or drinking more.

Recognizing that you are overstressed is the first step to regaining control of your emotional health.

HUMAN BODIES ARE designed to respond physically, rather than mentally, to a stressful situation. This immediate, primitive reaction is known as the "fight or flight" response. It prepares the body for any vigorous exertion, either in the form of violent conflict or a rapid escape to safety.

How the body reacts to stress

Even if the threat is emotional, rather than physical, these same physiological reactions occur – the heart beats faster, the muscles tense, and the skin sweats more. These changes, however, cannot protect the body against psychological pressure, such as frustration.

If an individual is constantly placed in threatening situations, where the body initiates this arousal response but there is no chance to escape from or conquer the source of the threat, he or she will become tense and overstressed.

Anyone can suffer from stress but some types of people are more vulnerable than others to suffering stress-related medical problems, such as peptic ulcers. By learning to recognize the signs of stress, anyone can reduce the day-to-day pressure of life before becoming ill.

IMMEDIATE ACTION

Do not ignore aches and pains – they may be a warning that you are under too much stress. Take steps to ease the pressure before a crisis occurs.

IS YOUR CHILD UNDER STRESS?

Children between the age of five and 12 who cling to an adult, so that they are unable to play with other children, cannot sleep alone, or cannot be left in a room on their own, are overanxious. Other signs of stress in children include:

• Frequently complaining of headaches or abdominal pains.
• Jumping or flinching easily when startled.
• Constantly asking for reassurance.
• Appearing nervous or frowning a lot.
• Experiencing difficulty falling asleep, having regular nightmares, or sleepwalking.

Adolescent angst
Teenagers have to cope with many stressful events. If your son or daughter shows signs of stress, talk to them, or consult your doctor.

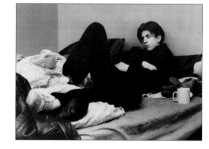

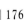

STRESS AND HEART RATE

Any stress raises the pulse by activating the body's fight or flight response. When a high pulse rate is linked to exercise this is an appropriate response – it allows the body to perform efficiently. It is when the body becomes aroused without any accompanying muscular response, such as being stuck on a train, that the stress is likely to be harmful. The chart below shows how the pulse rate reacts to stress during a typical working day.

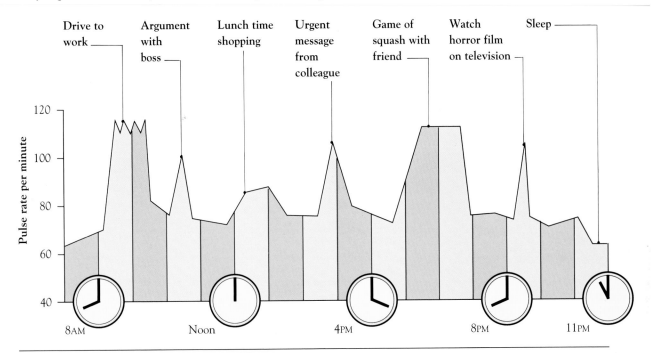

Drive to work — Argument with boss — Lunch time shopping — Urgent message from colleague — Game of squash with friend — Watch horror film on television — Sleep —

Pulse rate per minute

120 — 100 — 80 — 60 — 40

8AM — Noon — 4PM — 8PM — 11PM

FIGHT OR FLIGHT RESPONSE

The release of the hormones adrenaline, noradrenaline, and cortisol from the activated adrenal glands, and the stimulation of the sympathetic nerves, prepare the body to fight or flee. This response occurs in all animals, not just humans, as a reaction to a threat. It can be beneficial; for instance, it may improve sporting performance. Signs of this fight or flight response in the human body include:

• Heart begins to pound.
• Breathing is deeper and faster.
• Muscles receive greater blood flow.
• Blood sugar level rises to provide more energy.
• Eyes focus for distance vision.
• Pupils widen to let in more light.
• Sweating increases to cool the body.

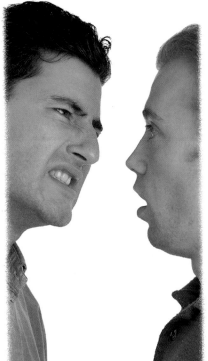

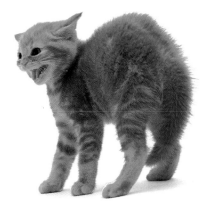

The fight or flight response in animals
Animals and humans react in the same way to stressful and threatening situations – their bodies both automatically invoke the fight or flight response. A cat, for instance, arches its back, bristles its fur and whiskers, flattens its ears, and enlarges its pupils.

STRESS AND ILLNESS

Too much stress increases your risk of suffering from an illness or accidental injury.

I T IS SIMPLY NOT possible to avoid all stressful situations and events. In fact to do so would not be healthy, for stress is an essential part of life. If it is kept under control, stress is a positive force that can improve your performance and efficiency and help to keep you alert and out of danger.

A prolonged period of severe stress, or several sources of minor stress, however, are not good for

WHAT EFFECT DOES STRESS HAVE ON THE BODY?

Research has demonstrated that as people become more and more stressed they become increasingly susceptible to both physical illness and mental problems. The reasons for this association are not yet completely understood, but the following areas of the body seem to be most affected by stress:

Hair
Some forms of baldness have been linked to high levels of stress.

Brain
Many mental and emotional problems may be brought on by stress. In extreme cases, long-term stress can cause a so-called nervous breakdown in which the person is no longer able to cope with day-to-day problems.

Heart
Stress can increase blood pressure which in turn increases the risk of a heart attack. However, tension is not the only, or even the most important, cause of high blood pressure. Other factors, such as your genes, diet, and level of exercise, play a vital role.

Immune system
Prolonged stress can weaken the immune system. Sufferers are therefore more susceptible to minor infections, such as colds and boils.

Digestive tract
Stress is known to cause or aggravate many diseases of the digestive tract, including gastritis, peptic ulcers, irritable bowel syndrome, and colitis.

Mouth
Mouth ulcers frequently develop in an individual who has become run down by being under too much stress.

Muscles
Minor muscle twitches and nervous tics become more noticeable when an individual is overstressed.

Skin
Attacks of eczema or psoriasis may suddenly flare up during periods of abnormal stress.

Lungs
Some asthmatics find their condition is aggravated by emotional upsets.

Reproductive organs
Stress may result in many types of menstrual disorder. For instance, periods may cease (known as amenorrhea). In men, stress is the most common cause of impotence and premature ejaculation.

Bladder
Many women, and some men, develop an irritable bladder as a direct response to stressful events.

your health. Excessive stress puts your body into a state of emotional turmoil. This agitation may affect a variety of organs and systems within the body and eventually produce many different types of disease.

A COMMON PROBLEM

It is thought that as many as 60 percent of visits to the doctor are directly related to stress. There are many different factors that can cause these stress-related symptoms but worries about work or money are the most common. Because the numbers of working women have increased, just as many women as men now suffer from symptoms that have been brought on by stress due to pressures at work.

CAN YOUR PERSONALITY INFLUENCE YOUR HEALTH?

Stress affects blood pressure, but it is not known whether your ability to cope with stress alters your risk of having a heart attack. It has been argued that aggressive people (type A) are more likely to develop heart disease than those who are relaxed (type B). Smoking and diet, however, are now thought to influence your health more.

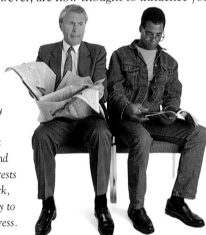

Type A personality
People who are very highly competitive, find it difficult to delegate, and have few interests outside of work, are more likely to suffer from stress.

Type B personality
People who are easy-going, able to relax, and are not over-competitive, are less likely to develop stress-related health problems.

ALL IN THE MIND?

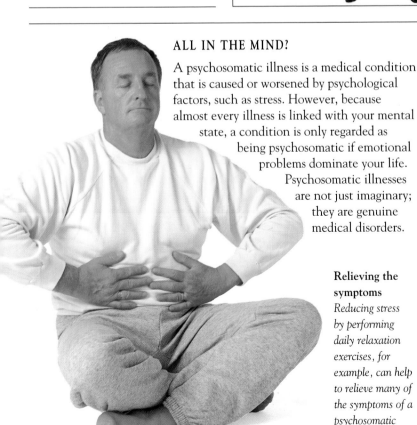

A psychosomatic illness is a medical condition that is caused or worsened by psychological factors, such as stress. However, because almost every illness is linked with your mental state, a condition is only regarded as being psychosomatic if emotional problems dominate your life. Psychosomatic illnesses are not just imaginary; they are genuine medical disorders.

Relieving the symptoms
Reducing stress by performing daily relaxation exercises, for example, can help to relieve many of the symptoms of a psychosomatic illness.

MIND OVER MATTER – THE PLACEBO EFFECT

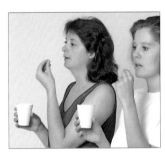

Your state of mind can influence your health. In 40 percent of people a tablet which contains only sugar (known as a placebo) will prove to be effective in relieving pain, anxiety, and other symptoms. The simple fact that an individual believes the tablet will work is enough to overcome many different symptoms.

CONTROLLING STRESS

Although you cannot avoid stress altogether, you can improve your ability to deal with it.

EVERYONE EXPERIENCES stress at certain times in their lives, often due to events beyond their control. Whatever the sources of stress in your life, however, you can learn to control its effects on you.

A number of simple measures, such as meditation or confronting the source of your problems, can be used to ease tension. Learning and carrying out these antistress techniques can improve your ability to cope with stressful situations.

Reducing your stress level

Identifying what is causing your stress is the first step to reducing it. Taking almost any action to relieve it will help because this is a sign that you are no longer prepared to endure an unacceptable level of pressure.

Sometimes it is not easy to see just what is putting you under stress. To help pinpoint the problem, every time you find yourself becoming anxious make a note of the circumstances, and then see whether a pattern emerges. As you dig deeper into the nature of your responses to people and situations, you will probably discover what is going wrong.

Taking control
Organize your time to reduce your stress levels – plan ahead, do not over-schedule yourself, and leave time for relaxation.

Make a list of all the things that have been troubling you, putting them in order of priority. Then, beginning with the problem that causes you the greatest irritation, anxiety, or stress, work out a way to solve it or deal with it. As you resolve each problem, move down your list, tackling only one source of stress at a time.

Talking through problems

Discussing what is bothering you is often a good way to find a solution. Once you have decided who or what is at the root of your anxiety, talk the issue over, either with a friend or with the person who is causing the problem.

Admitting that you cannot handle a problem alone may be an embarrassing or awkward confession to make, but involving another person in your troubles at an early stage can speed up the process of finding a constructive solution.

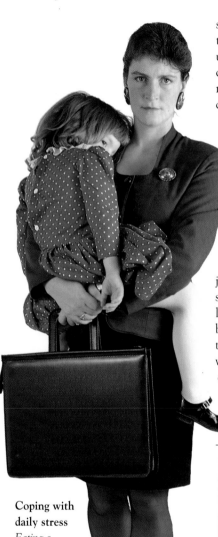

Coping with daily stress
Eating a balanced diet may help your body deal more effectively with stress. It is not necessary to take a "stress vitamin" supplement.

COPING WITH A LIFE CRISIS

No matter how well planned your life is, or how healthy your mind and body are, a crisis can bring on stress. The following strategies may help:

- Learn to recognize a crisis.
- Seek and listen to advice.
- Do not brood about past events or blame someone else.
- Do not worry over future events that are beyond your control.
- Consider each problem separately.
- Make a list of your worries; they will seem less overwhelming.

- Stick to a daily routine to create a greater sense of security.
- Take your mind off your worries through a leisure activity or exercise.
- Do not try to work out solutions to your problems just before bedtime.
- Consult a doctor or counselor before stress builds up to an intolerable level.

TRANQUILLIZERS

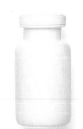

Although tranquillizers can prove helpful in cases of extreme stress, such as bereavement, they are not a long-term solution. Only take tranquillizers for the shortest possible time to avoid the problem of becoming dependent on them. This will also give you the chance to build up your own ability to live with and fight against the pressures you are under.

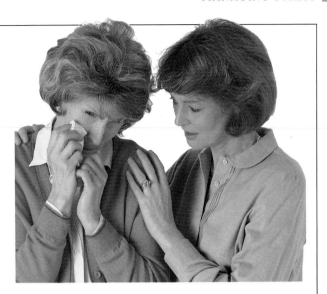

Giving and receiving comfort

Turning to friends and family for help and support can ease your difficulties, making them less stressful.

WAYS TO CONTROL STRESS

Stressful situations may be inevitable and beyond our control, but the anxieties that they arouse can be relieved by using the following antistress techniques.

These techniques work by helping you to avoid or reduce the stresses of daily life, to release accumulated stress, and to spot stress warning signs.

 Take regular breaks. A short rest period during the day will help to relieve pressure and refresh your mind after a session of concentrated mental or physical effort, or if you have become frustrated with a project.

 Plan each day. Listing what you need to accomplish in order of priority, setting realistic goals, saying no to unacceptable or impractical deadlines, and finishing one task before you move on to the next can help you feel in control.

 Be realistic. Try not to take on too much. Sometimes, to relieve a tight schedule, you may need to change ideas or arrangements; do not feel guilty about doing so.

 Take care of your social life. It is important to develop interests outside your career or family. Do not always neglect friends in favor of work or family commitments.

See your doctor. If the stress in your life has become intolerable or is causing physical symptoms or depression, counseling may help make your lifestyle less stressful.

 Exercise regularly. Physical activity reduces tension, helps you sleep better, releases pent-up emotions, and takes your mind off your worries. Choose an activity just for the enjoyment, not to satisfy a competitive desire to win.

 Relax. This will relieve warning signs of stress such as headaches, muscle pains, or difficulty sleeping. Progressive muscle relaxation, meditation, and yoga are all good ways to help you keep these symptoms of stress at bay.

 Talk about your problems. Your partner, a friend, or a family member may be able to help you find a solution, but even if not, just discussing your feelings can often help.

 Take vacations or short breaks to unwind. It is better to get away from home if you would otherwise begin stressful home activities, like spring-cleaning or redecorating.

 Avoid making too many changes at once. Major events that require you to change the way you live are easier to deal with if they do not happen close together.

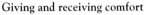

RELAXATION EXERCISES

Relaxation reduces muscular tension caused by stress and improves your health.

RELAXATION IS A SKILL that needs to be learned and mastered. When stress makes you tense from time to time, there a number of techniques that can help you relax.

Many relaxation exercises can be done anywhere, at any time. They are most successful if done regularly, not just when you feel you are close to breaking point. Acquiring the ability to relax without having to make a special effort will then be particularly helpful when you are under more pressure.

Relaxing to relieve pain

As well as making your muscles less tense, daily relaxation has been shown to relieve pain in some types of recurrent headache or backache. It may also lower the blood pressure of some people being treated for hypertension (abnormally high blood pressure). However, no one should stop taking medication for hypertension without their doctor's knowledge and agreement.

OTHER WAYS TO RELAX

- Slow your breathing. Take deep, even breaths for five minutes.
- Close your eyes and count backward from 20, saying each number silently as you breathe out.
- Shut your eyes and imagine a beautiful scene. For five minutes, explore the sights, sounds, and smells, savoring every detail of this picture.
- Get strenuous exercise to help reduce muscle tension and anxiety.

EXERCISES TO RELIEVE PHYSICAL TENSION

The following exercise routine can relax muscles made tense and tight by stress. Wear comfortable clothing that allows you to move freely. Remove your shoes and any glasses or contact lenses before you start.

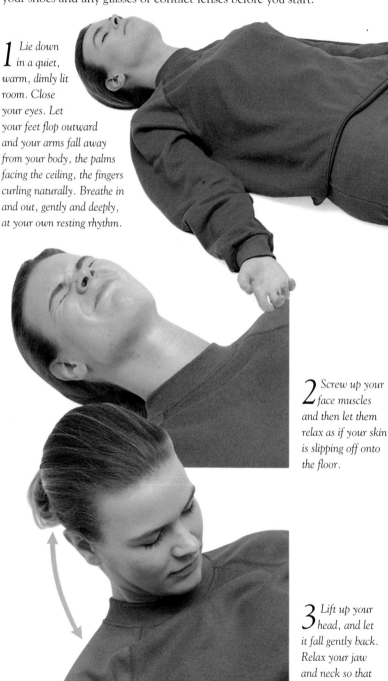

1 Lie down in a quiet, warm, dimly lit room. Close your eyes. Let your feet flop outward and your arms fall away from your body, the palms facing the ceiling, the fingers curling naturally. Breathe in and out, gently and deeply, at your own resting rhythm.

2 Screw up your face muscles and then let them relax as if your skin is slipping off onto the floor.

3 Lift up your head, and let it fall gently back. Relax your jaw and neck so that you can feel your throat opening.

Work through each stage; then repeat for at least 10 minutes. Your whole body should feel completely relaxed. Lie totally limp for a few more minutes. Before returning to normal activities, do some gentle stretching.

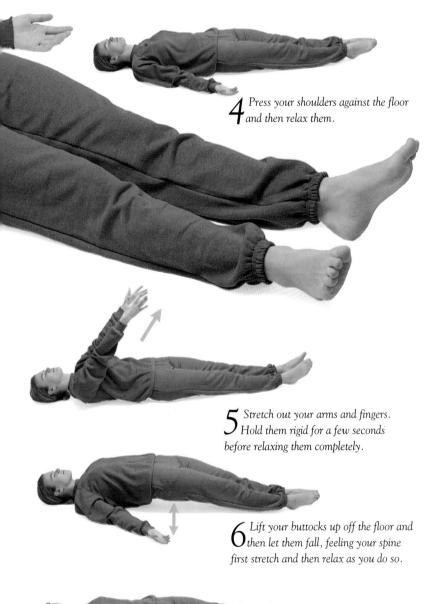

4 Press your shoulders against the floor and then relax them.

5 Stretch out your arms and fingers. Hold them rigid for a few seconds before relaxing them completely.

6 Lift your buttocks up off the floor and then let them fall, feeling your spine first stretch and then relax as you do so.

7 Keeping your heels together, stretch your legs and toes out; then relax them completely.

BREATHING EXERCISES

Breathing exercises can be used to help you relax. The habit of taking deep breaths is an effective weapon against the build-up of tension.

- Sit in a quiet room with your feet flat on the floor.
- Become aware of the chair supporting your full weight and let your shoulders relax.
- Breathe deeply and slowly, breathing out for twice as long as you breathe in (you can judge this by counting silently to yourself).
- Continue for five minutes, but stop if you begin to feel dizzy.
- While you are concentrating on your breathing, try to clear your mind of all other thoughts.
- Do this breathing exercise twice a day, everyday.

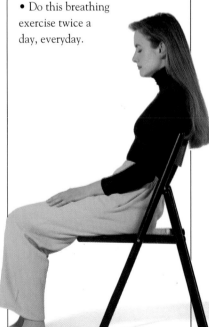

MEDITATION AND YOGA

MEDITATION HAS traditionally been a feature of many religions, particularly those based on Eastern philosophies. The goal of meditation is to find tranquillity by emptying the mind of distracting thoughts and worries.

A number of organizations teach meditation techniques. It is not, however, difficult to learn to meditate effectively on your own.

A simple meditation technique

To begin meditating, sit cross-legged (or if that is uncomfortable, in another relaxed position), with your back straight and eyes closed, in a quiet room where you will not be disturbed.

Once your breathing is regular, choose a word that has no emotional significance for you and, without moving your lips, repeat it silently to yourself. Pay full attention to the sound of the word, not to its meaning.

Alternatively, fix your gaze on a stationary object such as a wall pattern. But do not try to analyze its shape or form logically.

· If you find that your mind begins to wander, or that distracting thoughts intrude, gently bring

Many people have adopted meditation or yoga as a way of relaxing both the mind and body.

yourself back to the word, phrase, or object you have chosen. Do not strain to banish these intrusive thoughts and images. Simply try not to follow them or to worry about how well you are doing.

Transcendental meditation

In transcendental meditation, the instructor gives each individual a personal secret word or sound called a mantra to be repeated over and over again.

Meditate in this manner for five minutes, twice a day at first. Then, as you become more adept,

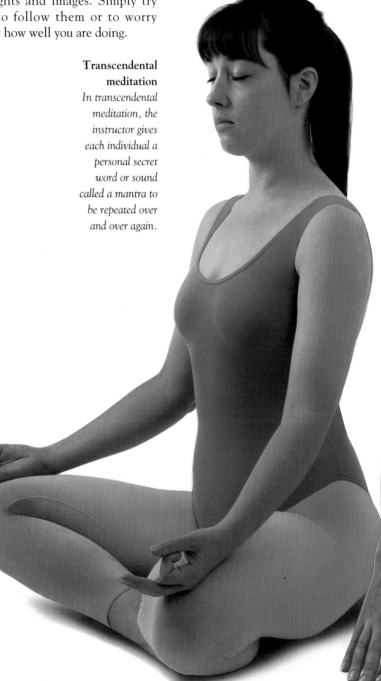

HATHA YOGA

Hatha yoga prepares you for higher forms of meditation by restoring health and balance to the body and mind, using physical movements and postures called asanas and breathing techniques called pranayamas to relax the body and calm the mind. It has become very popular in the US because in addition to its powerful relaxing effect it increases flexibility, strength, balance, and coordination.

gradually extend the meditation period until you can do about 20 minutes at each session.

Benefits of meditation

Clinical trials have shown that regular meditation can be a useful therapy for reducing stress levels and relieving many stress-related disorders. Although experienced meditators may use these techniques as a pathway toward spiritual experiences, for most people meditation is just a way of releasing inner tension and uneasiness.

During meditation, there may be a marked decrease in the body's oxygen consumption, as cell metabolism slows down. At the

Yoga
The spinal twist is an excellent position for improving flexibility in the spine and relieving back pain.

same time, measurement of the electrical activity in the brain demonstrates an increase in alpha waves, which are the slow brain waves associated with relaxation.

Both the pulse and the rate of breathing normally slow down. Blood pressure, however, is only lowered in those people who start with a slightly elevated reading.

Regular meditation can also help control alcohol abuse in those individuals who have been drinking to relieve tension and anxiety.

Benefits of yoga

Successful meditation is the final goal of yoga, a system of Indian philosophy and physical discipline which teaches coordinated movements and postures, relaxation and breathing control, and meditation techniques. The individual adopts positions that exercise almost every part of the body, while using controlled breathing techniques.

Correctly practiced, yoga is a useful method of relaxation which helps clear the mind and reduce physical tension. It also maintains body flexibility, promotes suppleness, and can increase both muscle strength and endurance.

WARNING

It is best to begin a yoga program in a supervised class, rather than by experimenting on your own. Some positions can cause overstretching and injury if done incorrectly. Certain positions are unsuitable or have to be modified to minimize the risk of injury in the elderly, or to avoid aggravating medical disorders, like glaucoma (raised pressure in the eye), high blood pressure, or back trouble.

THE BENEFITS OF MASSAGE

Having a relaxing massage is a useful way to reduce stress.

BACK MASSAGE

A soothing back rub can cure tension and muscular pain in the back, as well as imparting a feeling of peace and relaxation. Ask the person you are massaging to lie on his or her stomach, then kneel beside the base of the spine with one knee bent to support your weight. Alternate soft, soothing touches with long, deep strokes.

STROKING, RUBBING, kneading, and pummelling different areas of the body can increase blood flow, reduce pain, relax muscles, and make the skin more supple.

Massage can help treat painful muscle spasms, muscle injuries, and muscle tension caused by a build-up of stress. It can even combat stress by encouraging relaxation at the end of a busy day.

When giving a massage, use firm pressure on large muscles. On smaller areas, use either your thumbs or fingertips. You can apply deep pressure and release muscle tension with your thumbs. Kneading fleshy areas like the thighs will relax the muscles.

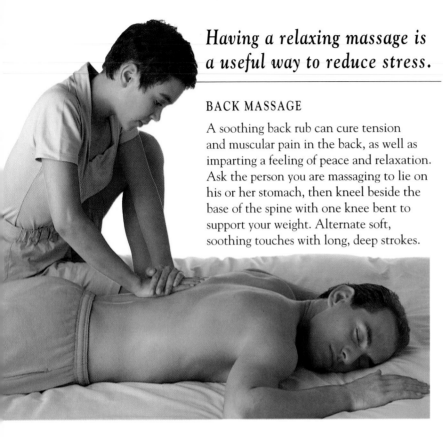

MASSAGE TECHNIQUES

• Choose a warm, peaceful, dimly lit room where you will not be disturbed by anyone.
• Remove all jewelry.
• Cover the body with towels; only expose the area being massaged.
• Give the massage on a firm, padded surface, such as thick blankets placed on the floor, rather than a soft bed.
• During the massage, concentrate on the movements; do not chatter.
• Keep one of your hands in contact with the body all the time.
• Use rhythmic motions.

1 Place your right hand on the lower back. Put your left hand on top and exert pressure. Slide up the back and over the shoulders.

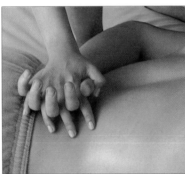

2 To lift the shoulder blade, place the forearm across the lower back. Hold it with one hand. Use the other hand to grip and gently rock the shoulder up and down. Replace the arm at the side.

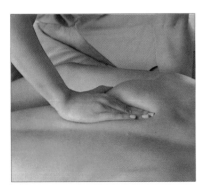

3 Slip one of your hands under the shoulder. Raise it to lift the shoulder blade a little. Press your other hand into and under the shoulder blade, up across the shoulder, then down the arm.

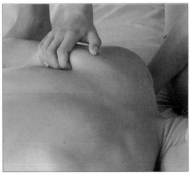

4 Keeping your hand under the shoulder, grip and rock the raised shoulder blade gently with your fingertips. Move up the blade and repeat. Then use soothing strokes to relax the area.

HEAD, NECK, AND SHOULDER MASSAGE

Tension can build up in the muscles of the neck and shoulders after long periods spent sitting at a desk. Massage is a simple way of easing it.

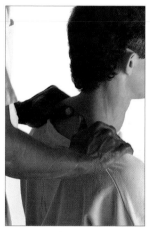

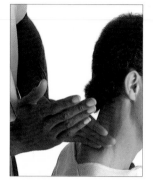

3 To stimulate circulation and relieve headaches, make chopping motions across the shoulders and between the shoulder blades. Keep your wrists loose and your hands relaxed.

4 To loosen the neck, clasp the fingers together behind the neck. Slide the heels of your hands together, scooping up the neck muscles.

1 To ease muscle tension and eyestrain, hold the head between your hands, fingertips across the forehead. Push gently, first to the left, then to the right, keeping the head in a straight line. You can also pull up gently to stretch the neck. Rub the scalp all over with small circular motions.

2 To relieve tension in the neck and shoulders, place your hands on the shoulders, then massage the muscles of the shoulders, neck, and upper back with your thumbs. Use small, circular motions; be firm.

FOOT MASSAGE

A foot massage not only keeps your feet flexible and healthy, but helps refresh and relax your whole body.

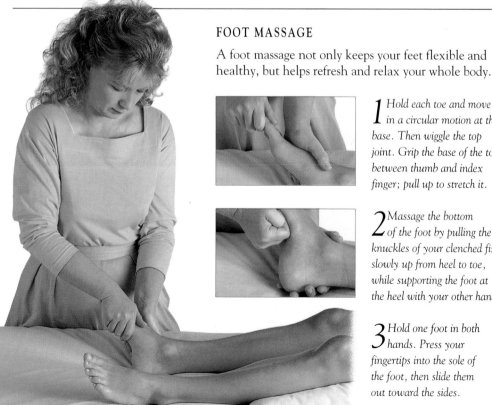

1 Hold each toe and move it in a circular motion at the base. Then wiggle the top joint. Grip the base of the toe between thumb and index finger; pull up to stretch it.

2 Massage the bottom of the foot by pulling the knuckles of your clenched fist slowly up from heel to toe, while supporting the foot at the heel with your other hand.

3 Hold one foot in both hands. Press your fingertips into the sole of the foot, then slide them out toward the sides.

USING A MASSAGE OIL

To help your hands glide smoothly over the skin, use a light vegetable oil or some talcum powder. If using oil, place a little oil (less than a teaspoonful) on one hand, then rub both hands together to warm the oil. If you prefer, the oils can be scented with essential oils.

187

COPING WITH STRESS AT HOME

In most homes there are tensions that may strain the emotional health of each member of the family.

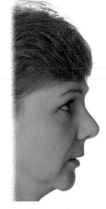

Dealing with teenage children
Having a child rebel against your authority or grow up and leave home can be very stressful.

THE STRESSES OF FAMILY life are far greater than many people realize. Stress can come just from the strain of juggling the demands of children and other family members or from a single event, such as coping with a death in the family.

Sources of domestic stress
Many parents do not appreciate how much stress they are under. For example, a child who demands attention at night can cause his or her parents to become exhausted, lose patience, and then feel guilty.

The individuals in any family have to adapt their behavior, attitudes, and emotions in response to changing roles and life events – both pleasing and distressing. A father may lose his job, a daughter may leave home, a grandparent may die, or a son may have a particularly turbulent adolescence.

If a family member has a serious problem, such as drug addiction, this can produce an intolerable amount of stress in the home. His or her relatives will be more likely to develop a stress-related illness.

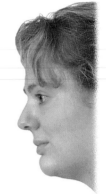

Growing up
Living with parents who treat you like a child or moving away from home, for example to start college, can be very stressful.

TROUBLED PARTNERSHIPS

Half of all marriages in the US end in divorce and most relationships have to overcome some difficulties.

A wide variety of different stressful situations and events can cause these problems.

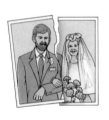

Sexual problems
An unsatisfying sex life can be both a cause and a sign of too much stress.

Illness
The diagnosis of a serious illness can cause high levels of stress for the whole family.

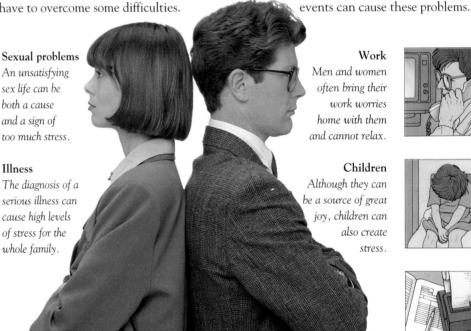

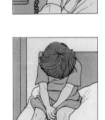

Work
Men and women often bring their work worries home with them and cannot relax.

Children
Although they can be a source of great joy, children can also create stress.

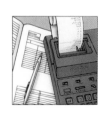

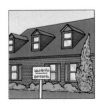

Moving
Buying or selling a house can put great stress on a marriage.

Money
Worries about mortgages and debts lead to many family rows.

MARRIAGE GUIDANCE

A relationship that is in difficulties may benefit from professional help. You can seek advice from a doctor. Most couples, however, talk to a professional marriage counselor.

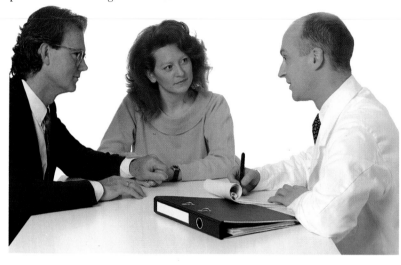

HOW TO REDUCE DOMESTIC STRESS

- Go away for a weekend outing.
- Make sure everyone in the family helps with the household chores.
- Contact your bank or financial adviser if you have money troubles. Work out a system of repayment.
- Discipline your children consistently and appropriately.
- Walk away and take time to calm down if you feel the urge to lash out.
- Seek professional counseling.

Talking the problems through
Therapy begins with an analysis of the good and bad aspects of the relationship. Talking openly, the partners discuss areas they would like to see improved.

STRESS MANAGEMENT PLANS

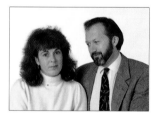

BOB AND GERALDINE FANSHAWE, a married couple in their 30s, have been unhappy in their relationship for the last six months. Both have been working long hours to pay their large mortgage. They recently went on vacation and had hoped that this would revive their marriage. Instead it was full of arguments and highly stressful. Friends persuaded them to go for counseling.

ANDREW DAVEY is a 17-year-old high school student studying for his S.A.T. examinations. Recently he has been having furious arguments with his parents over his appearance, the length of his hair, the fact that he has had his ears pierced, and his refusal to come home before midnight after he has been out with friends. The whole family has come for counseling because they cannot agree upon a set of house-rules that Andrew ought to live by.

Discussion

According to marriage counselors, vacations together often make a couple's difficulties worse rather than better. At home Bob and Geraldine can use their hectic daily routine to avoid each other and important decisions. On vacation they were forced into each other's company all the time and had to confront their conflicting attitudes and emotions.

Stress management plan

- *share the blame for their problems equally.*
- *start to discuss grievances with each other and not just bottle up their thoughts.*
- *find some form of relaxing leisure activity that they can both enjoy together on a regular basis.*
- *plan their next vacation more carefully, with more activities of mutual interest.*

Discussion

Most teenagers need to identify with their peer group as they struggle to find their own identity and come to terms with new emotions during the transition into adulthood. Extreme styles of behavior and dress help give a sense of belonging. They should only become a cause for parental concern if they are associated with drug abuse or other illegal activities.

Stress management plan

- *negotiate a reasonable curfew time. Allow him to come in late when there is no school the next day.*
- *ignore Andrew's appearance – his dress and behavior will probably tone down as he grows older.*
- *show an interest in him, his friends, and his activities.*
- *do not argue over minor and unimportant issues.*

COPING WITH STRESS AT WORK

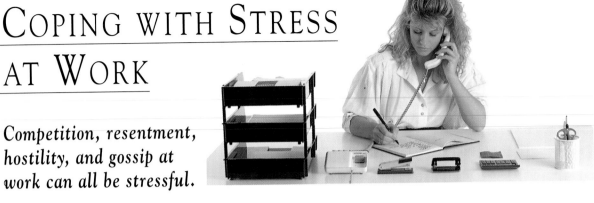

Competition, resentment, hostility, and gossip at work can all be stressful.

STRESS AT WORK is thought to be one of the main reasons for taking sick leave. The people who are most at risk are those who have a demanding job but no control over their workload, those who do not have enough work to do, and those who are frustrated because they have not been promoted. Unless these difficulties can be solved, finding a new job may be the only solution. Making life outside work more fulfilling may also help.

Stress factors at work

Many factors contribute to a build-up of stress at work and lead to physical or emotional ill-health. Too much work to do is a common cause of stress, often due to setting unrealistic deadlines. But work that is not stimulating may also be harmful. Workers who have no job satisfaction or who are facing redundancy may also feel stress.

Interpersonal problems such as conflict of loyalties, hostility from colleagues, sexual harassment, or confrontations with the public can also create stress. These conflicts are often aggravated by having no procedure to settle grievances. The working environment can be the source of other stresses too. A difficult journey to work raises blood pressure and may lead to stress, as will a forced relocation or crowded working conditions.

Are you a workaholic?
Working long hours, taking work home, cancelling vacations, and missing family occasions due to pressure at work are signs that you are working too hard and putting yourself under too much stress.

HOW TO DEAL WITH SEXUAL HARASSMENT

• Be more assertive.
• Make it clear that you find the behavior offensive.
• Keep a diary of the harassment.
• Ask your colleagues if they have had the same problem.
• If you cannot solve the problem yourself, make a formal complaint.

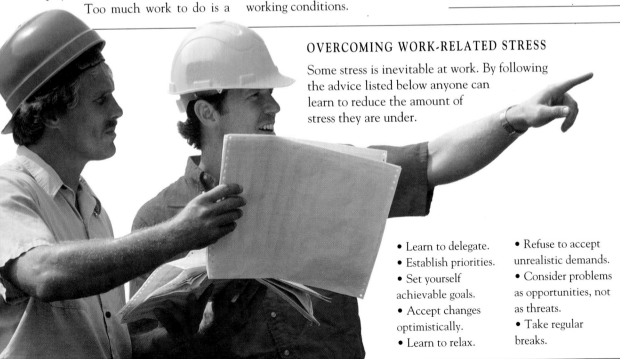

OVERCOMING WORK-RELATED STRESS

Some stress is inevitable at work. By following the advice listed below anyone can learn to reduce the amount of stress they are under.

• Learn to delegate.
• Establish priorities.
• Set yourself achievable goals.
• Accept changes optimistically.
• Learn to relax.

• Refuse to accept unrealistic demands.
• Consider problems as opportunities, not as threats.
• Take regular breaks.

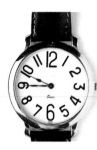

TIME MANAGEMENT

Learning to manage your time effectively at work is a good way of reducing the stress you are under. By following the tips listed below you will be able to control your stress levels.

• Every day, prepare a daily planner which lists the tasks you need to work on.
• Concentrate on the most difficult jobs first.
• Prioritize your tasks.
• Transfer all uncompleted tasks to the next day's action list.
• Divide large projects into manageable sections.
• Try to view unwelcome projects as a challenge.
• Reward yourself for work that is completed.
• Do not put things off.
• Make a note of anything that interfered with your work. Try to remove these interruptions.

KEY

✳	Urgent	Del.	Delegated	⇒	Carried over
Imp.	Important	✓	Completed		

Use the symbols in the key to indicate the priority of each task.

DAILY PLANNER		DATE	
Time	APPOINTMENTS AND SCHEDULED EVENTS		Place
1pm	Lunch with the marketing team to finalize contracts		The Bistro
5pm	Weekly planning meeting.		Board-room
9pm	Dinner party		Home

TO BE DONE TODAY (Prioritized daily action list)	
1. Check details of contracts.	✳ ✓
2. Telephone head office for new sales figures.	Imp. ⇒
3. Write report for new client.	✳ ✓
4. Arrange interviews for assistant.	Imp. Del.
5. Pick up glasses from optician.	⇒
6. Buy wine for dinner tonight.	Del.

INTERRUPTIONS
- Difficulty finding essential reference information; files need to be reorganized.
- Too many telephone calls.

STRESS MANAGEMENT PLANS

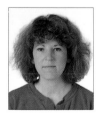

KAREN MILLER is a 32-year-old mother of two, who has recently been promoted. After three months in her new role she has begun to feel tired and lacking in energy. Her husband suggests that she have a checkup rather than hand in her notice, which she has been threatening to do.

Discussion

Although lethargy is a common symptom of stress, Karen's doctor examines her and orders some blood tests to exclude any underlying medical cause. The tests do not reveal any problems so her doctor suggests that she learns to manage her stress.

Stress management plan

• *organize daily workload better and learn to delegate.*
• *share the household chores with husband.*
• *take a proper lunch break each day.*
• *plan more family activities.*

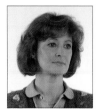

HILARY CHAMBERS, 42, is a doctor's receptionist. She frequently has to deal with patients who are annoyed or upset at delays in being seen by the doctor. At home, she is very short-tempered and has trouble sleeping. Hilary decides to ask her own doctor for some sleeping tablets.

Discussion

Hilary's insomnia and short temper are both clearly caused by work-related stress. Rather than just prescribing some sleeping tablets, her doctor encourages her to try to change some of the more troubling aspects of her job.

Stress management plan

• *if possible, improve the appointments system.*
• *remember to warn each patient in advance when delays are expected.*
• *improve the waiting room.*
• *try relaxation exercises.*

LIFE AFTER RETIREMENT

Retirement may account for one quarter of your adult life – planning ahead can make it less stressful.

ALTHOUGH RETIREMENT may be looked forward to as a well-earned rest, it can be a difficult time. Worries about money and the sudden change from the structured routine of the workplace to life at home can be highly stressful.

In the US more than two million people reach retirement age every year. Many plan ahead, outlining interesting projects to do and activities to try. Retirement is a good time to make changes in your lifestyle that will promote both health and wellbeing.

Maintaining a positive attitude

The common view of the elderly as frail and isolated is outdated. Social withdrawal and a gradual deterioration in health are not inevitable features of growing older. If you feel unwell, do not dismiss your symptoms as being just part of old age; see your doctor.

A positive attitude is important too. Believing that you can go on living life to the full – but perhaps at a gentler pace than before – should enable you to continue to enjoy your life.

Staying active and alert will help you retain the same quality of life after retirement that you had while you were working. It should

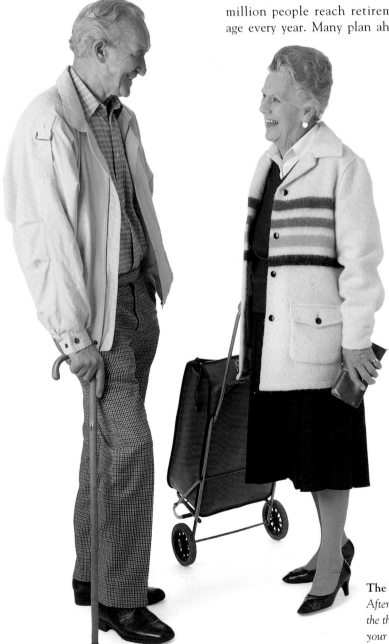

ACTIVE RETIREMENT

- Take up a new hobby.
- Learn a new language or skill.
- Sign up for community service or voluntary work.
- Join a political party or local or national pressure group.
- Start an evening class or Open University degree.
- Seek out new pleasures – travel, go to concerts, or visit museums.
- Keep up close ties with friends and family – emotional support is important for your wellbeing.
- Set your financial affairs in order.

The benefits of retirement
After retirement, you will have the opportunity to do all the things you may not have been able to find time for in your working years. Friendships and family ties often become more important.

also minimize any physical discomfort caused by aging and help you make the most of your retirement.

Looking towards the future

Responsibilities tend to decrease with age which may make you less willing to take on new projects or tasks. But since future goals and expectations are needed to keep your mind sharp, you should continue to seek out new challenges.

Write down all the things you would like to achieve or experience over the next five years, including social or artistic goals, new places you have always wanted to visit, and people you want to meet. Try to accomplish at least one of these ambitions each year.

In addition to this long-term plan, a shorter, more specific list of objectives should be drawn up to cover the next few months.

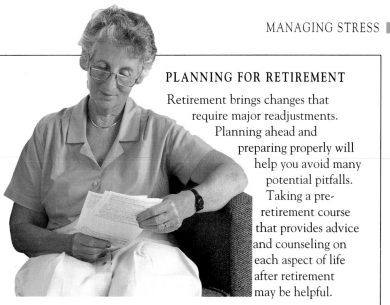

PLANNING FOR RETIREMENT

Retirement brings changes that require major readjustments. Planning ahead and preparing properly will help you avoid many potential pitfalls. Taking a pre-retirement course that provides advice and counseling on each aspect of life after retirement may be helpful.

Moving to a retirement home. Think carefully first: friends may be harder to make when you are older and less active in the community.

Alternative work. Part-time or voluntary work can ease the transition from full-time work. A part-time job can also provide extra income.

Income and assets. A financial adviser can help you budget for your retirement and manage your pension and any investments wisely.

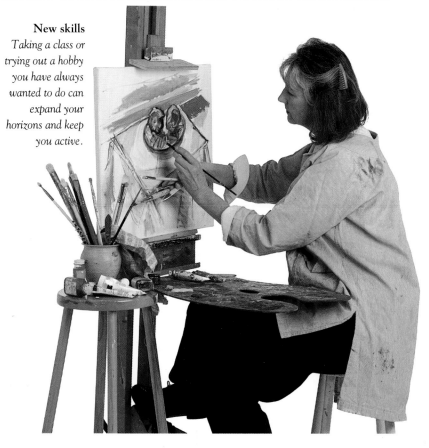

New skills
Taking a class or trying out a hobby you have always wanted to do can expand your horizons and keep you active.

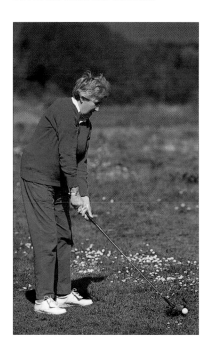

Exercise and independence
Getting regular physical exercise will help you remain supple, active, and physically fit. Golf, which allows you to set your own pace, is well-suited to older people.

SLEEP AND INSOMNIA

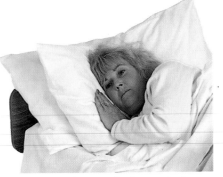

At some time in their lives, one in three people are likely to complain that they suffer from insomnia or sleeping problems.

MANY PEOPLE FIND that they have problems getting enough sleep. This, however, is often just a misconception about how much sleep is really needed. The amount of sleep that people require varies a lot. Some people manage on less than four hours' sleep a night, others need over 10 hours. The typical adult needs between seven and eight hours a night.

Children and the elderly usually have different sleep patterns. Infants normally sleep for at least

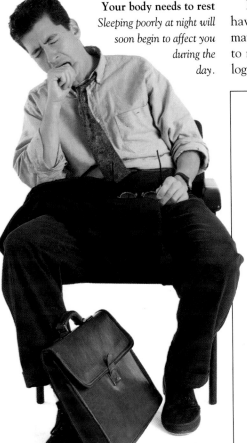

Your body needs to rest
Sleeping poorly at night will soon begin to affect you during the day.

14 hours a day – adult sleep patterns are not adopted until around the age of 12. Later in life, sleep tends to become broken up into shorter periods and most elderly people start to wake up earlier and earlier in the morning.

What is insomnia?

Insomnia is the inability to get to sleep. Sleeplessness can take different forms. The sufferer may find it hard to fall asleep initially, keep waking up during the night, or lie awake for long periods.

Disrupted sleep patterns may have many different causes. They may be due to worry and stress or to more serious medical or psychological problems like depression.

Are you kept awake by worries?
Lying awake and worrying is not going to solve anything. Take steps to cure the problem and your insomnia will disappear.

SLEEPING PILLS

Sleeping pills are among the most frequently prescribed drugs in the US. They are addictive and should, therefore, be taken in the smallest effective dose, for the shortest possible time. They can also cause daytime side effects such as poor concentration. You should not drive or operate machinery while taking them. Sleeping pills are only given when all possible self-help measures have failed.

CAUSES OF INSOMNIA

Many factors can lead to insomnia. Worrying, drinking too much caffeine, or withdrawing from tranquillizers or alcohol can all disturb your normal sleeping patterns. Other more serious factors, such as depression or physical disorders, may also affect your sleep. See your doctor if self-help measures do not cure your insomnia.

Caffeine
Since caffeine is a stimulant, it can keep you awake.

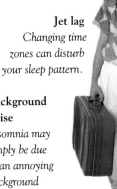

Jet lag
Changing time zones can disturb your sleep pattern.

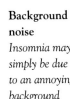

Background noise
Insomnia may simply be due to an annoying background noise, such as a partner snoring.

SLEEP PATTERNS

The brain does not rest completely during sleep. Electrical activity, which can be measured by an electroencephalogram (EEG), continues. Sleep is divided into two distinct phases known as REM (rapid eye movement) and non-REM. There will be four or five periods of REM (dream-sleep) in an average night's sleep. Non-REM sleep, however, makes up about 80 percent of the sleeping pattern.

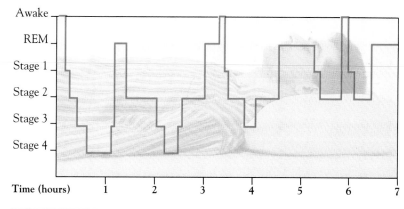

Awake
REM
Stage 1
Stage 2
Stage 3
Stage 4

Time (hours)   1   2   3   4   5   6   7

WHY DO WE SLEEP?

Sleep rests and restores our bodies. The brain and the body's metabolic processes require regular periods of rest to recover. Growth hormone is released while you sleep to renew tissues and produce new bone and red blood cells. Dreaming may also help the brain sort out information stored in the memory during waking hours.

Electrical activity during REM sleep

The stages of sleep
These EEGs show the brain's electrical activity during sleep. There are four progressive stages of non-REM activity. The deepest sleep, stage 4, is thought to be the most restorative. In REM sleep, the brain is more active and the eyes move rapidly. People woken in this phase of the sleep cycle often report dreams.

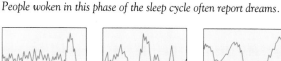

Stage 1   **Stage 2**   **Stage 3**   **Stage 4**

HOW TO GET YOUR CHILD TO SLEEP

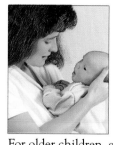

If a full stomach does not settle your baby down for sleep you could try gentle rocking or a lullaby. Setting a regular sleeping pattern is important too. Do not overstimulate your baby during night-time feedings; keep the lights low.
For older children, establish a bedtime routine, such as a story before bed.

Sleeping through the night
For you and your child to get a full night's sleep you need to make sure that his or her day is full of activity. Children will only sleep if they are actually tired.

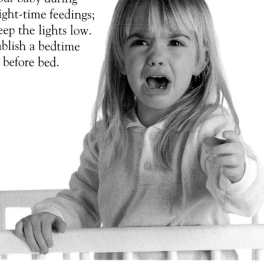

HOW TO BEAT INSOMNIA

Before asking your doctor for sleeping pills, there are many things you can do to help you beat your insomnia:

• Reduce your consumption of tea, coffee, and alcohol.
• Do not eat a big meal late at night.
• Have a hot, milky drink shortly before you go to bed.
• Get some exercise during the day.
• Do not allow your bedroom to become too hot or cold.
• Wear earplugs if there is a lot of background noise.
• Sleep on a comfortable mattress.
• Get up at the same time every day.
• Avoid having a mid-afternoon nap.
• Try to stop worrying about not sleeping – just resting in bed will do you some good.

COPING WITH ANXIETY

Anxiety is a perfectly normal reaction to a stressful situation – it only becomes an illness if it is not controlled.

ANXIETY BECOMES AN illness when feelings of unease, fear, or impending doom surface without any obvious threat; if they are out of all proportion to an event; or when psychological and physical symptoms begin to disrupt everyday activities completely.

A common problem

Anxiety disorders affect roughly four percent of the population. These distressing problems occur most frequently in young adults.

In addition to the general disorder, there are a number of specific types of anxiety. Panic attacks are outbursts of unreasonable fear and anxiety that occur for no apparent reason. Phobias are irrational fears of particular situations or objects. Post-traumatic stress may follow a serious incident – sufferers develop a feeling of detachment.

What causes anxiety?

Many theories exist to explain the underlying cause of anxiety. Some anxious individuals appear to have a raised level of arousal in their brain, which makes them react more excitedly and adapt more slowly to stressful events. Psychoanalytical ideas, developed by Freud, hold that anxiety originates from repressed, unresolved childhood experiences. Behavioral psychologists believe that anxiety is a deeply conditioned habit.

Search for a solution
With a little help, nearly all anxiety sufferers can overcome their fears and regain full control of their lives.

OBSESSIVE AND COMPULSIVE BEHAVIOR

Many people exhibit some degree of obsessional thought and compulsive behaviour, such as double-checking that a window is shut. This is only a problem if it starts to interfere seriously with daily living. Someone suffering from a hand-washing compulsion, for instance, may admit to worrying about infection but the true cause is often an unrelated psychological issue. This type of repetitive, ritualized behavior is performed to allay fears and relieve anxiety.

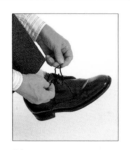

Obsessions
Anxiety can cause ritualistic behavior, such as always dressing in the same order.

Compulsions
Hand washing, counting, and checking that doors and windows are locked are some of the most common compulsions developed by anxious people.

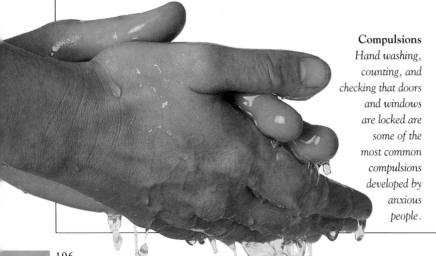

MONITORING YOUR HEALTH
If you develop several of the following symptoms you may be suffering from anxiety:

- Palpitations and chest tightness.
- Overbreathing.
- Feeling of suffocation.
- Tension headaches.
- Unexplained muscle aches.
- Restlessness or insomnia.
- Diarrhea.
- Irritability.
- Trembling.
- Sexual problems.
- Sweaty palms.

DRUGS TO REDUCE ANXIETY

There are two main types of drug that are prescribed to relieve the wide range of symptoms that accompany anxiety:

• **Benzodiazepines**. These drugs promote relaxation by reducing nerve activity in the brain. Although they are an effective short-term treatment, they do not resolve the underlying causes of an anxiety disorder. Also, if they are taken for longer than two weeks, there may be withdrawal symptoms.

• **Beta blockers**. These may be prescribed when anxiety causes physical symptoms such as palpitations, shaking, or chest tightness. These symptoms are the result of overactivity in the nervous system. By stopping this overactivity from affecting the heart, beta blockers can prevent palpitations occurring.

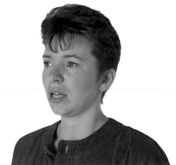

Short-term relief
A prescribed drug is often the best form of treatment to control anxiety symptoms during periods of intense emotional upset.

PHOBIAS

Many people have minor phobias, such as a fear of heights, snakes, or spiders. These phobias may cause occasional distress but they do not interfere with the ability to lead a normal life. However, there are some phobias that are so disabling that the sufferer is unable to leave the house. Most of these phobics can be successfully treated by behavior therapy and, sometimes, a course of antidepressants.

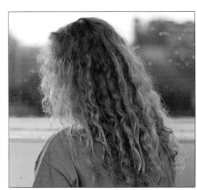

Agoraphobia
The fear of open spaces or entering a crowded place is the most common phobia for which treatment is sought.

HOW TO OVERCOME YOUR ANXIETY

• **Remove the source of the stress**. For example, if work is causing the problem, change to a less demanding job.
• **Get regular exercise**. Swimming or jogging may help relieve stress.
• **Relax**. Muscle-relaxation exercises or meditation can help to reduce anxiety.
• **Visit your doctor**. A short course of an anti-anxiety drug may relieve your symptoms.
• **Try behavior therapy**. With the emotional support of a trained therapist you can confront your phobias, control your obsessional behavior, or learn relaxation methods.

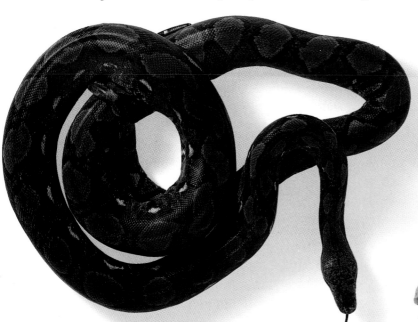

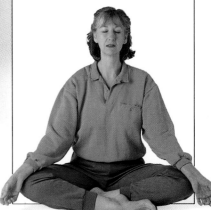

ENHANCING YOUR SELF-ESTEEM

A positive self-image and a healthy attitude to life will increase your resistance to stress-related illness.

SELF-DOUBT AND A SUDDEN lack of confidence in your ability to perform a particular task is normal. Every single person, no matter how confident they may appear to be, is bound to have the occasional doubt about whether they are up to the challenge that lies ahead of them. This is usually a defensive reaction to a high-pressure event.

It is when this loss of self-esteem continues, and starts to influence the way you perceive your own personality and capabilities, that stress builds up. Emotional, mental, or physical problems are then bound to occur.

Self-image and stress
Many mental health specialists believe that neurotic disorders – such as anxiety and depression – stem from a basic incompatibility between your self-image and the way other people see you. Therefore, if you cannot reduce your anxiety or depression, and decide to seek professional help, the primary aim of the therapist will be to bring out a positive change in your own self-perception. Once you regain your sense of worth, your level of stress should fall, and your symptoms disappear.

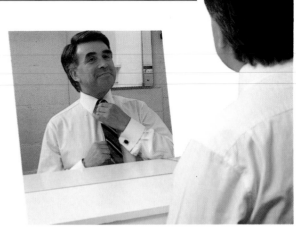

What do you see when you look in the mirror? *Do you look carefree and relaxed or do you look worried and tense? A positive self-image is a sign that your level of self-esteem is high.*

BOOST YOUR SELF-ESTEEM

If you think carefully, you are bound to be able to find some aspects about yourself and your life that are good. The following measures are designed to give your ego a boost and enhance your wellbeing. If you are still unhappy with your level of self-esteem, consider seeking professional help.

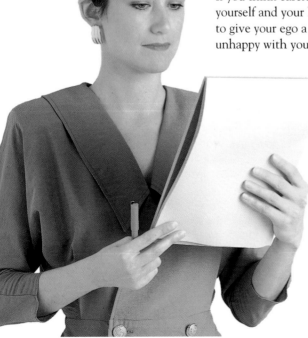

Assessing yourself
Writing down all your good points and all the things you have been successful at can improve your self-esteem by making you focus on the positive aspects of your life.

• Get to know yourself better; make a list of all your positive characteristics.
• Think positively about those things you have succeeded in doing.
• Choose one aspect of your life at a time and work on changing it.
• Set yourself achievable and measurable targets.
• Do not try to change too many aspects of your life too quickly.
• Find a suitable role model to emulate, not an unrealistic ideal.
• Stop brooding about past failures and errors of judgment.
• Do not use alcohol to boost your self-esteem.

ASSESSING YOUR SELF-ESTEEM

To evaluate your current level of self-esteem, try answering the following questions. These questions are very general and cannot provide all the answers, but they will help you to think about your self-image and your overall attitude to life. Because self-esteem represents only one area of your mental and emotional fitness, do not draw any firm conclusions about your state of mind from this questionnaire alone.

 How much success have you had in life?

- I am proud of my achievements.
- I have done fairly well at some things.
- I have failed at most things I have ever tried.

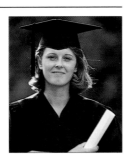

Your perception of your own ability to manage specific tasks tends to be influenced by your past performance. If you feel you have been a failure in the past, your self-confidence is likely to need a boost.

 How do you feel about the way you look?

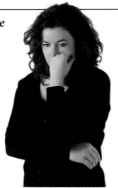
- I would not want to change my appearance.
- Photographs never do me justice.
- There are a lot of things about my body I would change if I could.

Wishing you looked different or could be transformed into someone else reveals that you have a low opinion of yourself. Work on improving your self-image.

 Is your personality attractive to other people?

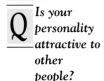

- I am generally well-liked.
- I wish I could be more popular.
- I feel that nobody likes me.

The way you feel about your personality is a reliable indicator of your current level of self-esteem, so try to lose any negative feelings you have about yourself.

 Do you have any regrets about your past?

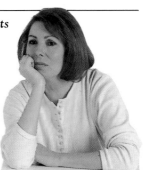
- If I had to live my life again I would do it in the same way.
- I have made a few bad decisions.
- I am ashamed of things I have done.

Most people have a few regrets. If you brood about previous mistakes, however, you will erode your self-esteem. Do not dwell on the past; it cannot be altered.

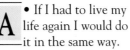 *Do you think you play a useful role at work or at home?*

- I am well satisfied with my contribution.
- I find it difficult to gain the approval of others.
- I never seem to do anything right.

Thinking that others do not approve of you, or that you cannot get anything right, reveals that you suffer from feelings of inferiority. You should take positive steps to enhance your self-esteem.

What is your attitude to criticism?

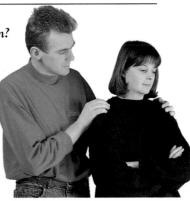
- I feel I benefit from constructive criticism.
- I get very upset if I am criticized.
- I do not voice my opinions as I worry that people will criticize them.

Being unable to seek out and accept criticism from other people is a sign of insecurity and a lack of self-confidence. Try to look at your good points in order to boost your self-esteem and improve your outlook.

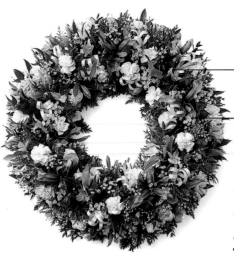

OVERCOMING
DEPRESSION

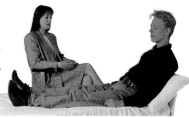

Depression is more than just being sad; it is an unshakeable feeling of despair.

Bereavement and depression
The loss of a loved one may trigger intense, long-term grief, producing severe symptoms of depression. Working through feelings of grief and loss with the support of friends and relatives can help.

DEPRESSION IS THE most common serious mental illness. Around five percent of the population suffer from a depressive episode at some time in their lives that is severe enough to require treatment. Although depression can occur at any age, it is most common between the ages of 35 and 55 in women, and 10 years later in men.

Talk to a professional
If you think you may be depressed, go and see you doctor. He or she may then refer you to an expert who can help you talk your problems through, explore your feelings, and conquer your depression.

Who are the sufferers?
Women appear to be more prone to depression than men. One in six women seeks help compared to only one in nine men. It is not known if this is due to differences between the sexes. Women may just be more willing to admit their feelings of sadness to a doctor, while men may turn to alcohol,

MONITORING YOUR HEALTH
If you develop several of the following symptoms you may be suffering from depression:

- Early morning wakening.
- Being tearful.
- Lack of energy.
- Bingeing or loss of appetite.
- Feeling isolated and disconnected from the world.
- Becoming withdrawn and apathetic.
- Having a lot of unexplained aches and pains.
- Feeling worthless.
- Poor concentration.
- Difficulty making decisions.
- Losing interest in sexual activity.

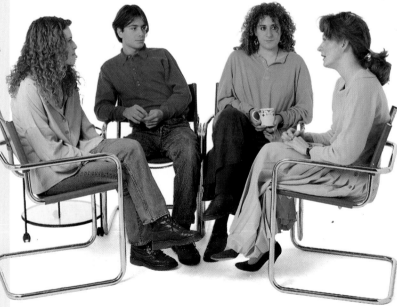

Group therapy
Talking with other people, who may be going through similar emotional problems, can help. The group usually meets once or twice a week for an hour. A therapist leads the discussion, helping group members to express and understand their feelings.

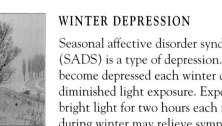

WINTER DEPRESSION
Seasonal affective disorder syndrome (SADS) is a type of depression. Sufferers become depressed each winter due to diminished light exposure. Exposure to bright light for two hours each morning during winter may relieve symptoms.

violence, or some other means of expressing their feelings of despair.

Types of depression

There are two basic categories of depression. Exogenous or reactive depression is caused by a major upset in your life, such as divorce or bereavement. This form of depression only becomes an illness when the period of grief is excessive or prolonged, making the person disinterested in life and unable to cope with daily activities.

Endogenous depression, where the symptoms of misery and feelings of helplessness are not linked to any external event, is more common. There is no ready explanation for the depression, so friends and relatives often find it harder to offer help and sympathy.

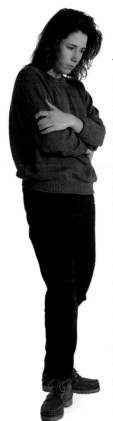

SUICIDE

Each year about 4,800 people in the US commit suicide – most of them are suffering from depression. For every successful suicide, there are at least another 10 failed attempts. Nobody can predict reliably who is likely to commit suicide, so all threats to do so should be taken seriously. There are, however, a number of risk factors and warning signs to be on the lookout for:

- Stating an intent to commit suicide.
- Sudden, inexplicable lifting of mood.
- Setbacks, like being laid off.
- Diagnosis of an incurable illness.
- Suicide by a friend or relative.
- Abuse of alcohol or drugs.
- A previous attempted suicide.
- Loss of a partner.
- Lack of social support.

POSTNATAL DEPRESSION

Over half of all mothers go through a period of mild depression after their baby is born. Known as "baby blues," this depression causes women to feel miserable and emotional and have tearful outbursts. Symptoms typically appear between four and five days after the birth and usually only last for a day or two. Hormonal changes may be the cause, but other factors can also be responsible, such as a sense of anticlimax after all the anticipation and apprehension; minor worries, such as early feeding difficulties; and physical exhaustion.

Severe depression
Starting a few days after coming home, one in 10 mothers may experience restlessness, fatigue, inability to cope, exaggerated fears about the baby's health, irritability, and even hostility to the baby. Treatment with antidepressants may help.

RECOVERING FROM DEPRESSION

Most people who suffer from depression will recover completely if they receive appropriate help.

- **Plenty of support**. Reassurance from friends and family is essential.
- **Antidepressants**. These drugs restore appetite, energy, and sleep patterns. They take over two weeks to start working, however, and can cause dizziness or drowsiness.
- **Psychotherapy**. This treatment is most helpful for people whose personality or life experiences are the main causes of their depression.
- **Cognitive-behavioral therapy**. This therapy teaches positive thinking to enhance self-esteem.
- **Electroconvulsive therapy** (ECT). Sufferers who do not respond to other treatments may have an electric shock passed through the brain for a few seconds. Dramatic improvements do occur and side effects are minimal.

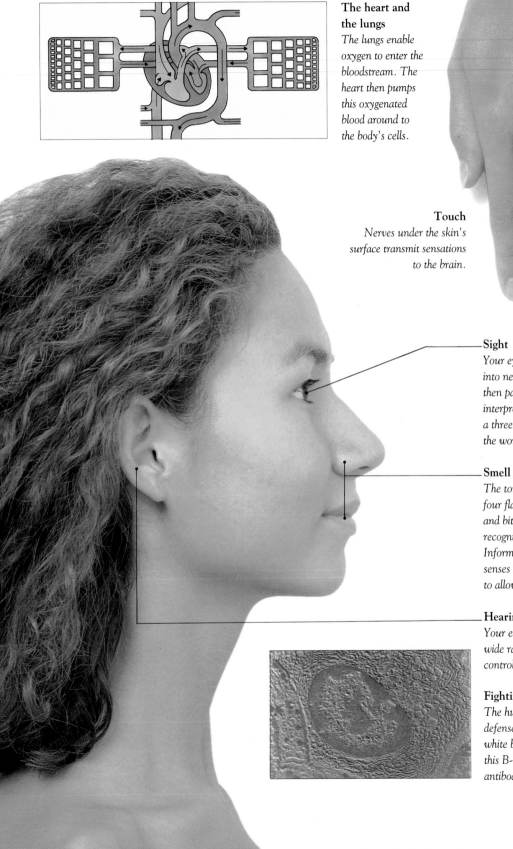

The heart and the lungs
The lungs enable oxygen to enter the bloodstream. The heart then pumps this oxygenated blood around to the body's cells.

Touch
Nerves under the skin's surface transmit sensations to the brain.

Sight
Your eyes transform rays of light into nerve impulses which are then passed on to the brain and interpreted to provide you with a three-dimensional image of the world around you.

Smell and taste
The tongue can only taste four flavors (sweet, sour, salty, and bitter) while the nose can recognize thousands of odors. Information from these two senses is combined in the brain to allow you a full range of tastes.

Hearing
Your ears enable you to hear a wide range of sounds and also control your sense of balance.

Fighting infection
The human body has many defenses. For instance, white blood cells, such as this B-lymphocyte, make antibodies to fight infections.

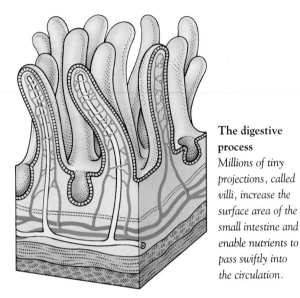

CHAPTER SEVEN

The digestive process
Millions of tiny projections, called villi, increase the surface area of the small intestine and enable nutrients to pass swiftly into the circulation.

THE HEALTHY BODY

KNOWING HOW YOUR body works will help you safeguard and protect it. For example, learning how the heart pumps blood around the body through the circulatory system will help you understand why keeping your arteries clear by eating a low-fat diet is best for you and your family. Knowing your body will also help you communicate better with your doctor.

The body's systems work together in harmony. The heart pumps out blood to the lungs to collect oxygen and to the intestines to become enriched with nutrients, which are then distributed to the rest of the body via the circulatory system. The cells use these nutrients to produce energy. This energy then fuels the muscles which move bones and joints in response to orders from the nervous system. The endocrine system triggers long-term activities like growth and the immune system keeps the body healthy.

The body is always changing. It grows from a single cell at conception to a million-celled organism in adulthood. Puberty transforms children into adults. Adulthood is a plateau during which the body changes very little externally. Yet all the while, the tissues are being repaired and regenerated. In women, pregnancy brings about great and obvious changes that result in new life. Aging produces the final great physical changes of human life.

Making the right choices for health will help you and everyone in your family feel better and be healthier at every one of life's stages.

The foot
Each foot has 26 bones – the feet contain one quarter of the bones in the entire body. A complex network of muscles and tendons act on the bones, positioning each foot during standing, walking, and running.

HEART AND CIRCULATION

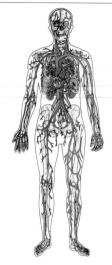

The cardiovascular system *is made up of the heart and the blood vessels.*

THE CIRCULATORY SYSTEM ensures that every living cell in your body is supplied with life-giving blood, rich in oxygen from the lungs and nutrients from the digestive system. The beating of the heart keeps the blood moving and heart valves ensure that it travels in the right direction. Blood flows around the body in a continuous double circuit, going from the heart to the lungs to take on oxygen, then back to the heart where it is pumped to the rest of the body.

Veins, arteries, and other blood vessels form a network of tubes that is thousands of miles long. But the power of the heart means that the blood takes only about one minute to travel round the system.

Located just to the left of the center of your chest, the heart can change its rate to suit your body's need for oxygen, beating slowly at rest and rapidly during exertion. If the heart stops beating for as little as four minutes, brain damage or death will occur.

The heart chambers *consist of two thin-walled upper chambers, the atria, and two thick-walled lower ones, the ventricles. They are divided by the septum, a wall of muscle. Blood from the right and left sides does not mix.*

Trachea (windpipe)_____

Aorta_____

Superior vena cava_____

Right lung_____

Right atrium_____

HOW THE BLOOD CIRCULATES

The heart pumps the blood round the circulatory system. Deoxygenated blood (blue) enters the right side of the heart and is pumped to the lungs to take up oxygen. Now full of oxygen (red), it returns to the left side of the heart and is pumped round the body, bringing oxygen to the cells. It then returns to the right side of the heart, where the process begins again.

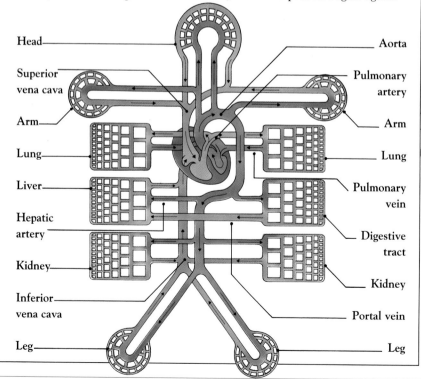

Head — Aorta

Superior vena cava — Pulmonary artery

Arm — Arm

Lung — Lung

Liver — Pulmonary vein

Hepatic artery — Digestive tract

Kidney — Kidney

Inferior vena cava — Portal vein

Leg — Leg

KEEPING YOUR HEART HEALTHY

- Lose any excess weight.
- If you smoke, stop.
- Eat less saturated fat and more fiber.
- Exercise three times a week for 20 minutes.
- Have your blood pressure checked regularly.
- Drink less alcohol.

Pulmonary valve_____

Tricuspid valve_____

Right ventricle_____

Heart muscle *consists of a branching network of muscle fibers. The heart needs a plentiful supply of oxygen and nutrients to continue beating spontaneously, rhythmically, and completely automatically.*

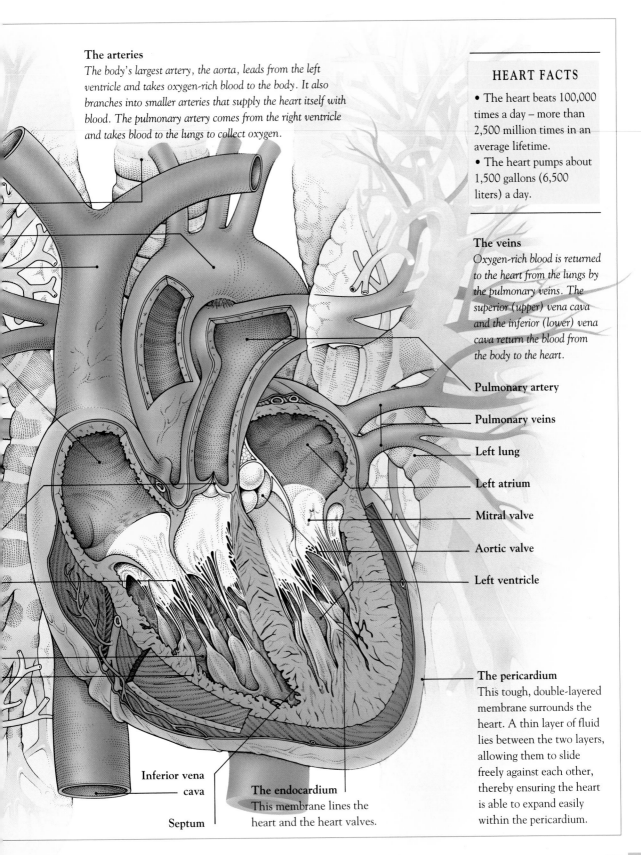

The arteries
*The body's largest artery, the aorta, leads from the left
ventricle and takes oxygen-rich blood to the body. It also
branches into smaller arteries that supply the heart itself with
blood. The pulmonary artery comes from the right ventricle
and takes blood to the lungs to collect oxygen.*

HEART FACTS
• The heart beats 100,000
times a day – more than
2,500 million times in an
average lifetime.
• The heart pumps about
1,500 gallons (6,500
liters) a day.

The veins
*Oxygen-rich blood is returned
to the heart from the lungs by
the pulmonary veins. The
superior (upper) vena cava
and the inferior (lower) vena
cava return the blood from
the body to the heart.*

Pulmonary artery

Pulmonary veins

Left lung

Left atrium

Mitral valve

Aortic valve

Left ventricle

The pericardium
This tough, double-layered
membrane surrounds the
heart. A thin layer of fluid
lies between the two layers,
allowing them to slide
freely against each other,
thereby ensuring the heart
is able to expand easily
within the pericardium.

**Inferior vena
cava**

Septum

The endocardium
This membrane lines the
heart and the heart valves.

RESPIRATORY SYSTEM

THE RESPIRATORY SYSTEM allows you to take oxygen into your body and exhale carbon dioxide. Oxygen, from the air you inhale, is absorbed into the blood and circulated to the body cells so that they can produce energy. Carbon dioxide is a waste product of this energy production.

The lungs are the center of the respiratory system. Air enters the lungs through the upper respiratory tract which consists of the nose, throat, and trachea (windpipe). Inside the chest, the trachea divides into two bronchi, one going to each lung. These bronchi branch still further into bronchioles which terminate as balloon-like cavities called alveoli. Here, oxygen is exchanged for carbon dioxide through the walls of tiny blood vessels that run over the alveoli.

Muscles between the ribs, and the diaphragm, suck air into the chest when they contract. When they relax, the diaphragm moves up and the lungs spring back to push air out through the nostrils and mouth.

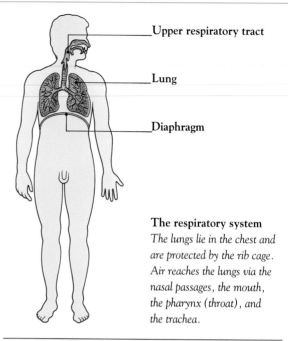

The respiratory system
The lungs lie in the chest and are protected by the rib cage. Air reaches the lungs via the nasal passages, the mouth, the pharynx (throat), and the trachea.

Labels: Upper respiratory tract / Lung / Diaphragm

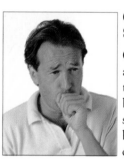

COUGHING AND SNEEZING

Coughing is a reflex action which unblocks the airways. Foreign bodies, mucus, and sputum (phlegm) are brought up. If you are coughing up sputum, do not take a cough suppressant as it will stop your airways from being cleared.

Sneezing is an involuntary attempt by your body to clear your nose and upper respiratory tract. The common cold often starts with sneezing when the lining of your nose becomes inflamed.

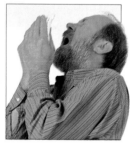

COUGHING UP BLOOD

Bright or rusty streaks or clots of blood in coughed-up sputum can be a sign of a serious disorder. Consult your doctor immediately.

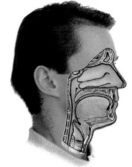

BREATHING

You normally breathe through your nose. The nasal passages allow air to enter your lungs and also warm it up. Tiny hairs inside the nose filter out foreign bodies, such as dust particles.

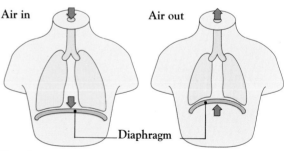

Air in / **Air out**

Diaphragm

Breathing in
You breathe in because your diaphragm contracts. Also, the muscles between your ribs contract, pulling your rib cage upward and outward and making your chest larger. Your lungs expand to fill the space, sucking air into them.

Breathing out
You breathe out because the muscles of your chest and diaphragm relax. When the diaphragm is relaxed it pushes up against the lungs, squeezing the air out. Healthy lungs are very elastic and expand and contract easily.

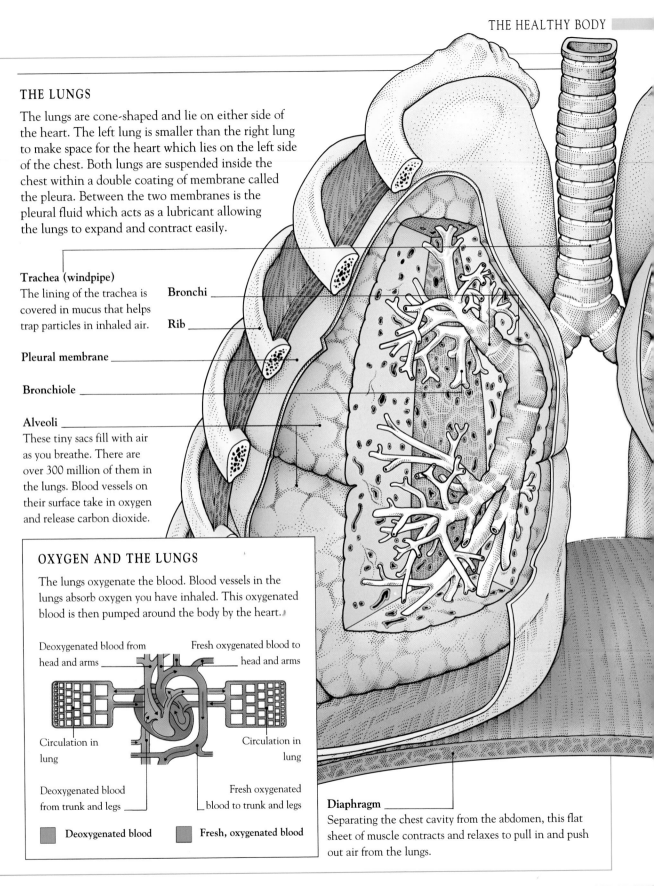

THE LUNGS

The lungs are cone-shaped and lie on either side of
the heart. The left lung is smaller than the right lung
to make space for the heart which lies on the left side
of the chest. Both lungs are suspended inside the
chest within a double coating of membrane called
the pleura. Between the two membranes is the
pleural fluid which acts as a lubricant allowing
the lungs to expand and contract easily.

Trachea (windpipe)
The lining of the trachea is
covered in mucus that helps
trap particles in inhaled air.

Bronchi

Rib

Pleural membrane

Bronchiole

Alveoli
These tiny sacs fill with air
as you breathe. There are
over 300 million of them in
the lungs. Blood vessels on
their surface take in oxygen
and release carbon dioxide.

OXYGEN AND THE LUNGS

The lungs oxygenate the blood. Blood vessels in the
lungs absorb oxygen you have inhaled. This oxygenated
blood is then pumped around the body by the heart.

Deoxygenated blood from
head and arms

Fresh oxygenated blood to
head and arms

Circulation in
lung

Circulation in
lung

Deoxygenated blood
from trunk and legs

Fresh oxygenated
blood to trunk and legs

■ **Deoxygenated blood**   ■ **Fresh, oxygenated blood**

Diaphragm
Separating the chest cavity from the abdomen, this flat
sheet of muscle contracts and relaxes to pull in and push
out air from the lungs.

THE DIGESTIVE SYSTEM

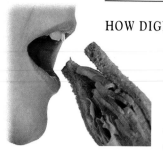

HOW DIGESTION WORKS

1 In the mouth, food mixes with the saliva, whose enzymes break down starch. The food is then ground into smaller pieces by the teeth before moving down the esophagus to the stomach.

2 Physical breakdown continues in the stomach. In addition, the food is mixed with acidic gastric juices that are secreted by glands in the stomach lining. This begins the breakdown of proteins and reduces the food to a thick liquid which is then gradually passed into the duodenum.

3 As soon as the food enters the duodenum it is bathed in bile and enzymes. Bile is produced in the liver and stored in the gallbladder. It aids the digestion of fats. Enzymes secreted by the pancreas are essential for the breakdown of proteins, fats, and carbohydrates. The duodenum leads directly into the rest of the small intestine.

4 The final stage of digestion takes place in the small intestine. Additional enzymes combine with the bile and pancreatic juices to reduce the food to molecules. These are small enough to pass through the wall of the small intestine. Here, nutrients are carried by the bloodstream to the liver for storage and distribution. Undigested food residues pass into the large intestine.

5 Water and undigested remains, arriving from the small intestine, are carried along the large intestine. Here, most of the water and salt is absorbed back into the body through the thin wall of the colon. Waste material passes directly into the rectum, ready to be discharged through the anus. Fiber cannot be digested and forms the bulk of the feces.

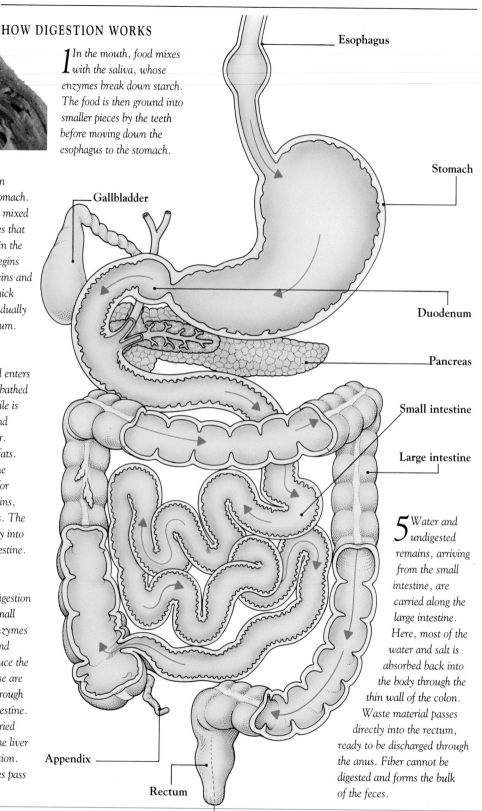

Esophagus

Stomach

Gallbladder

Duodenum

Pancreas

Small intestine

Large intestine

Appendix

Rectum

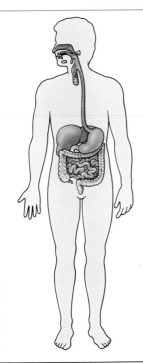

INDIGESTION

Indigestion, brought on by eating, can cause nausea, pain in the upper abdomen, and heartburn. The following measures will help to prevent indigestion, but visit a doctor if symptoms persist for over four hours.

- Do not rush your food.
- Avoid rich, spicy meals.
- If you smoke, stop.
- Reduce alcohol intake.
- Eat smaller meals.
- Avoid strenuous exercise after a meal.

FOOD PROVIDES THE energy for life. But before your body can use this energy to create new cells and to power chemical reactions within the body, your food must be digested, or broken down. The proteins, carbohydrates, and fats in the food are broken down chemically into smaller, simpler forms so that they can pass directly, via the bloodstream and lymphatic system, into the liver to be processed, and then to the body cells. Vitamins and minerals do not need digesting; they can be absorbed as they are.

The digestive tract is basically a 30-foot-long (9 m) muscular organ that is open to the outside at both ends. Food goes in at one end and, after being physically ground into smaller pieces, is put through a series of complex chemical processes in the stomach and intestines. Once the food reaches the end of the small intestine it has been reduced to molecular level and its nutrients will have been absorbed into the bloodstream. Undigested matter is then simply pushed out at the other end of the digestive tract.

HOW IS FOOD ABSORBED SO QUICKLY?

Most nutrients are absorbed through the wall of the small intestine in a few hours. They pass swiftly through millions of tiny projections, called villi, that massively increase the surface area of the intestine.

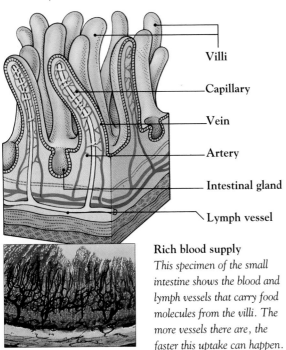

- Villi
- Capillary
- Vein
- Artery
- Intestinal gland
- Lymph vessel

Rich blood supply
This specimen of the small intestine shows the blood and lymph vessels that carry food molecules from the villi. The more vessels there are, the faster this uptake can happen.

HOW LONG DOES DIGESTION TAKE?

The approximate period of time that food spends in each part of the digestive system is shown below. The length of time that any particular food spends in the stomach varies: liquids pass through more quickly than solids.

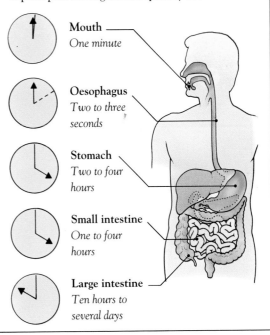

Mouth
One minute

Oesophagus
Two to three seconds

Stomach
Two to four hours

Small intestine
One to four hours

Large intestine
Ten hours to several days

THE SKIN, HAIR, AND NAILS

YOUR SKIN, HAIR, and nails mirror your state of health. Since most people notice slight changes in the condition of these areas very rapidly, they often provide the first warning signs of ill-health.

Although the hair and nails have little practical function, the skin is vital. It is a supple, elastic tissue that covers and protects the body. It is waterproof, bacteria-proof, self-repairing, and the largest organ in the body. It has two layers: the epidermis or outer layer and the dermis or inner layer.

The skin manufactures vitamin D, tans to protect the body against ultraviolet rays, regulates body temperature, and is embedded with nerves that provide the sensations of touch, pressure, and pain.

SKIN CARE

- Clean your skin with water and mild soap.
- Remove all make-up every night.
- Do not squeeze pimples – this will spread infection.
- Visit your doctor if your skin changes appearance.
- When sunbathing use high-factor sunscreens.
- Remove dead skin on your feet with a pumice.
- Always dry between your toes thoroughly.

Epidermis
The surface of the skin is formed of a layer of flat, dead cells which contain a protein called keratin; these cells make the skin waterproof. This layer acts as a protective coating and is thickest in areas of the body that are subject to the most wear and tear, such as the palms of the hands and the soles of the feet. The remainder of the epidermis consists of an intermediate layer and a basal cell layer.

Basal cell layer
Cells at the base of the epidermis grow, divide, and mature. They move upwards to replace those worn away at the surface. Replacement takes about two months. This layer also contains melanocytes that make melanin to color your skin and hair.

Dermis
The thicker dermis lies beneath the epidermis and contains most of the skin's living structures. Embedded in connective tissue within the dermis are specialized structures such as hair follicles, nerve endings, and sebaceous (oil) and sweat glands which open to pores on the surface of the skin. This region also contains the blood vessels. Below the dermis is a layer of fat known as subcutaneous fat.

Blood vessels
Small blood vessels in your skin dilate in hot weather to help you lose heat. This increase in blood flow may make you appear flushed.

Collagen fibers
Skin's strength and elasticity depends on these fibers. As you age, collagen is broken down, leading to wrinkles and sagging.

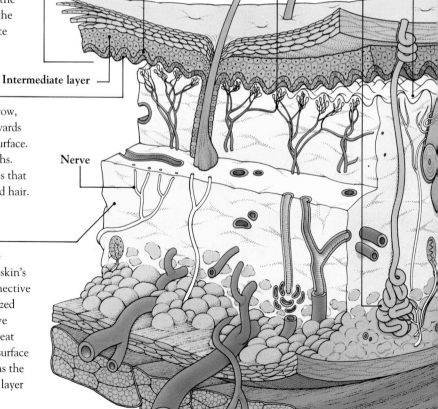

Melanocyte

Sweat gland

Intermediate layer

Nerve

HAIR CARE

Hair consists of dead cells. It grows for three years and then falls out to be replaced by a new hair. In any one day you will lose between 150 and 300 hairs. You can control your hair's condition, but not the amount you lose.

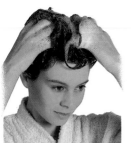

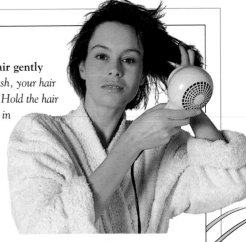

Removing the oil and dirt
Shampoo and condition your hair regularly to keep it healthy.

Treat your hair gently
Comb, not brush, your hair when it is wet. Hold the hair dryer at least 6 in (15 cm) away from your hair to avoid heat damage, such as split ends. Leave hair slightly damp.

Sebaceous (oil) gland
These glands produce an oil that keeps the skin supple and free of infection. This oil also makes hair greasy.

Hair

Hair follicle (root)

Pore

NAILS

Fingernails increase dexterity. Both fingernails and toenails grow from a fold of skin at their base. The nails are formed by a protein called keratin, which is made up of dead cells and gives nails their hardness. A fingernail takes about six months to grow from base to tip; toenails take twice as long. There are many simple, practical things you can do to keep your nails healthy:

• Wear rubber gloves if you have to immerse your hands in water for long.
• Keep nails short to stop them splitting.
• Trim your nails after a bath as they are then at their softest.
• File with an emery board from the side towards the center.
• Cut toenails in a straight line to prevent ingrowing toenails.

Subcutaneous fat

BONES, MUSCLES, AND JOINTS

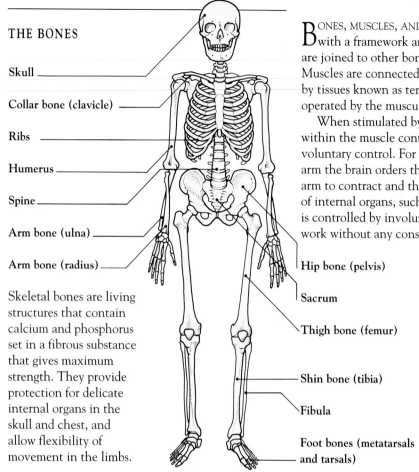

THE BONES

Skull

Collar bone (clavicle)

Ribs

Humerus

Spine

Arm bone (ulna)

Arm bone (radius)

Skeletal bones are living structures that contain calcium and phosphorus set in a fibrous substance that gives maximum strength. They provide protection for delicate internal organs in the skull and chest, and allow flexibility of movement in the limbs.

Hip bone (pelvis)

Sacrum

Thigh bone (femur)

Shin bone (tibia)

Fibula

Foot bones (metatarsals and tarsals)

BONES, MUSCLES, AND JOINTS provide the body with a framework and a means of support. Bones are joined to other bones by cords called ligaments. Muscles are connected to bones either directly, or by tissues known as tendons. Bones and joints are operated by the muscular system to produce motion.

When stimulated by motor nerves, fibers within the muscle contract and relax rapidly to give voluntary control. For example, to straighten your arm the brain orders the triceps muscle in your upper arm to contract and the biceps to relax. Movement of internal organs, such as the beating of the heart, is controlled by involuntary muscles, which normally work without any conscious control.

BONE COUNT

An adult's skeleton has 206 separate bones – 32 in each arm, 31 in each leg, 29 in the skull, 26 in the spine, and 25 in the chest. A few people have another pair of ribs, making 13 pairs. Many people have an extra bone in their hands or feet.

JOINTS

Joints are junctions between bones. There are several types and they are capable of different ranges of movement. Fixed joints, like those in the skull, hold bones together and do not move once they fuse in childhood. Joints in the spine are only partially movable, but over the whole spinal column this adds up to considerable flexibility. Freely movable joints, also termed synovial joints, contain lubricating fluid between the bones and allow the most movement.

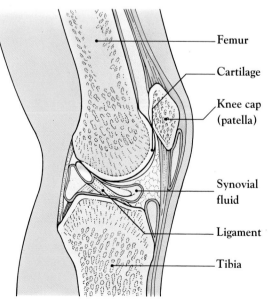

Femur

Cartilage

Knee cap (patella)

Synovial fluid

Ligament

Tibia

Joint movement
All the movable joints have a similar structure, as shown by this diagram of a knee joint, but each allows a different type of movement. Pivot joints, such as the neck, move in a rotational plane; hinge joints, like the knee, move in only one direction; ball and socket joints, like the hip, allow the most motion.

MUSCLES

Skeletal muscles contract and relax to create movement and are classified according to the action they perform. Extensors open a joint, flexors close it. Adductors draw part of the body inwards, abductors move it outwards; levators raise it and depressors lower it.

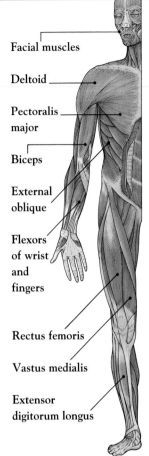
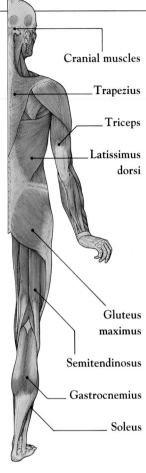

Facial muscles

Deltoid

Pectoralis major

Biceps

External oblique

Flexors of wrist and fingers

Rectus femoris

Vastus medialis

Extensor digitorum longus

Cranial muscles

Trapezius

Triceps

Latissimus dorsi

Gluteus maximus

Semitendinosus

Gastrocnemius

Soleus

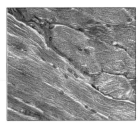

Muscle fibers
Viewed under a microscope, skeletal muscles are striped in appearance, made up of many thousands of long, thin muscle fibers.

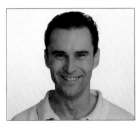

Smiling and laughing
The zygomaticus major muscle enables you to smile and laugh. Other muscles around the head control a vast range of facial expressions.

MUSCLE BOUND

There are over 600 named muscles in the human body. Skeletal muscles account for 40 to 45 per cent of body weight. Each is made up of bundles of fibres – some, like ciliary fibres in the eye, are tiny, while the buttock muscles are over 1 ft (30 cm) long.

CLEVER HANDS

Hands enable you to grip and manipulate objects: they are the most versatile part of your body. Forearm muscles operate most of the hands' movements, but short muscles in the palms control the more delicate actions.

OPPOSING THUMBS

Humans and other primates are the only creatures to have fingers and thumbs that move independently. This enables the hand to grip.

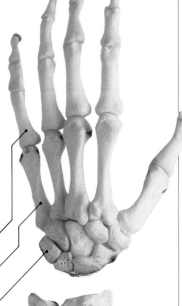

Bone

Tendon

Muscle

Finger bones (phalanges)

Palm bones (metacarpals)

Wrist bones (carpals)

THE KIDNEYS AND URINARY SYSTEM

THE URINARY TRACT is the system that removes waste chemicals and excess water from your body. It consists of the kidneys, which turn chemicals and water removed from the blood into urine, the ureters which drain the urine from the kidneys, the bladder which stores the urine until it can be passed out of the body, and the urethra, the tube through which the urine is expelled. Chemical waste is produced in the body from the breakdown of worn-out tissues, nutrients, and medications. The kidneys filter out these waste chemicals from the blood.

 The urinary system is subject to various problems. For example, in women the urethra is only 1 in (2.5 cm) long, so their urinary tracts are prone to infections introduced from outside the body. Kidney infections can scar the tissue, reducing the efficiency of the filtering process. Kidney or bladder stones can form, causing great pain as they are passed.

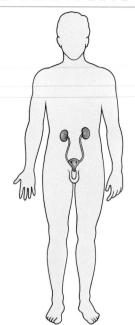

The urinary tract
The organs of the urinary tract are located in the torso. The kidneys lie just above the waist on either side of the spine; the bladder is located behind the pubic bone.

WARNING

See your doctor if you have any of the following symptoms: blood in the urine, pain or difficulty passing urine, discharge of pus, or an offensive smell to your urine.

HOW THE URINARY TRACT WORKS

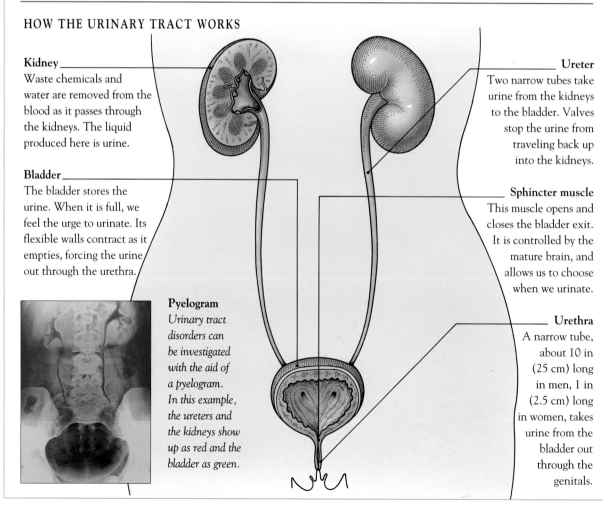

Kidney
Waste chemicals and water are removed from the blood as it passes through the kidneys. The liquid produced here is urine.

Bladder
The bladder stores the urine. When it is full, we feel the urge to urinate. Its flexible walls contract as it empties, forcing the urine out through the urethra.

Pyelogram
Urinary tract disorders can be investigated with the aid of a pyelogram. In this example, the ureters and the kidneys show up as red and the bladder as green.

Ureter
Two narrow tubes take urine from the kidneys to the bladder. Valves stop the urine from traveling back up into the kidneys.

Sphincter muscle
This muscle opens and closes the bladder exit. It is controlled by the mature brain, and allows us to choose when we urinate.

Urethra
A narrow tube, about 10 in (25 cm) long in men, 1 in (2.5 cm) long in women, takes urine from the bladder out through the genitals.

CYSTITIS

Cystitis is an inflammation of the inside of the bladder, usually due to a bacterial infection. Bacteria that are harmless inside the bowel may cause cystitis if they find their way into the urinary tract. The infection may spread on upwards into the kidneys through the ureters.

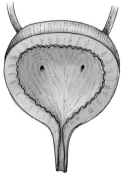

Bladder infection
The bladder lining becomes irritated and inflamed.

Urethral infection
The bacteria multiply in the urethra and travel up into the bladder.

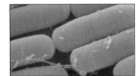

***Escherichia coli* bacteria**
This electron microscope photograph shows E coli bacteria, which are a common cause of cystitis.

PREVENTING CYSTITIS IN WOMEN

- Drink at least three pints of fluid each day.
- Wear cotton underwear.
- After a bowel action, wipe from front to back.
- Do not use perfumed soaps, deodorants, or powders in the genital area.
- Urinate before and after sexual intercourse.

KIDNEY FUNCTION AND AGE

The kidneys become less efficient as you age. In young people there are about one million nephrons, or tiny filters, within the kidney. With increasing age the number of working nephrons decreases gradually.

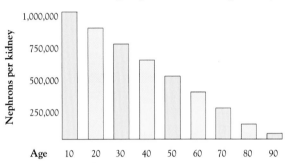

URINARY INCONTINENCE

Passing urine when you did not intend to is called incontinence. It is more common among older people than among the young, and affects more women than men. It has many causes, including urinary infections, obstruction of the outflow of the bladder, and dementia. Weakness in certain muscles, either of the sphincter muscle that controls the flow of urine out of the bladder or of the pelvic floor muscles after childbirth, may also cause incontinence. Although it can be very embarrassing to talk about, it is vital to discuss this problem with your doctor, who can often find the cause and cure it. Even when incontinence cannot be cured, there are many aids that can make it easier to live with.

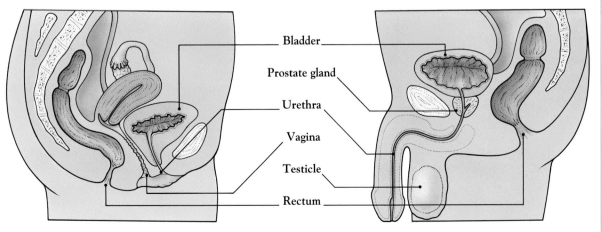

Bladder
Prostate gland
Urethra
Vagina
Testicle
Rectum

THE ENDOCRINE SYSTEM

THE ENDOCRINE SYSTEM controls body processes such as metabolism, growth, response to stress, and sexual development and function. The glands of the endocrine system secrete dozens of chemical messengers known as hormones. The pituitary gland, located at the base of the brain, is often called the master gland because it triggers the production of hormones by many of the other glands.

Hormones activate and control many different aspects of mental and physical function. They are manufactured in numerous hormone-secreting glands, as well as in other body organs and tissues including the kidneys, lungs, skin, and intestines. Within these glands, hormone-producing cells are clustered around blood vessels which can then transport the hormone, through the bloodstream, around the body. Although hormones circulate throughout the entire body, they are only triggered into action when they come into contact with the specific tissues and organs which are "programmed" to respond to them.

The more of a particular hormone there is circulating in the blood, the stronger its effect will be. If necessary, synthetic hormones can replace naturally occurring hormones within the body to keep it functioning normally. Hormone imbalance can result from an infection or from excessive stress, both of which are able to influence a gland's production of hormones.

SYMPTOMS OF A HORMONE DISORDER

The symptoms associated with hormone disorders are extremely varied, reflecting the many different bodily functions under the control of hormones. Because hormones can be measured in the blood, a simple blood test will usually reveal if you are suffering from an endocrine disorder. Common symptoms include: fatigue, thirst, excess urine production, slow or premature sexual maturation, excess body hair, weight gain or loss, changes in body fat distribution, anxiety, and skin changes. Consult your doctor if you have any of these symptoms.

THE HORMONE-PRODUCING GLANDS

Thyroid gland —————
Hormones that stimulate metabolism and maintain body temperature are produced in this gland.

Pancreas —————
This gland produces digestive enzymes and also controls the body's use of sugar by producing insulin and glucagon. Deficient insulin production causes diabetes and can be controlled by injections of synthetic insulin.

Adrenal gland
By producing hormones such as hydrocortisone, this gland helps control blood pressure, metabolism, and the body's salt balance.

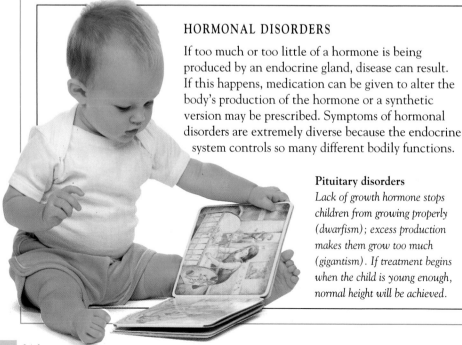

HORMONAL DISORDERS

If too much or too little of a hormone is being produced by an endocrine gland, disease can result. If this happens, medication can be given to alter the body's production of the hormone or a synthetic version may be prescribed. Symptoms of hormonal disorders are extremely diverse because the endocrine system controls so many different bodily functions.

Pituitary disorders
Lack of growth hormone stops children from growing properly (dwarfism); excess production makes them grow too much (gigantism). If treatment begins when the child is young enough, normal height will be achieved.

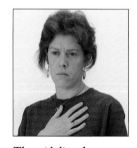

Thyroid disorders
Underproduction of hormones by the thyroid causes hypothyroidism, leading to symptoms like lethargy, weight gain, and dry skin. Most overweight people, however, do not have a thyroid problem.

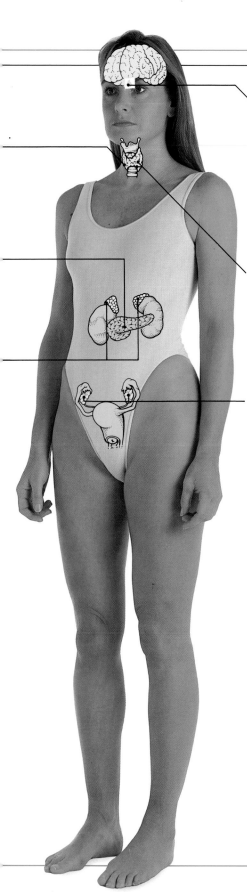

Pituitary gland
The pituitary gland regulates other glands and secretes hormones that control growth and the concentration of urine. In addition, it stimulates labor and milk production in women.

Parathyroid glands
These small glands are located within the thyroid gland. Parathyroid hormone regulates the level of calcium in the blood.

Ovaries
The female sex hormones, oestrogen and progesterone, are produced in the ovaries in response to stimulation by the pituitary gland. They control ovulation, menstruation, fertility, and sexual characteristics.

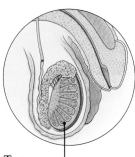

Testes
The male sex hormone, testosterone, is produced in the testes in response to stimulation by the hormone gonadotrophin, released by the pituitary. It controls sperm production and sexual characteristics.

HORMONE PRODUCTION

Feedback mechanisms help each gland produce the right amount of hormone. The hypothalamus detects hormone levels in the blood and orders glands to alter their hormone production in response. This can be illustrated by the control of the thyroid:

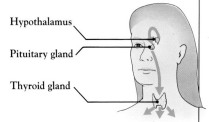

Hypothalamus

Pituitary gland

Thyroid gland

1 The body is functioning normally. Hormones produced by the thyroid and the pituitary are in balance.

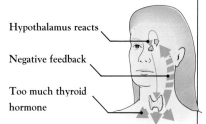

Hypothalamus reacts

Negative feedback

Too much thyroid hormone

2 Hormone production by the thyroid increases. The hypothalamus detects this change and signals the pituitary gland to produce less of the hormone that stimulates thyroid activity.

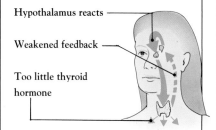

Hypothalamus reacts

Weakened feedback

Too little thyroid hormone

3 If hormone production by the thyroid drops, the hypothalamus signals the pituitary to produce more thyroid-stimulating hormone.

THE BRAIN AND NERVOUS SYSTEM

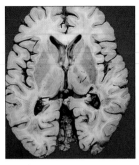

Nerve cell concentrations
Formed by nerve cells, gray matter "houses" your intellect, talents, and emotions.

THE BRAIN IS THE BODY'S control center and the largest organ of the central nervous system (CNS). It receives, sorts, interprets, and stores sensations and information from the nerves that extend from the CNS to every part of the body.

Two cerebral hemispheres make up nearly 90 percent of the brain tissue. Made up of nerve tissue, they have a folded surface that increases the brain's surface area. The hemispheres govern thought processes, senses, and movement. The brain stem connects the brain to the spinal cord and contains the nerve centers that control breathing and other vital functions. The cerebellum is concerned with balance, coordination of muscles, and posture.

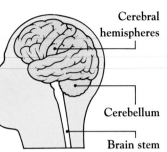

Cerebral hemispheres

Cerebellum

Brain stem

Structure of the brain
The brain consists of the brain stem, the cerebellum, and the cerebral hemispheres.

THE BRAIN MAP

The two cerebral hemispheres are divided into lobes. Arteries and veins run in the grooves between the lobes and supply oxygen and nutrients to the brain.

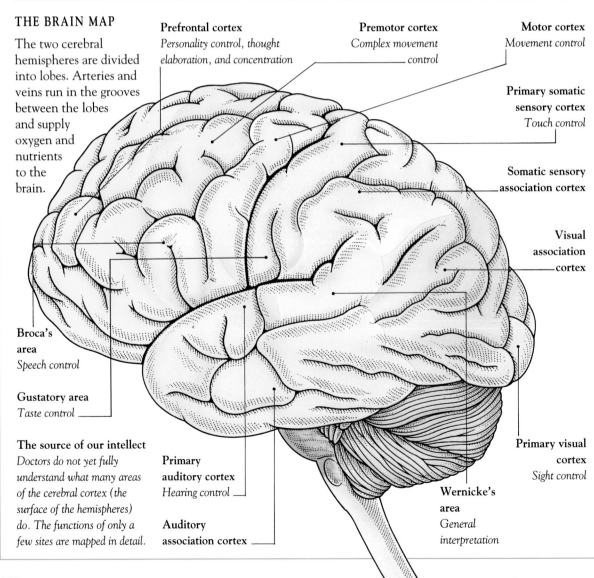

Prefrontal cortex
Personality control, thought elaboration, and concentration

Premotor cortex
Complex movement control

Motor cortex
Movement control

Primary somatic sensory cortex
Touch control

Somatic sensory association cortex

Visual association cortex

Broca's area
Speech control

Gustatory area
Taste control

The source of our intellect
Doctors do not yet fully understand what many areas of the cerebral cortex (the surface of the hemispheres) do. The functions of only a few sites are mapped in detail.

Primary auditory cortex
Hearing control

Auditory association cortex

Wernicke's area
General interpretation

Primary visual cortex
Sight control

MATTER OF FACT

The average human brain weighs 3 lb (1.4 kg) and contains about 100 billion neurons (nerve cells). These billions of cells are involved in forming memories and are essential components of the learning process. Men's brains are bigger than women's but this difference in size has no effect on intelligence. The left side of the brain controls the right side of the body and vice versa.

INTELLIGENCE

Many definitions of intelligence exist, but it is basically a measure of your ability to grasp and reason out concepts. It increases up to about six years of age and then stabilizes. Intelligence quotient (IQ), measured by intelligence tests, rises till the age of about 26 and gradually falls after 40. IQ's continue to increase because day-to-day experiences teach you how to apply your intelligence.

Logical reasoning
Test your powers of reasoning by studying the shapes shown above. Can you work out what should be next in the series?

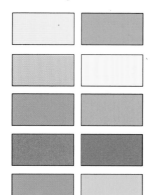

Short-term memory
Starting from the top, concentrate on each pair of colors for about 10 seconds. Now cover the left-hand column, expose one rectangle at a time, and try to recall the matching colours. Repeat the test half an hour later. After doing the test a few times you should be able to remember all the colors.

THE NERVOUS SYSTEM

The central nervous system (CNS) comprises the brain and spinal cord. It analyses and initiates responses. Sensory nerves around the body gather information and carry response signals through nerve cells back to the CNS. Motor nerves take instructions from the brain and spinal cord out to muscles to initiate movement. Autonomic nerves control functions like sweating, heart rate, and sexual arousal.

Nervous system in action
Complex processes that need precise movements, such as playing a guitar, are made possible by the sophistication of the nervous system.

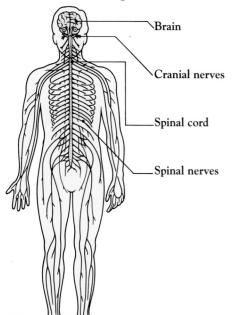

- Brain
- Cranial nerves
- Spinal cord
- Spinal nerves

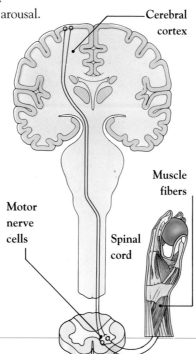

Cerebral cortex

Motor nerve cells

Muscle fibers

Spinal cord

How do you grasp an object?
When you have decided to pick up an object impulses are sent from the brain, through the motor nerves in the spinal cord, to the group of muscles in the forearm and the hand. Various muscles then either contract or relax to allow you to grasp the object.

219

BLOOD, BONE MARROW, AND LYMPH

BLOOD, BONE MARROW, and lymph are all part of an intricately balanced transport and defense system that provides the body's tissues with oxygen and nutrients, and protects against infection.

New blood cells are constantly created in the bone marrow to replace old cells which are destroyed in the spleen. These new cells pass into the bloodstream and are pumped around the body.

Red blood cells transport oxygen to body cells and platelets enable blood clotting to take place. White blood cells are created in both the bone marrow and the lymph glands. They rove around the body between the bloodstream, the lymph glands, and the lymphatic vessels, fighting infections.

Plasma

Plasma is a yellowish fluid in which the blood cells are suspended. It contains salts, nutrients, enzymes, antibodies, and dissolved blood-clotting factors.

Red blood cells

These disk-shaped cells are the most numerous type in the blood, with about five million in one cubic millimeter. They are filled with the oxygen-carrying red pigment, haemoglobin. Their shape gives them a large surface area which lets them combine with more oxygen in the lungs and transport it around the body.

White blood cells

There are several types of white blood cell which play different roles in fighting infection. Some directly attack invading microbes, others produce antibodies that attack microbes and provide immunity. They are larger than red blood cells but less numerous; there are only about 7,500 in a cubic millimeter.

Platelets

Produced in the bone marrow, these particles are the smallest type of blood cell. There are approximately 250,000 per cubic millimeter of blood. Platelets gather at the site of an injury in a blood vessel and plug the hole.

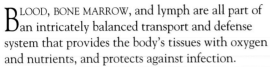

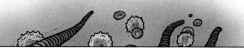

HOW DOES THE BLOOD CLOT?

Blood clotting is achieved by the solidification of blood. It reduces or controls blood loss by sealing damaged blood vessels. Generally clots only form at the site of an injury. But clotting is not always beneficial: abnormal clots (thrombi) can block blood vessels and lead to heart attacks and strokes.

Platelets are activated

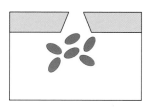

Coagulation occurs

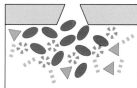

Damaged vessel is plugged

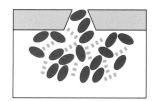

KEY

 Platelets

 Blood-clotting factors

 Fibrin

 Fibrinogen

1 *Platelets from the blood in contact with the damaged area become sticky, and adhere to the blood vessel wall.*

2 *Platelets release chemicals that turn blood-clotting factors into, first, fibrinogen, and then the protein fibrin.*

3 *Fibrin filaments link with the platelets and the red and white blood cells to form a solid blood clot.*

BLOOD TURNOVER

The normal life span of a red blood cell is about 120 days. Blood in blood banks must therefore be discarded after a few weeks as it contains too many dead cells. White blood cells survive in the blood for between nine hours and 10 years, depending on the type. Platelets only remain active for about nine days.

THE ROLE OF THE LYMPHATIC SYSTEM

The lymphatic system consists of a network of lymph glands (or nodes) found mainly in the neck, groin, and armpits, which are connected by lymphatic vessels. It drains tissue fluid (lymph) back into the bloodstream and helps to combat infection.

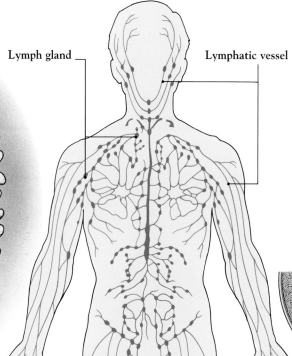

Lymph gland

Lymphatic vessel

BONE MARROW

The central cavity found in some flat bones, and the spaces in spongy bone, contain a fatty tissue called bone marrow. All platelet-forming and red blood cells, and most white blood cells, are made in the bone marrow by a series of divisions from a stem cell. New cells are then released into the blood circulation.

Bone marrow

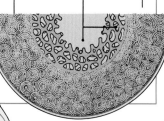

THE IMMUNE SYSTEM

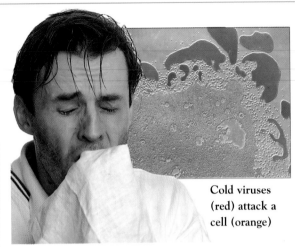

Cold viruses
(red) attack a
cell (orange)

The common cold
After each cold, the body produces antibodies against that specific type of cold virus. However there are many different cold viruses, so it is impossible to be immune to all of them.

T HE IMMUNE SYSTEM protects the body from being damaged by the millions of harmful chemicals and microorganisms that bombard it over a lifetime.

There are two different types of immunity. Innate immunity consists of physical barriers like the skin, and substances (usually enzymes) that are present in the mucous membranes (the linings of the mouth, throat, eyes, intestines, vagina, and urinary tract) which destroy microorganisms. Infants are also protected by antibodies received from their mothers in the uterus and through breast milk.

Adaptive immunity develops over time as the body is exposed to microorganisms. Antibodies fight off any invading organisms. Later these invaders are remembered by white blood cells, so the body can fight them off more quickly if they are encountered again. Immunity to diseases, such as polio, can also be conferred artificially through immunization.

BARRIERS TO INFECTION

The body is protected from infection by most microorganisms because of physical barriers such as the skin and chemical barriers such as enzymes.

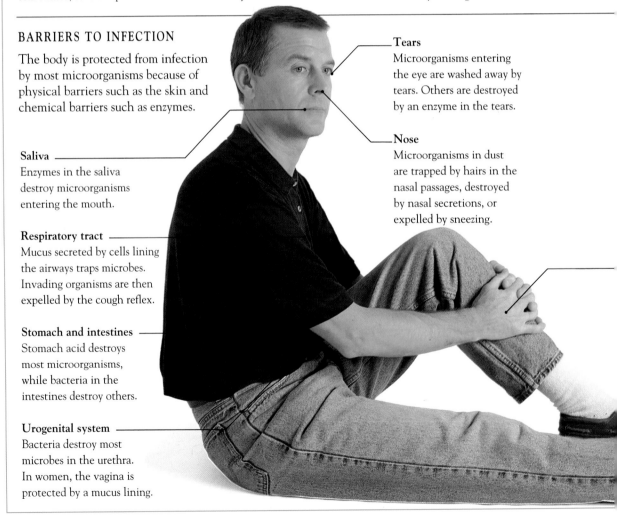

Saliva
Enzymes in the saliva destroy microorganisms entering the mouth.

Respiratory tract
Mucus secreted by cells lining the airways traps microbes. Invading organisms are then expelled by the cough reflex.

Stomach and intestines
Stomach acid destroys most microorganisms, while bacteria in the intestines destroy others.

Urogenital system
Bacteria destroy most microbes in the urethra. In women, the vagina is protected by a mucus lining.

Tears
Microorganisms entering the eye are washed away by tears. Others are destroyed by an enzyme in the tears.

Nose
Microorganisms in dust are trapped by hairs in the nasal passages, destroyed by nasal secretions, or expelled by sneezing.

HOW CELLS DEFEND THEMSELVES

Microorganisms that slip through the innate immune system and invade the body are then attacked by white blood cells in the adaptive immune system.

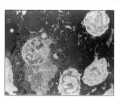

Phagocytes
go to the site of an infection where they "eat" bacteria. Dead phagocytes form pus.

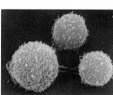

Killer T-cells
multiply quickly to destroy infections and tumors. They are a type of T- lymphocyte.

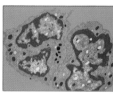

B-lymphocytes
in the bloodstream and lymph nodes make antibodies to destroy foreign organisms.

B-memory cells
are made from B-lymphocytes after an infection. They make antibodies against that virus.

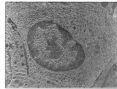

IMMUNIZATION

Some infectious diseases can be prevented by immunization with a vaccine. Vaccines are made from dead or modified microorganisms. They no longer cause the disease itself, but confer immunity by making the body produce antibodies. Immunization has led to the eradication of smallpox, while polio and diphtheria are almost unknown in the West.

BOOST YOUR IMMUNE SYSTEM

• Eat a balanced diet rich in vitamins and minerals.
• Get regular exercise, but do not overdo it.
• Try not to become run down by chronic mental or physical stress.
• Avoid alcohol and tobacco.

Skin

Skin provides a barrier against microbes. Sebum, an oil secreted by sebaceous glands, is acidic and toxic to many bacteria. Sweat glands also secrete antimicrobial substances.

ORGANS OF THE IMMUNE SYSTEM

The immune system consists of the bone marrow, thymus, lymph nodes, and other lymphoid tissues, blood vessels, spleen, and lymphatic vessels.

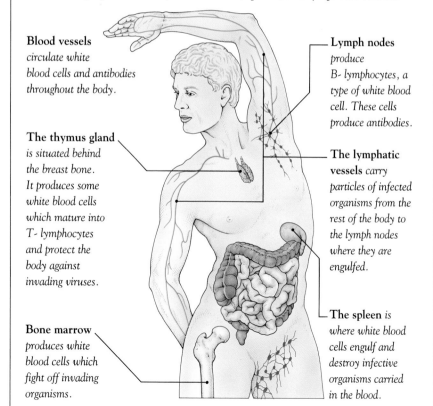

Blood vessels
circulate white blood cells and antibodies throughout the body.

The thymus gland
is situated behind the breast bone. It produces some white blood cells which mature into T- lymphocytes and protect the body against invading viruses.

Bone marrow
produces white blood cells which fight off invading organisms.

Lymph nodes
produce B- lymphocytes, a type of white blood cell. These cells produce antibodies.

The lymphatic vessels *carry particles of infected organisms from the rest of the body to the lymph nodes where they are engulfed.*

The spleen *is where white blood cells engulf and destroy infective organisms carried in the blood.*

THE FEMALE REPRODUCTIVE SYSTEM

A WOMAN'S REPRODUCTIVE organs consist of the ovaries, fallopian tubes, uterus, vagina, and vulva. The ovaries are about the size and shape of unshelled almonds, contain thousands of eggs, and lie one on each side of the uterus. Next to each ovary is the opening to one of the fallopian tubes. Once an egg has ripened in the ovary, it enters the fallopian tube. The fallopian tubes are about 4 in (10 cm) long, with a thin muscle wall and a central canal the thickness of a very fine needle. The uterus is a powerful muscular organ that stretches during pregnancy to hold the growing baby.

The cervix leads from the uterus to the vagina. Slightly acidic secretions keep the vagina clean and moist and help reduce the risk of infection. The amount of these secretions varies according to the woman's age and the stage of her monthly cycle. After menopause the vaginal secretions diminish.

ROUTINE CARE OF YOUR REPRODUCTIVE ORGANS

- Keep a record of your monthly cycle so that you can get to know what is normal for you.
- After a bowel action, wipe yourself from front to back to reduce the risk of contamination.
- If you are having an x-ray make sure that your ovaries are shielded from unnecessary exposure to radiation by wearing a protective apron.

- Make sure that you have a cervical smear at least every three years after you become sexually active.
- See a doctor if blood loss during menstruation becomes heavier or irregular; if you lose blood between your periods or after sexual intercourse; if you have any unusual discharge or irritation, abdominal or pelvic pain, or pain during intercourse.

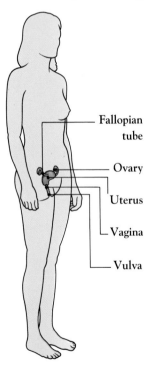

The reproductive system *is in the lower part of the abdomen. Each of the ovaries lies close to the opening of a fallopian tube which joins at its other end to the uterus. The vagina runs from the uterus to the vulva.*

Fallopian tube

Ovary

Uterus

Vagina

Vulva

HOW EGGS ARE PRODUCED

During a woman's fertile years, from the onset of menstruation to the menopause, the hormones estrogen and progesterone trigger the release of an egg by one of the ovaries each month. The egg travels slowly down the fallopian tube to the uterus. If it is fertilized by a sperm along the way, it begins to divide and implants into the wall of the uterus, resulting in a pregnancy. Unfertilized eggs, together with the soft, thick uterine lining, are expelled at the end of each cycle. This is known as menstruation, usually called a period, and occurs roughly once a month during a woman's fertile years.

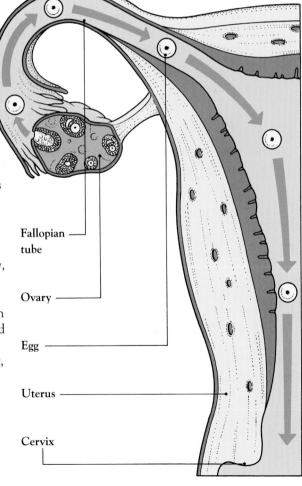

Fallopian tube

Ovary

Egg

Uterus

Cervix

The uterus

The uterus is a flexible bag of muscle. Its walls are lined with a mass of thick, soft tissue. This is either shed each month in menstruation or provides the "nest" for the fertilized egg. The uterus is pear-sized, except during pregnancy, when it expands as the fetus grows.

The ovaries

The ovaries release eggs and sex hormones. They lie on either side of the uterus, just below the openings of the fallopian tubes. Each ovary has numerous follicles in which the eggs develop. An egg is released each month by one of the ovaries during a woman's fertile years.

The fallopian tubes

These tubes run from the ovaries to the uterus and are 4 in (10 cm) long. At the end near the uterus they are very thin, while the end near the ovaries is funnel-shaped. Fertilization takes place in the fallopian tubes. The fertilized egg continues down the tube to the uterus.

The cervix

The cervix is at the bottom of the uterus and sticks out into the vagina. It is soft and round. A narrow canal (the os) in its center connects the cavity of the uterus with the vagina and allows menstrual blood to escape. When a woman goes into labor, the os opens fully to allow the baby to be born.

The urethra

This tube runs from the bladder to the outside of the body, allowing urine to be expelled. In women it is about 1½ in (4 cm) long.

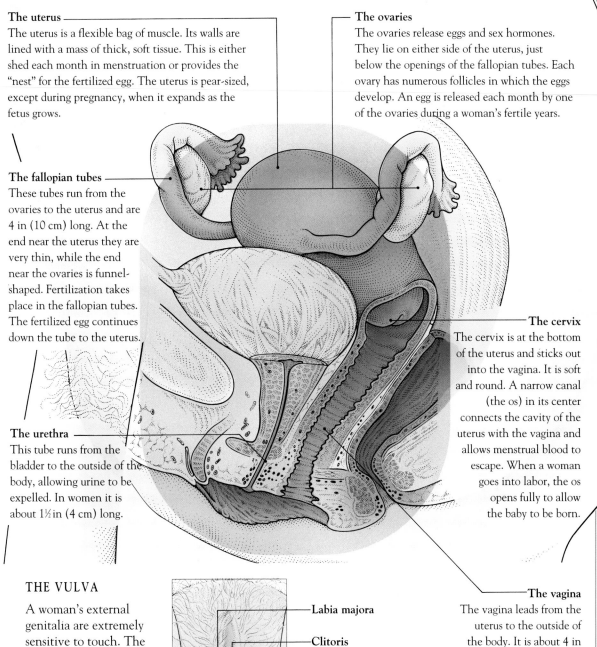

THE VULVA

A woman's external genitalia are extremely sensitive to touch. The labia, the outer lips of the vulva, protect the clitoris and the entrance to the urinary tract and vagina. In young girls, a thin layer of skin, the hymen, partly covers the entrance to the vagina.

Labia majora

Clitoris

Urinary (urethral) opening

Labia minora

Entrance to the vagina

The vagina

The vagina leads from the uterus to the outside of the body. It is about 4 in (10 cm) and secretes fluids that keep it clean and moist. The entrance to the vagina is situated behind the urethra and in front of the anus.

THE MALE REPRODUCTIVE SYSTEM

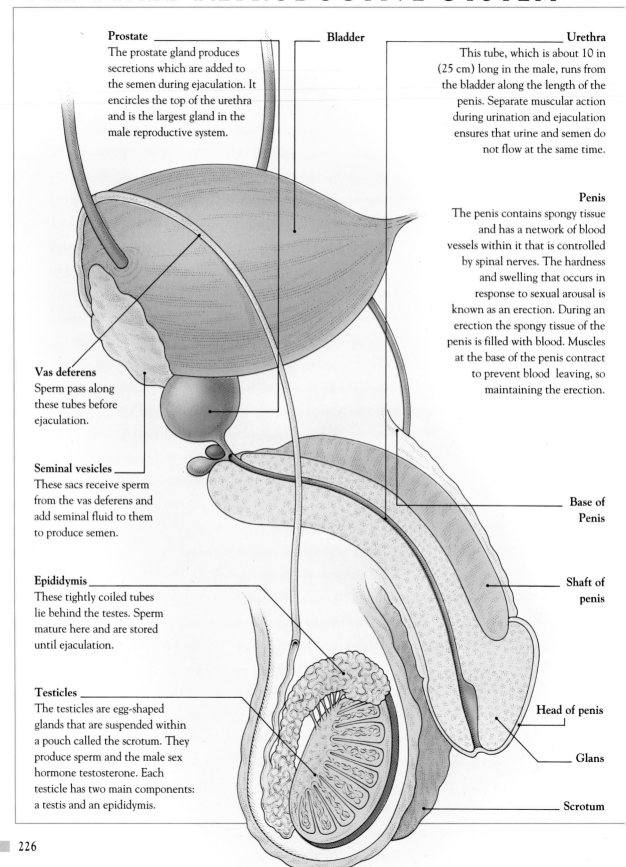

Prostate
The prostate gland produces secretions which are added to the semen during ejaculation. It encircles the top of the urethra and is the largest gland in the male reproductive system.

Bladder

Urethra
This tube, which is about 10 in (25 cm) long in the male, runs from the bladder along the length of the penis. Separate muscular action during urination and ejaculation ensures that urine and semen do not flow at the same time.

Penis
The penis contains spongy tissue and has a network of blood vessels within it that is controlled by spinal nerves. The hardness and swelling that occurs in response to sexual arousal is known as an erection. During an erection the spongy tissue of the penis is filled with blood. Muscles at the base of the penis contract to prevent blood leaving, so maintaining the erection.

Vas deferens
Sperm pass along these tubes before ejaculation.

Seminal vesicles
These sacs receive sperm from the vas deferens and add seminal fluid to them to produce semen.

Epididymis
These tightly coiled tubes lie behind the testes. Sperm mature here and are stored until ejaculation.

Testicles
The testicles are egg-shaped glands that are suspended within a pouch called the scrotum. They produce sperm and the male sex hormone testosterone. Each testicle has two main components: a testis and an epididymis.

Base of Penis

Shaft of penis

Head of penis

Glans

Scrotum

CIRCUMCISION

The foreskin of the penis may be surgically removed either for religious reasons or for reasons of hygiene (it stops secretions accumulating). The operation is also performed if the foreskin is too tight or if it regularly becomes infected and painful.

THE MALE REPRODUCTIVE organs consist of the penis and testicles. Within each testicle is a gland, called a testis, and a long tube called an epididymis. Sperm are continually produced in each testis and then passed into the epididymis, where they are stored. They mature over two or three weeks. Shortly before ejaculation, sperm are propelled from the epididymis, through a long tube called the vas deferens, into the seminal vesicles where seminal fluid is manufactured and added to the sperm to produce semen, which is also known as ejaculate.

During sexual excitement, spongy tissue in the penis fills with blood causing an erection. When orgasm occurs semen travels along ducts, which pass through the prostate gland, into the urethra. It is then ejaculated from the urethra through the penis. On average there is about 3-6 ml of fluid in ejaculate.

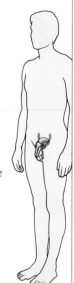

Sex organs
The male sex organs consist of the visible genitalia and internal organs such as the prostate gland, urethra, the vas deferens, and the seminal vesicles.

SPERM AND FERTILITY

Each sperm consists of a long whip-like tail that propels it along and a head that contains the heredity material. Only about 0.05 mm in length, there are up to 600 million sperm in just one milliliter of ejaculate (semen). Semen can be analysed to give an accurate indication of fertility. The number of sperm are counted and their mobility measured.

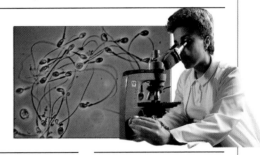

SELF-EXAMINATION

Men under 40 should examine their testicles at least once a month. Cancer of the testes is the most common cancer in young men, but, if detected early enough, it has a 90 per cent cure rate. Examine each testicle by rolling it between your thumbs and fingers. Go to your doctor if you find a lump, a change in texture, any swelling or tenderness, or if you find ulcers on your scrotum. The epididymis at the back of testicles may feel firm – do not mistake it for a tumour.

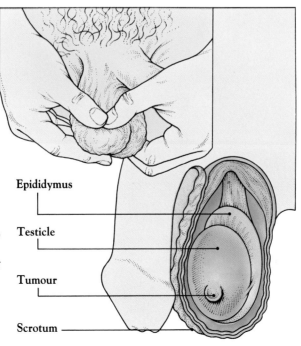

Epididymus

Testicle

Tumour

Scrotum

ROUTINE CARE

There are several simple measures that you can take to help ensure that your genital area remains healthy and problem-free.

• Regularly retract your foreskin and clean underneath it as infections often occur under the foreskin.
• A penile discharge, pain during intercourse, or sores, blisters, spots, or lumps on your genitals may be symptoms of a sexually transmitted disease. Consult your doctor immediately.

THE EYE

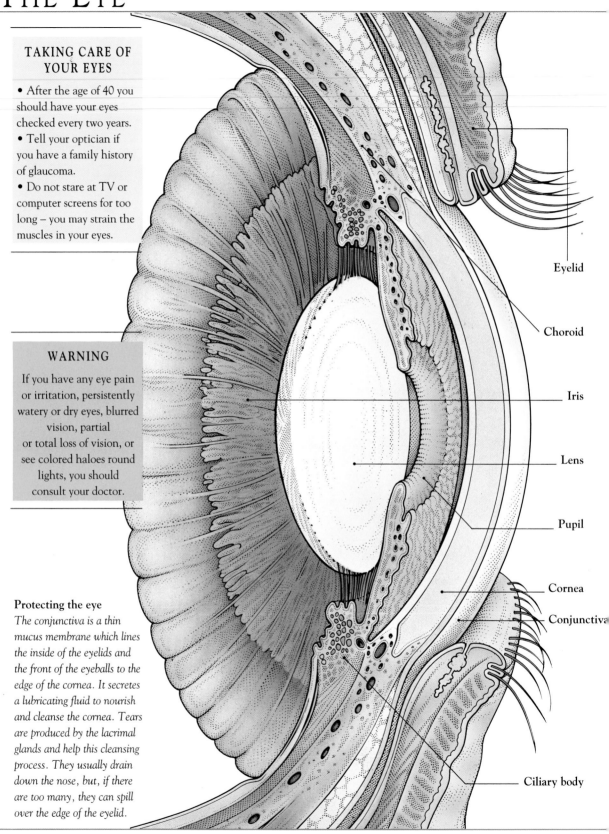

Protecting the eye
The conjunctiva is a thin mucus membrane which lines the inside of the eyelids and the front of the eyeballs to the edge of the cornea. It secretes a lubricating fluid to nourish and cleanse the cornea. Tears are produced by the lacrimal glands and help this cleansing process. They usually drain down the nose, but, if there are too many, they can spill over the edge of the eyelid.

Eyelid

Choroid

Iris

Lens

Pupil

Cornea

Conjunctiva

Ciliary body

HOW YOU SEE

1 The cornea is transparent and covers the front of the eye. The iris lies behind the cornea and has a space at its centre called the pupil. Tiny muscles in the iris alter the pupil's size and thus the level of light that reaches the retina.

2 A lens located behind the iris provides the eye with focusing power. This lens is suspended within a round ring of muscle, the ciliary body. By contracting, this muscle changes the shape of the lens and allows the eye to focus.

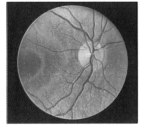

View of the retina

3 The focused image falls on to the retina at the back of the eye, which is made up of nerve tissue and supplied with oxygen and glucose by blood vessels within the choroid.

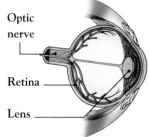

Optic nerve

Retina

Lens

4 The optic nerve carries electrical impulses from the nerves of the retina to the visual cortex in the brain, where they are interpreted.

THE EYE IS THE organ of vision. It transforms rays of light into a pattern of nerve impulses that can be transferred to the brain and interpreted. The two eyes work together to provide the brain with a three-dimensional view of the world.

Two very different systems operate together to process these images. The first is an optical system made up of the cornea at the front of the eye and the internal lens. This system directs light, from objects before you, onto the retina which lines the back of the inside of the eye. The second is the neurological system. Nerves transmit a wealth of information from the retina, along the optic nerve, to the back of the brain where it is interpreted. When the information reaches the brain it is assembled and processed to enable us to view the outside world.

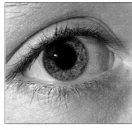

The outer eye
The eye is a delicate, jelly-filled ball, protected by bony sockets. The whites of the eyes (sclera), the colored part of the eye (iris), and the dark centre (pupil) are visible on the front of the eyeball.

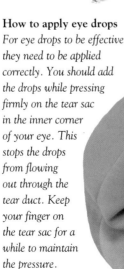

PROTECT YOUR EYES

Your eyes are already well protected by the skull, the lids, the lashes, and the tears that constantly bathe them. But by treating your eyes gently and respecting how delicate they are, you can avoid harming them. Wear protective goggles when swimming in chlorinated water, and always wear goggles when using dangerous chemicals, high-speed machinery, power tools, and even when using a trimmer in the garden. Try to avoid rubbing your eyes since this can easily spread infection from your hands to your eyes.

How to apply eye drops
For eye drops to be effective they need to be applied correctly. You should add the drops while pressing firmly on the tear sac in the inner corner of your eye. This stops the drops from flowing out through the tear duct. Keep your finger on the tear sac for a while to maintain the pressure.

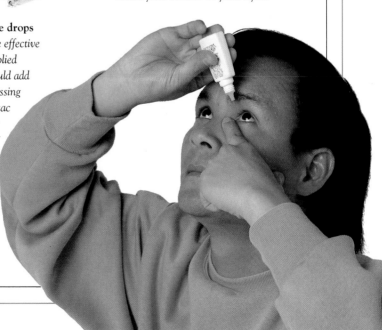

THE EAR

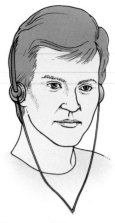

Listen carefully
Personal stereo systems should not be played too loudly. Eventually the noise could harm your hearing.

SOUND TRAVELS THROUGH the air in waves. These waves reach the outer ear and are then channeled by the pinna down the ear canal. When they strike the eardrum, they make it vibrate. Three small, movable, interlinked bones in the middle ear (the hammer, stirrup, and anvil) convey these vibrations to the inner ear where they reach the cochlea. The cochlea is shaped like a snail's shell and has hairs along its length which are vibrated by the incoming sound waves. The movement of each hair sets off a nerve impulse that is sent to the brain along the auditory nerve. The brain then processes these signals, comparing them to sounds you have heard before that are stored in your memory. This enables you to recognize sounds you have heard before.

NOISE LEVELS

The decibel (dB) scale is used to measure sound. Every increase of 10 dB means a doubling of sound intensity, so 90 dB is twice as loud as 80 dB. At the lowest point, 0 dB, nothing can be heard by the human ear. Noise causes pain and immediate damage to the ear at around 130 dB, while noise of 90 dB can be tolerated for about two hours before it harms your ears. You should wear headphones if you work on a building site where pneumatic drills are used, at an airport near jets, or in a noisy factory.

The sound barrier
The ears hear many levels of noise. Close to the ear, a ticking watch is 30 dB, a personal stereo 80 dB, while a jet is over 130 dB.

dB	30	80	130

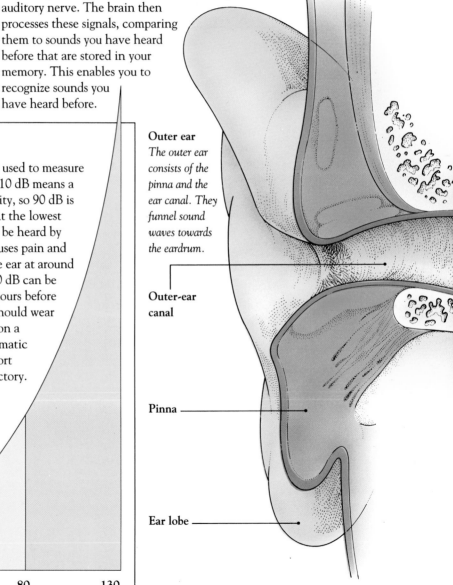

Outer ear
The outer ear consists of the pinna and the ear canal. They funnel sound waves towards the eardrum.

Outer-ear canal

Pinna

Ear lobe

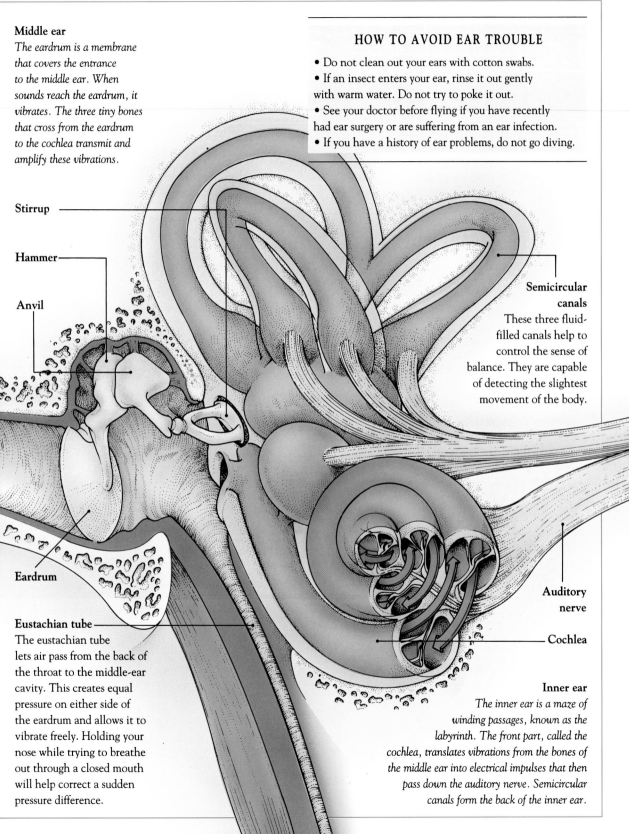

Middle ear
The eardrum is a membrane that covers the entrance to the middle ear. When sounds reach the eardrum, it vibrates. The three tiny bones that cross from the eardrum to the cochlea transmit and amplify these vibrations.

Stirrup

Hammer

Anvil

Eardrum

Eustachian tube
The eustachian tube lets air pass from the back of the throat to the middle-ear cavity. This creates equal pressure on either side of the eardrum and allows it to vibrate freely. Holding your nose while trying to breathe out through a closed mouth will help correct a sudden pressure difference.

HOW TO AVOID EAR TROUBLE

- Do not clean out your ears with cotton swabs.
- If an insect enters your ear, rinse it out gently with warm water. Do not try to poke it out.
- See your doctor before flying if you have recently had ear surgery or are suffering from an ear infection.
- If you have a history of ear problems, do not go diving.

Semicircular canals
These three fluid-filled canals help to control the sense of balance. They are capable of detecting the slightest movement of the body.

Auditory nerve

Cochlea

Inner ear
The inner ear is a maze of winding passages, known as the labyrinth. The front part, called the cochlea, translates vibrations from the bones of the middle ear into electrical impulses that then pass down the auditory nerve. Semicircular canals form the back of the inner ear.

THE FIVE SENSES

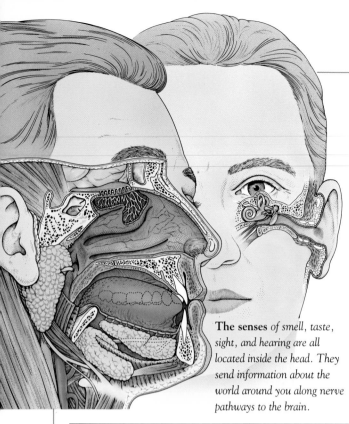

EACH OF YOUR senses provides you with information about one aspect of the world around you. Specially developed systems within the eye, ear, nose, tongue, and skin translate sensory information into electrical signals which are passed along the nervous system to the brain. The brain can then understand and process this information, enabling you to see, hear, smell, taste, and feel.

Although the senses work independently of one another, they can also work together, compensating for each other or adding to the information the brain receives. The senses of smell and taste, for instance, are closely linked. By itself, the tongue can only distinguish four tastes – sweet, sour, bitter, and salty. The nose, however, can distinguish tens of thousands of scents. Food odors pass through the back of the throat and enter the nose. These odors determine how foods taste. Because smell influences taste so much, people are unable to taste food properly when their noses are blocked.

The senses *of smell, taste, sight, and hearing are all located inside the head. They send information about the world around you along nerve pathways to the brain.*

SIGHT

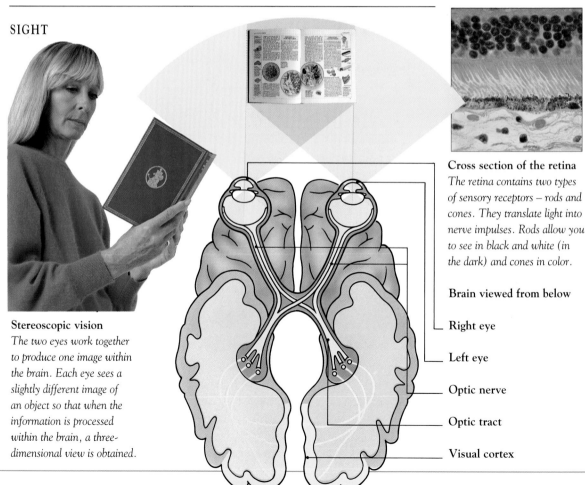

Stereoscopic vision
The two eyes work together to produce one image within the brain. Each eye sees a slightly different image of an object so that when the information is processed within the brain, a three-dimensional view is obtained.

Cross section of the retina
The retina contains two types of sensory receptors – rods and cones. They translate light into nerve impulses. Rods allow you to see in black and white (in the dark) and cones in color.

Brain viewed from below

— **Right eye**

— **Left eye**

— **Optic nerve**

— **Optic tract**

— **Visual cortex**

TASTE

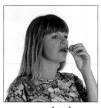

Chemicals in food and drink dissolve in saliva inside the mouth. They then enter pores in the tongue which contain the four types of taste buds – sweet, sour, bitter, and salty. In the brain, information from the taste buds and nose are combined, allowing us to experience taste.

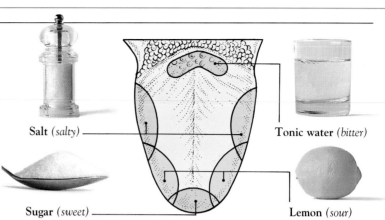

Salt (*salty*)

Sugar (*sweet*)

Tonic water (*bitter*)

Lemon (*sour*)

TOUCH

Thousands of specialized sensory nerve cells under the skin's surface respond to external stimulation. They are sensitive to touch, pain, heat, cold, and pressure. The sensations from each part of the body are received by different areas of the brain's cerebral cortex. The most sensitive parts of the body, such as the lips and hands, are represented by larger areas of the cerebral cortex.

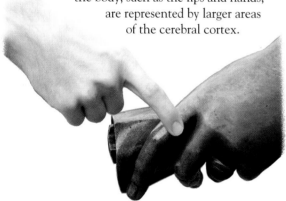

SMELL

Within the nose, air passes over sensitive, hairlike nerve endings, which are stimulated by scent in the inhaled vapors. This information is sent to the olfactory bulb, which relays it via the olfactory nerve to the brain for interpretation. The sense of smell may be temporarily lost when a disorder of the respiratory system produces a stuffy nose.

Olfactory bulb

Olfactory nerve

HEARING

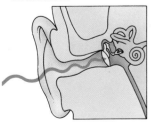

Hair

Hair cell

Basilar membrane

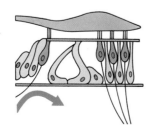

Auditory cortex

Nerve fibers of the cochlea

Sound wave

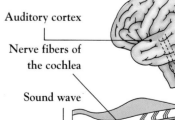

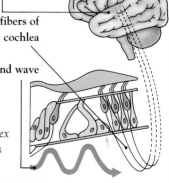

1 *Sound waves enter the ear and make the eardrum vibrate. These vibrations are transmitted via tiny bones in the middle ear to the cochlea.*

2 *In the cochlea, the vibrations set the basilar membrane in motion, which in turn moves the hair cells that line this sound receptor.*

3 *Sensory nerve fibres are stimulated, sending impulses to the auditory cortex in the brain, which interprets them as sounds.*

CHANGES IN THE BODY

FROM CONCEPTION TO BIRTH

The journey from conception to birth involves an incredible sequence of changes. A single cell continuously divides and multiplies to form a tiny embryo; first the brain develops, then the spine and nervous system. Next the fetus buds arms and legs. After just nine months the baby is fully formed.

T HE BODY IS NOT a static unit, proceeding through life unchanged. From the moment of conception, the body's cells multiply, divide, and multiply again. At certain times, such as in infancy and during pregnancy, these changes are rapid. At other times, for instance during adulthood, the changes are often not visible from the outside. But activity within the cells allows for the regeneration and repair of tissue, the growth of bones, nails, and hair, and increases in muscle bulk. As we age, our body clocks run down and the physical changes of aging begin.

Pregnancy

The most rapid changes in the human body occur in a developing fetus. The mother's body also changes. She gains weight and her pelvis and breasts change in preparation for birth and breast-feeding. A good, well-balanced diet and regular health checks are vital for both her health and that of her baby throughout the 40 weeks of pregnancy.

Childhood and adolescence

In the first year of life, a baby triples his or her birth weight. For the next two decades, the child continues to grow. The long bones in the arms and

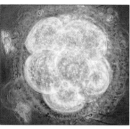

One month
After just 28 days most of the primitive organs are formed: the embryo's heart is already beating and there is a simple brain, spine, and nervous system. The embryo is now about ⅕ in (5 mm) in length.

The first few hours
The ripe egg starts to divide just two or three hours after fertilization. First it divides into two, then into four; after three days it has split into 32 cells. A week later it implants into the lining of the uterus.

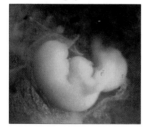

Three months
The embryo now looks much more human. Sexual differentiation has taken place, the eyes are migrating to the sides of the head, and the fingers are visible. The fetus is 1½ in (4 cm) long.

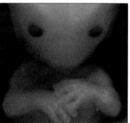

Five months
After just five months the nose, mouth, and eyes are all well-developed. The fetus is now 10 in (25 cm) long and can make a fist, suck a thumb, move around, and kick the mother.

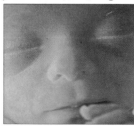

Birth
After an average of 266 days the baby is fully developed. Just a few minutes after birth the baby is able to see colors and lights, sense people touching his or her skin, and latch onto the breast.

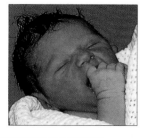

FROM CHILDHOOD TO OLD AGE

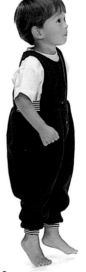

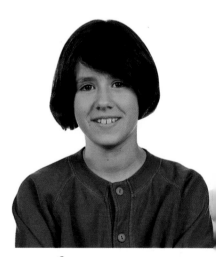

2 years
At two, the rapid growth of infancy is complete and the baby has become a child.

9 years
During the years between infancy and puberty, the rate of growth is slow and steady.

legs have caps of cartilage on top which enable the child to grow to adult height. When growth is complete this cartilage fuses onto the bone shaft. As well as growing taller and heavier, children change their body proportions, with the trunk and limbs catching up with the head, which is three quarters of its adult size at birth.

Rapid physical changes occur during the years of puberty (from about age 13 to 19). The teenager needs greater help and guidance than ever as he or she struggles to deal with the issues of independence, sexuality, and peer group pressure.

Adulthood and old age

From the age of about 20 to 50, the body does not change much outwardly. Then, with the menopause in women and the onset of the physical changes of old age in both women and men, comes a series of rapid changes caused mainly by a progressive loss of the elastic tissues of the body, leading to wrinkling of the skin and loss of flexibility in the joints. But there is still a third of life left to live and the challenge of retirement to be met. A good diet, regular health checks, and continued physical and mental activity can help people make the most of growing older.

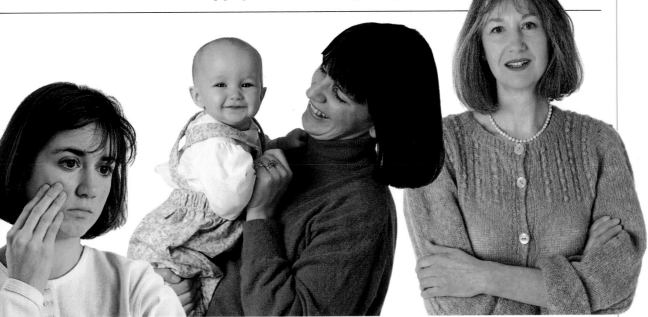

16 years
Puberty is a period of rapid growth and development which continues until full adult height is reached.

30 years
From 20 to 50, few external changes are visible – height and weight remain constant.

50 years
After 50, the changes of aging become more obvious, for example increased wrinkles and graying hair.

ADOLESCENCE

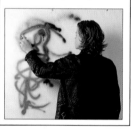

HEALTH TIPS

- Do not start smoking. Of those who do, 85 percent become addicted.
- Restrict your alcohol intake – it can seriously damage your health.
- Many drugs of abuse are addictive, all are illegal. Refuse all drugs – they can harm your physical and emotional health.
- If you are not old enough or do not feel that you are ready for sex, ignore pressure from friends. If you do have sex, be sure to use a condom to protect yourself from AIDS, other sexually transmitted diseases, and pregnancy.

ADOLESCENCE IS THE time when a boy or girl develops into a man or woman. It is a time of rapid change, both physically and emotionally, so it is often a stressful and awkward few years. The physical changes of adolescence are called puberty. Girls begin puberty a little earlier than boys, at about 10 to 12 years of age, while puberty begins in boys between the ages of 12 and 14.

Puberty begins when hormones from the pituitary gland signal the body to begin the process of changing from child to adult. About two years later, boys begin to notice outward physical changes. In girls, the physical changes start before menstruation begins. In three or four more years, all the changes are complete and the teenager has an adult body.

The emotional changes, however, often take longer. Separating from parents and becoming an adult can be a difficult process.

ADVICE FOR PARENTS

- Listen to what your son or daughter says.
- Discuss sex openly.
- Do not be distressed by arguments – they are a part of growing up.
- Talk to your child about their feelings of anxiety and depression – it may help.
- Try to reach a compromise about rebellious behavior.

THE ADOLESCENT GIRL

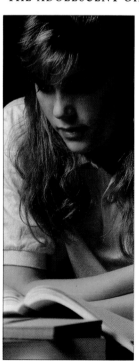

Around age 9, *the pituitary gland secretes hormones that start the changes of puberty.*

Around age 11, *girls start to get taller and weigh more. The nipples enlarge as the breasts begin to get bigger.*

By age 14, *most girls are menstruating. Underarm hair grows; sweat glands under the arms, in the groin, and around the nipples become active.*

By age 17, *body fat increases around the hips and tops of thighs, and the hips become wider. Menstruation is now usually regular.*

The first sign of puberty is usually the enlargement of your nipples and breasts; then hair will grow under your arms and in your pubic area. Your periods will start and you will grow taller – most girls reach their full height by age 16. In 95 percent of girls, periods start before the age of 15. Consult your doctor if your periods have not started by age 16. Early periods tend to be irregular and vary in length, but they are usually painless. Remember you can get pregnant soon after your periods begin.

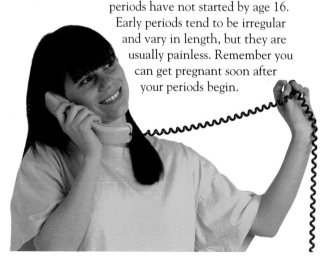

ACNE ACTION

Many teenagers suffer from pimples because androgen hormone levels are high during puberty. They are caused when the hair follicles and sebaceous glands become inflamed. Thorough washing and application of benzoyl peroxide can help control pimples, but picking may make them worse and can cause scarring. If your acne is severe, see a doctor.

A clean face
Washing with soap and water should remove excess oil, preventing spots. If acne does occur, try using a preparation from the chemist which has benzoyl peroxide in it.

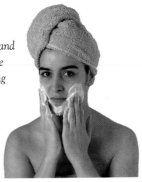

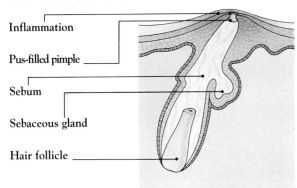

Inflammation

Pus-filled pimple

Sebum

Sebaceous gland

Hair follicle

Skin surface

How a pimple develops
When a follicle is blocked by sebum, an oily substance secreted by the sebaceous glands, bacteria are trapped and multiply. The follicle becomes reddened, inflamed, and sometimes filled with pus.

THE ADOLESCENT BOY

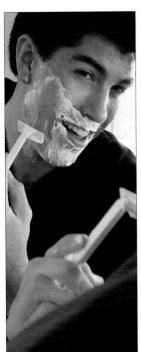

Around age 10, *the pituitary gland secretes hormones that trigger the bodily changes.*

At age 12, *some boys begin to grow pubic hair and their testes increase in size.*

By age 14, *boys are becoming taller and heavier, with broader shoulders and chests and a visible Adam's apple. As the voice box enlarges, the voice breaks and deepens.*

By age 17, *the changes are almost complete. The skin of the scrotum darkens, the penis lengthens, pubic and underarm hair is thick and coarse, and most boys need to shave.*

The age at which puberty is complete varies but it will not begin until a year or two after girls your age. Rapid growth can occur from 13, but usually does not start until 15. Growth in height continues until age 18, but the bones keep getting broader until age 20. Sexual maturity varies too. Your genitals may be mature at 14, while others your age may still have immature genitals.

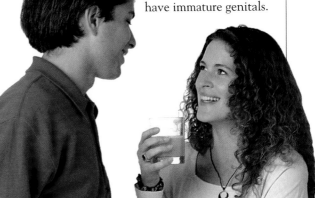

THE MENSTRUAL CYCLE

MENSTRUATION IS THE monthly bleeding that occurs in women of child-bearing age when the lining of the uterus is shed. Women usually begin menstruating between the ages of nine and 16 and continue until menopause at around the age of 50. The whole process is regulated by the complex interaction of hormones in the body.

During menstruation, most commonly known as a period, the lining of the uterus (the endometrium) is shed through the cervix into the vagina. A period continues for about five days on average. About three tablespoons of blood, as well as some other liquid and mucus, is lost. The uterus makes an anti-clotting substance that keeps the blood liquid. If you are losing a lot of blood or notice small or large clots, you should see your doctor.

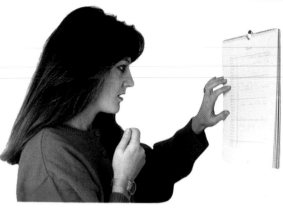

Keeping a record
Record when your period arrives each month. Be aware of the amount of blood you lose, and of any premenstrual symptoms or period pain; then you can see your doctor if changes occur.

PREMENSTRUAL SYNDROME

Premenstrual syndrome (PMS) may occur any time in the two weeks before your period begins. The exact cause is not yet known. Some of the symptoms are: irritability, tension, depression, fatigue, breast tenderness, fluid retention, and backache.

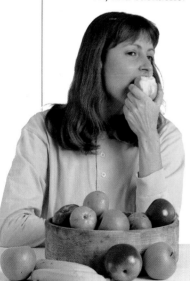

BEATING PMS

- Record your periods and symptoms of PMS for three months to see if they are really cyclical.
- Try vitamin or dietary supplements. Capsules of oil of evening primrose or vitamin B6 taken for 10 days before your period may help.
- Exercise aerobically by jogging or swimming.
- Take aspirin for cyclical breast pain. A supportive bra worn all the time can protect sensitive breasts.
- Visit your doctor – hormone or vitamin therapy may help.

Watch what you eat
Avoiding salt, caffeine, and chocolate in the two weeks before your period may reduce symptoms of PMS.

PERIOD PAIN

Severe pain before and during a period may be due to hormonal changes. A doctor may recommend an anti-inflammatory drug to relieve pain, or prescribe oral contraceptives to regulate hormone levels. Pain can also be due to an underlying disorder of the reproductive system such as pelvic inflammatory disease or endometriosis. Any new period pain should be reported to your doctor.

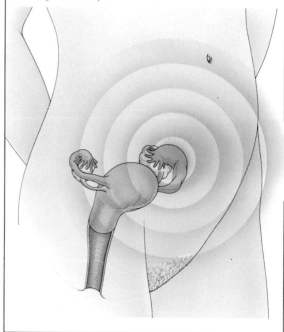

HOW HORMONES TRIGGER MENSTRUATION

Two hormones from the pituitary gland and the sex hormones, estrogen and progesterone, interact throughout the menstrual cycle. They trigger the development and release of an egg, the thickening of the endometrium, and then the shedding of this uterine lining during menstruation.

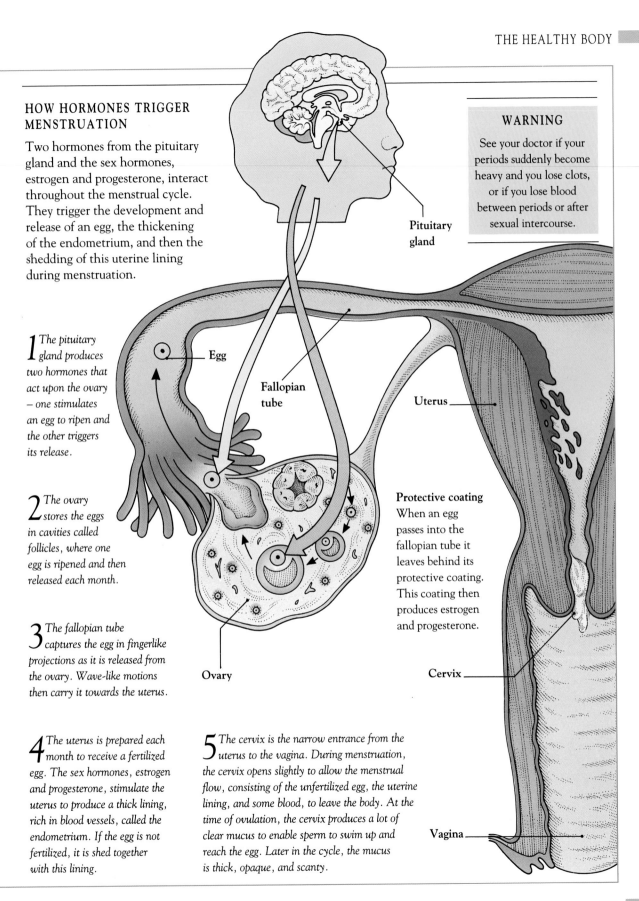

Pituitary gland

Egg

Fallopian tube

Uterus

Ovary

Cervix

Vagina

Protective coating
When an egg passes into the fallopian tube it leaves behind its protective coating. This coating then produces estrogen and progesterone.

1 The pituitary gland produces two hormones that act upon the ovary – one stimulates an egg to ripen and the other triggers its release.

2 The ovary stores the eggs in cavities called follicles, where one egg is ripened and then released each month.

3 The fallopian tube captures the egg in fingerlike projections as it is released from the ovary. Wave-like motions then carry it towards the uterus.

4 The uterus is prepared each month to receive a fertilized egg. The sex hormones, estrogen and progesterone, stimulate the uterus to produce a thick lining, rich in blood vessels, called the endometrium. If the egg is not fertilized, it is shed together with this lining.

5 The cervix is the narrow entrance from the uterus to the vagina. During menstruation, the cervix opens slightly to allow the menstrual flow, consisting of the unfertilized egg, the uterine lining, and some blood, to leave the body. At the time of ovulation, the cervix produces a lot of clear mucus to enable sperm to swim up and reach the egg. Later in the cycle, the mucus is thick, opaque, and scanty.

PREGNANCY

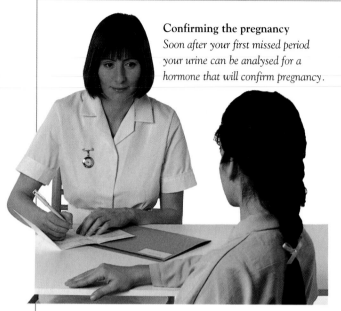

Confirming the pregnancy
Soon after your first missed period your urine can be analysed for a hormone that will confirm pregnancy.

A HEALTHY, YOUNG WOMAN who uses no form of contraception and has sexual intercourse twice a week, has a 90 percent chance of conceiving within one year. The average pregnancy lasts for 266 days.

A time of emotional turmoil

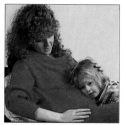

Changes in your physical and mental state are triggered by an increase in hormone levels as your body prepares to nurture your baby. Although these changes may make you feel worse rather than better, they are all for a good cause – each plays a vital part in the complex process of making your baby.

Being pregnant is not an illness and most women can continue with their everyday activities. Regular

THE THREE STAGES OF PREGNANCY

The nine months of pregnancy are traditionally divided into three stages of three months, known as trimesters. Each stage is characterized by particular developments in mother and baby.

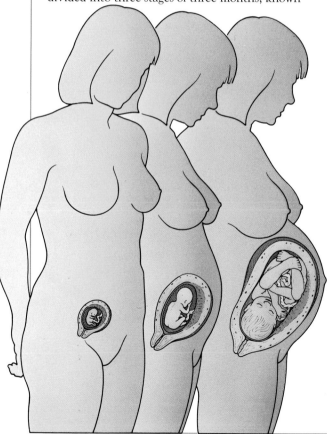

1 *In the first three months the embryo grows to about 2 in (5 cm) in length and all the major organs develop. Your breasts begin to swell and you will gain about 10 percent of your total pregnancy weight gain.*

2 *Most women are full of energy in the second trimester. The fetus grows rapidly and is recognizably human. Your abdomen swells and your naval may protrude. You will gain about 50 to 60 percent of your total pregnancy weight gain.*

3 *In the last three months the fetal organs mature. Stretch marks may develop. If your total weight gain is under 30 lb (13 kg) you should easily return to your original weight.*

RUBELLA

Commonly known as German measles, this normally mild illness can cause birth defects and miscarriages if it develops in a pregnant woman. The risks are particularly high in the first four months of pregnancy when the baby's internal organs are still developing. Ask your doctor whether you are immune. Vaccination is effective, but it is best to avoid becoming pregnant for three months afterwards. If you are already pregnant and not immune, you should avoid contact with anyone who has rubella.

exercise, especially walking or swimming, will help you stay fit and feel well (see p90).

A healthy lifestyle for a healthy pregnancy

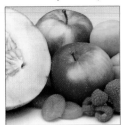

The fetus's tissues are formed inside your body using nutrients and energy from the foods you eat. It is therefore essential that you eat regular, well-balanced meals (see p60). Do not, however, be tempted to "eat for two" during pregnancy; your daily energy requirements only increase by about 300 Calories. You will find that your appetite increases, but try to avoid filling up on high calorie snacks that are low in nutrients.

Remember that the placenta not only carries nutrients to your baby, but can also allow harmful chemicals through. Avoid tobacco, alcohol, and any type of drug that could harm your baby.

Ideally you should be leading a healthy way of life even before you conceive, but no matter what stage of pregnancy you are in, it is never too late to start.

The importance of antenatal care

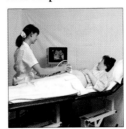

Regular medical care is essential throughout your pregnancy to help keep you and your baby healthy. Visit your doctor for checkups once a month for the first seven months. After this stage you should see your doctor or midwife more frequently. Following their advice will help to ensure that you have a safe, healthy, and enjoyable pregnancy.

COMMON MINOR AILMENTS

Every pregnancy is different. Some women do not have any difficulties at all, but others do. Minor problems that can happen at any time during pregnancy include: constipation, vaginal discharge, sleeping difficulties, bleeding gums, varicose veins, and morning sickness. In the last trimester some women suffer cramps, hot flushes, faintness, leaking urine, breathlessness, rashes, swollen ankles, back pain, and tiredness.

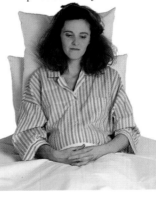

Take it easy
Pregnancy can make sleeping and getting comfortable in bed difficult. Try placing extra pillows behind your back.

Morning sickness
Often one of the first signs of pregnancy, morning sickness is not restricted to the morning – it can happen at any time of day. Eating dry biscuits or toast first thing in the morning may help relieve symptoms.

MISCARRIAGE

Miscarriages occur in about one in five pregnancies, generally in the first 12 weeks. Most women who suffer a miscarriage eventually carry a pregnancy to full term and have a normal, healthy baby. After the first trimester you should immediately report any bleeding to your doctor; at this later stage of pregnancy a significant number of possible miscarriages can be successfully treated.

DANGERS

Two to three percent of birth defects are thought to be caused by drugs or chemicals passing from the mother to the fetus. You can minimize the risk by avoiding all the following:

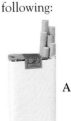

Alcohol

Tobacco   Cough medicines

All drugs, unless they are prescribed

MENOPAUSE

MENOPAUSE IS the term for the cessation of the menstrual periods. It happens when the ovaries become exhausted and gradually shrink, producing less estrogen as a result.

These changes are not sudden. Most women go through a premenopausal stage for two or three years. Initially the cycle may become shorter, sometimes by a full week. Next, it tends to lengthen, with lighter bleeding. The periods then stop, sometimes to resume again for a few months.

Pregnancy is less likely, but still possible, during the premenopausal stage. You should continue to use some form of contraception until you have not had a period for more than 24 months if you are under 50, or more than 12 months if you are over 50. If you suspect that you are pregnant you should see a doctor immediately. Pregnancy carries greater risks for both you and the baby as you approach menopause.

Some women dread menopause, fearing that they will experience unpleasant symptoms. However, there is no need for this worry – many women experience no symptoms at all and for those women who do there are effective treatments available.

SYMPTOMS AND SIGNS

Menopausal symptoms are due to a fall in the body's estrogen levels. Some women have no symptoms; the most common complaints are night sweats and hot flushes.

- Night sweats can cause profuse sweating, disturb your sleep, and leave you tired and irritable.

- The cells lining the vagina shrink as the estrogen level decreases. The vagina becomes drier and more prone to infection. Sexual intercourse may be painful.

- Falling estrogen levels make the pituitary gland produce more hormones that affect temperature and blood flow through the skin, causing hot flushes.

- Social, domestic, and work changes, rather than estrogen loss, may be the cause of depression during menopause.

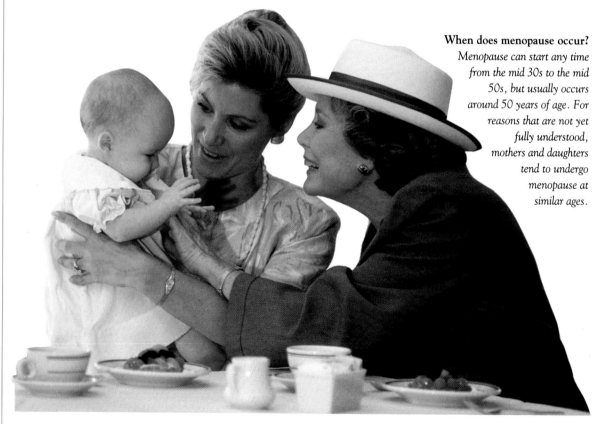

When does menopause occur?
Menopause can start any time from the mid 30s to the mid 50s, but usually occurs around 50 years of age. For reasons that are not yet fully understood, mothers and daughters tend to undergo menopause at similar ages.

VAGINAL BLEEDING

In the years leading up to menopause, your menstrual periods begin to change, sometimes becoming lighter, sometimes heavier. Keep a careful record of any bleeding. If periods become very frequent or heavy or if you lose blood between periods or after sex, consult your doctor. Irregular bleeding may be due to contraceptive methods such as the pill or the coil. If you are not sure what is causing the bleeding, talk to your doctor.

SURGICAL MENOPAUSE

If you have a hysterectomy, your uterus (womb) will be removed and your periods will stop at once. If your ovaries are left, you will continue to make hormones until your natural menopause would have occurred. However, if your ovaries are removed, and you do not have hormone replacement therapy, you will undergo a sudden menopause.

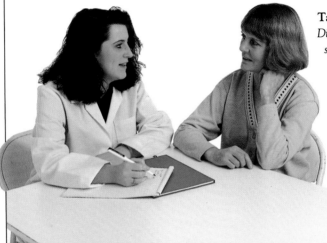

Talk to your doctor
Discuss all the various surgical options, and their consequences, with your doctor.

HORMONE REPLACEMENT THERAPY

Hormone replacement therapy (HRT) may be used by some women to reduce the severity of the physical and psychological symptoms of menopause. HRT replaces the estrogen your body no longer produces. It also protects against osteoporosis, which one in four women will develop, and heart disease.

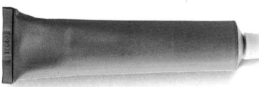

Creams *and ointments containing estrogen are sometimes used to prevent dryness and thinning of the vaginal skin.*

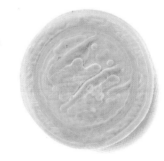

Skin patches *containing estrogen may be applied to the skin of the shoulder, lower abdomen, or thigh. The hormones are absorbed through the skin into the bloodstream. A new patch must be applied every three days in a different area.*

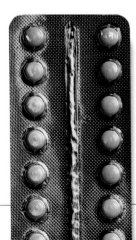

Tablets *containing estrogen are the most common method of hormone replacement.*

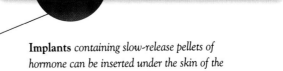

Implants *containing slow-release pellets of hormone can be inserted under the skin of the abdomen and usually last about six months.*

THE AGING PROCESS

As you age, your mental and physical abilities change. But ill health or reduced vitality need not occur. Eating well and exercising regularly can slow down the physical changes of aging, while mental changes can be combatted by keeping up an interest in new ideas and the world around you.

Everyone slows down as they grow older. Tissues become less elastic, making the skin wrinkle and the joints become stiffer. The bones thin and become more prone to fractures. Memory is less reliable.

But these changes vary from person to person; those who have kept their bodies in good condition and who are not ill show few signs of aging until well into their 60s. In their 70s, many people are still fit enough to run marathons, play a vigorous game of tennis, and lead a rewarding intellectual life.

CHANGES IN THE BODY

Brain and nervous system
Reduced blood flow to the brain and loss of nerve cells impair memory and mental abilities may decline.

Heart and circulation
The heart becomes less efficient and blood pressure tends to rise. Circulation slows down. Less exercise can be tolerated.

Lungs
The lungs become less elastic and so less efficient. At 75, the efficiency of the lungs is 40 percent less than at 30 years of age.

Liver
Toxins present in the blood are not processed as efficiently by the liver. Older people may therefore tolerate alcohol less well.

Joints
The joints become stiffer, causing a decrease in mobility. Over the years, as the disks and bones in the spine are compressed, there is a loss of height.

Muscles
Muscles start to lose their bulk and strength.

The human body undergoes a series of biological changes as the years pass. The senses may deteriorate – the hearing becoming less acute, the eyes less keen, and balance less stable. Short-term memory becomes unreliable and the body is more susceptible to illness and infection.

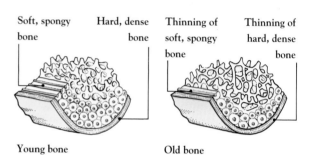

Soft, spongy bone | Hard, dense bone | Thinning of soft, spongy bone | Thinning of hard, dense bone

Young bone   Old bone

Changes in the bones
Bones lose density with age. In women, decreased estrogen production after menopause speeds bone thinning. As the bones thin, spaces develop in the bone tissue where protein and calcium have been lost. Thin bones are more likely to fracture.

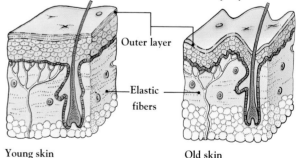

Outer layer

Elastic fibers

Young skin   Old skin

Changes in the skin
The skin of elderly people has a thin top layer and bruises more easily due to weakened capillaries. There are fewer collagen fibers, which give skin its elasticity, making the skin more prone to injury and giving it a wrinkled appearance.

JOINTS

Joints that have become diseased or damaged can be replaced by artificial substitutes made of metal or plastic. Joint replacement is of great benefit to people with degenerative arthritis, which gets more common with age. It is sometimes also used for severe cases of rheumatoid arthritis. Joints in the shoulders, elbows, hips, fingers, knees, and ankles can be replaced to relieve pain and restore movement. They are usually cemented into position, although cementless joints are being developed. Artificial joints do not have the same range of motion as healthy joints, but they are much more mobile than worn, arthritic joints.

Shoulder

Elbow

Hip

Finger joints

Knee

Ankle

Joints that can be replaced
Hip and knee joints damaged by arthritis are most frequently and successfully replaced, but other joints can also be treated this way.

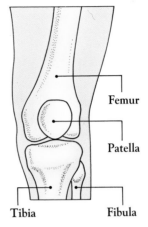

Femur

Patella

Tibia   Fibula

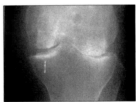

Before replacement
This x-ray shows an arthritic knee joint. The bone and cartilage are severely worn.

Femoral component
Fitted to the femur after cutting, shaping, and drilling.

Tibial component
Fitted to the upper end of the tibia during surgery.

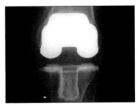

After replacement
This x-ray shows the two parts of the artificial knee joint in place.

PREVENTING HYPOTHERMIA

Serious loss of body heat may occur in sick, old people who are immobile. Signs are drowsiness, confusion, and pallor. Untreated, hypothermia may lead to unconsciousness and even death. Call a doctor immediately if you suspect someone is suffering from hypothermia.

To avoid hypothermia, keep the room you are in at a temperature of 68°F (19°C) even if you do not feel cold. Hot drinks and warm clothes will also keep you warmer. Be sure to eat well to maintain your body heat and health. Do not sleep in a cold bedroom.

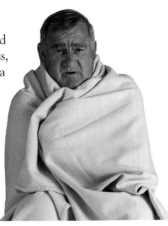

GRACEFUL AGING

• Stimulate your mind – take classes or read.
• Compensate for any loss in short-term memory by writing down facts and making lists.
• Eat a healthy diet.
• Keep supple and fit by exercising regularly.
• Plan your retirement.
• Keep senses keen with a hearing aid or glasses.

245

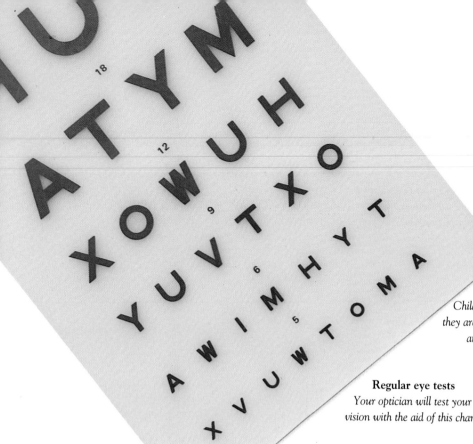

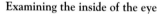

Monitoring development
Children are checked regularly to see that they are acquiring physical and mental skills at the right stage in their development.

Regular eye tests
Your optician will test your vision with the aid of this chart.

Blood samples
Blood tests can diagnose many different disorders, such as a hormone imbalance, an infectious disease, a deficiency of a vitamin or mineral, or some genetic disorders.

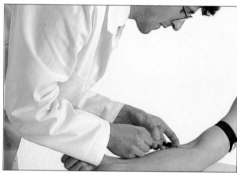

Examining the inside of the eye
Your doctor may use an ophthalmoscope to examine your eyes. A light source and a series of lenses allow the eye to be seen in great detail.

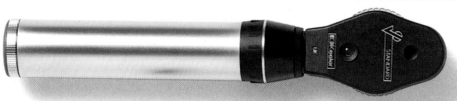

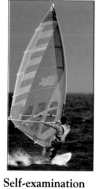

Self-examination
Exposure to sunlight increases your risk of cancer, check your skin regularly.

Testing the reflexes
A hammer may be used to check your reflexes. This test is usually done as part of a routine physical.

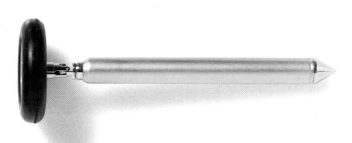

CHAPTER EIGHT

BODY WATCH

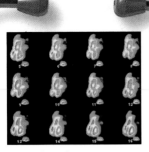

Blood pool imaging
Some tests your doctor may carry out are highly sophisticated. These scans show the heart's pumping action through one complete heart cycle.

EARLY DIAGNOSIS is the key to treating cancer and other disorders successfully. Many tests can be done to assess the state of your health. Some, such as measuring your pulse rate, are simple; others, like cardiac blood pool imaging, are at the frontiers of modern medical technology. This chapter will tell you about the tests your doctor may order and help you understand what these tests are and what they can tell you.

Different tests are recommended for different people. Selected diagnostic tests, such as an EEG, are performed only if your doctor suspects that something is wrong and needs more information. Some, like measuring your blood pressure, are part of a routine physical. Others, like cervical smears, are done as part of a nationwide screening program on all sexually active women under 65 years of age.

The tests that you can do by yourself at home may be the most important. You are the most likely person to find cancer warning signs – 90 percent of breast tumors, for example, are discovered by the woman herself. You know your own body best and so will be able to spot changes in your skin, breasts, testicles, bowel habits, or state of health that your doctor should know about.

It is vital that if you notice any of the changes discussed in this chapter you seek medical advice – some may be caused by cancer. Bringing them to the attention of your doctor could literally save your life.

Examining a cervical smear
Abnormal cells can be identified microscopically.

Listening for clues
The stethoscope is simply a convenient substitute for placing an ear to the human body. Different disorders, in the heart and lungs, produce different distinctive sounds.

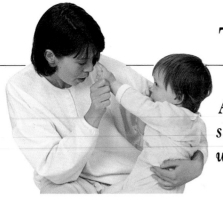

THE GROWING CHILD

All children develop new mental and physical skills in much the same order, but the rate at which they do so varies enormously.

BABIES UNDERGO A thorough physical examination soon after birth. During the first five years of life, each child is checked regularly to see that new skills are being acquired at about the right time so that the small minority of children who are showing signs of developmental delay may be helped.

By identifying any problems at an early stage, the necessary treatment can be started before a child has fallen too far behind others of the same age. Things that might be recommended to help a child include: wearing glasses to correct a visual defect or a hearing aid to treat deafness; physiotherapy may help a clumsy child; speech therapy can assist a child with a specific language disability.

Visual skills

Newborns cannot focus, but at six weeks babies respond to faces and objects that are 2 ft (60 cm) away. When a toy is dangled around 8 in (2 cm) away from a three-month-old baby, the baby's eyes should follow its movement.

By six months, babies look intently at everything. Not only do they follow moving objects, but they reach out for them, transfer them from hand to hand, and put them in their mouths.

At nine months a baby's grasp involves mostly the index and middle fingers. The grasp will be strong but he or she may find it difficult to release an object. All babies will use both hands equally at first – definite right or left-handedness is

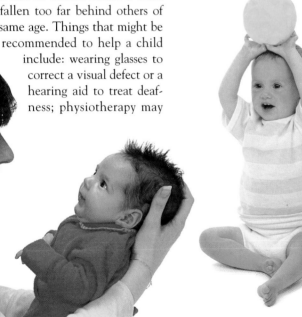

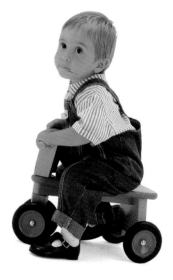

At six weeks
All babies are nearsighted during the first weeks of life, but at about six weeks your baby should smile or stare if you bring your face to within about 2 ft (60 cm). The irregular sleep patterns of the first weeks should be starting to settle into a regular pattern of sleeping for a long period at night and napping during the day.

At eight months
An eight-month-old baby will be able to roll over from a face-down position onto his or her back, remain unsupported in a sitting position when put there, and babble without meaning, producing a wide range of sounds. During mealtimes, babies of this age will want to use spoons or fingers to try to feed themselves.

At two years
Most two-year-old children will be walking unaided, climbing onto furniture, talking in simple sentences, playing imaginatively, and throwing the odd tantrum. They are beginning to have control over their bladders and bowels, but often still wear diapers, particularly at night. Fear of the dark and eating fads may be a problem.

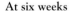

not clearly established until at least the age of three.

As your child's coordination and skills improve, a greater number of bricks can be balanced in a tower and drawings will evolve from scribbles to recognizable shapes.

Developing speech

A crying three-month-old baby should react to a loud noise by temporarily becoming quiet and still. At four months, the baby should turn towards a sound. Six-month-old babies make a variety of sounds; they laugh and squeal with delight.

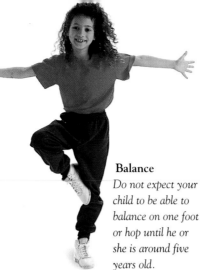

Balance
Do not expect your child to be able to balance on one foot or hop until he or she is around five years old.

At around nine months, a baby will start to use sound to attract your attention. The first meaningful words may come at any time from one year onwards, with a steady build-up in vocabulary over the next two years. Children will start to understand simple instructions by the age of two.

Walking

Most children learn to walk between the ages of nine and 15 months. Those children who learn to crawl early and efficiently may not start walking until much later, whilst others may walk right away and skip the crawling stage.

Bladder and bowel control

The age at which children can control their bladders and bowels varies. Bowel control is almost always acquired first, any time from 20 months onwards. Most children start to be dry during the day at around two years of age, but they will not be able to give up diapers at night for at least one more year.

At three years

Three-year-old children have large vocabularies, speak clearly in sentences, constantly ask questions, feed themselves, and start to share their toys with others. At this age it becomes easier to reason with them, and they have fewer tantrums. They are usually toilet trained and wear diapers only at night, if at all.

At five years

A five-year-old boy or girl enjoys singing and repeating nursery rhymes, telling stories, and looking at books. At this age, children can hop and skip, and draw recognizable figures rather than scribbles. They will be independent and adept at dressing, undressing, washing, and using the toilet by themselves.

MONITOR YOUR CHILD'S DEVELOPMENT

If you have any worries about your child's sight, hearing, speech, height, weight, or physical development, discuss them with your health visitor or family doctor. It may be difficult to spot a particular problem your child is having, especially if you have more than one child at home, so make sure you keep all appointments for their regular developmental check-ups.

THE ROUTINE PHYSICAL

Health screening looks for signs of disease and lets you know just how healthy your lifestyle really is.

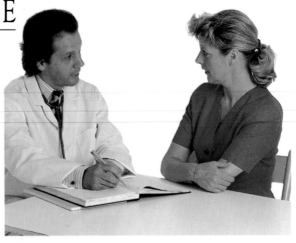

THERE ARE A number of different reasons why people undergo a routine physical. They may be worried about their lifestyle; perhaps someone they know has been taken ill suddenly; or maybe they want to be screened for a particular hereditary disease. Whatever the reason for the examination, the doctor will use a wide variety of tests in making his or her assessment. Regular screening can help to detect many disorders in their early stages, when treatment will be more successful.

COMPONENTS OF THE ROUTINE PHYSICAL

Many doctors recommend that all adults should have the following tests at these regular intervals. Of course, the more frequently you are tested the earlier your doctor will be able to detect problems.

TEST	HOW OFTEN?	WHY IS IT DONE?	WHEN TO TEST MORE OFTEN
Weight	Whenever you have any other type of test.	Being over or underweight is linked to many diseases.	If you have an unplanned or rapid change in weight.
Blood pressure	Once at senior school and then every one to three years.	Checks the health of the heart and blood vessels.	At least once a year if taking the oral contraceptive pill or more often if your doctor advises it.
Urine	Whenever you have any other type of test.	Can reveal kidney disease, diabetes, or an infection.	You will be tested if you have any urinary symptoms.
Blood sugar	Whenever you have any other type of blood test.	When fasting, high blood sugar can indicate diabetes.	If you are known to be diabetic.
Blood fats (cholesterol test)	Every one to five years.	It is one indicator of your risk of suffering from a heart attack.	If you have a family history of high cholesterol levels or are being treated for high cholesterol.
Cervical smear	Every one to three years for women aged 18 to 64 who have ever had sex.	Reveals abnormal cells that could develop into cancer of the cervix.	If you have had any previous abnormalities or your doctor advises it.
Mammography (breast x-ray)	Every one to three years, starting at age 40 to 50.	Detects the early stages of many breast cancers.	If you have had breast cancer or a family history of this disease.

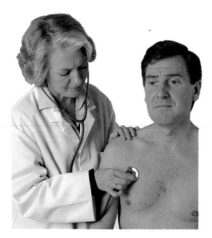

Listening for clues
Using a stethoscope to listen to your chest allows a doctor to assess the function of your heart and lungs. If placed over an artery, it can detect turbulence due to altered blood flow.

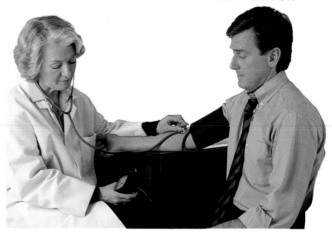

Measuring blood pressure
Blood pressure is the force of blood flow through the arteries. It gives information about the condition and function of your heart and circulation. Having high blood pressure when you are at rest is a common sign of arterial disease. If it remains untreated it increases the risk of suffering from a heart attack or stroke.

FEELING AND TAPPING FOR CLUES

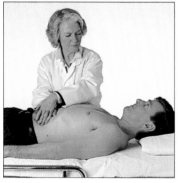

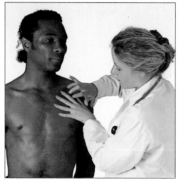

Palpation – feeling for clues is an important part of the physical examination. By exerting firm pressure with the flat of the hand, the doctor feels for any areas of tenderness or swelling. Palpation may detect enlargement of the lymph glands, of internal organs such as the liver, spleen, or kidneys, and of the heart.

Percussion – by tapping over the chest and abdomen the doctor checks for dullness or resonance of the sounds. Excess gas in the abdomen will increase resonance and if the liver is enlarged there will be a wider expanse of dull notes over the right side below the ribs. This procedure can also detect signs of a tumour or emphysema.

PHYSICAL APPEARANCE

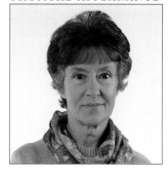

Your general appearance will provide clues to your health. Do you look fit and relaxed or tired and worried? Do your skin, hair, and nails appear healthy? Simply by looking at you a doctor can gain an overall impression of your health. A slight blue discoloration around your lips could be a sign of a heart, circulation, or lung disorder, while a flushed face might be due to alcohol abuse, a skin problem, or heart disease.

TESTING REFLEXES

Striking a tendon with a rubber hammer should cause the connecting muscles to tighten automatically. Damage to nerves in the spinal cord may cause this reflex to fail and damage to the brain may cause the reflex to be excessively brisk or violent.

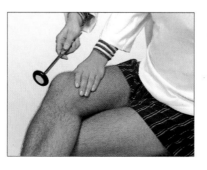

EYE TESTS

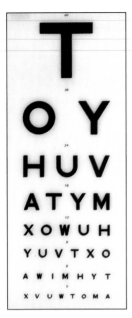

Snellen's chart
The sharpness of your distance vision can be tested by reading a Snellen's chart that is positioned 20 ft (6 m) away from you. This chart has eight rows of letters of diminishing size. A person with normal vision can read the second-to-bottom row.

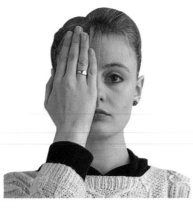

Monitoring your own vision
Check your own vision by taking the tests shown on the opposite page. If you notice any deterioration in your sight you should go to have your eyes tested professionally. Early detection of eye problems helps to minimize any permanent loss of vision.

GLAUCOMA IN THE FAMILY

Glaucoma is an eye disease that tends to run in families. It is caused by a build-up of pressure inside the eye and can lead to blindness. Therefore, if any member of your family has suffered from this condition you should have your eyes checked regularly. An ophthalmic optician, using a slit lamp (a high-powered binocular microscope) and a sensitive pressure gauge, can test for glaucoma.

Even if you think your sight is perfect you should have your eyes tested periodically.

EYE TESTS ARE essential for the very young, when a specific problem such as a squint can be corrected before it causes permanent damage. For older people, eye tests will detect any deterioration due to advancing age, so that treatment can be prescribed to preserve their eyesight. Everyone over the age of 40 should have their eyes tested at least every two years.

People with a medical condition that can affect the eyes, such as high blood pressure or diabetes, should have their sight checked at least once a year. If you suffer from a pain in the eye or a sudden change in vision, such as blurring, double vision, spots before your eyes, colored haloes around lights, or flashes of light, you should see your doctor as soon as possible.

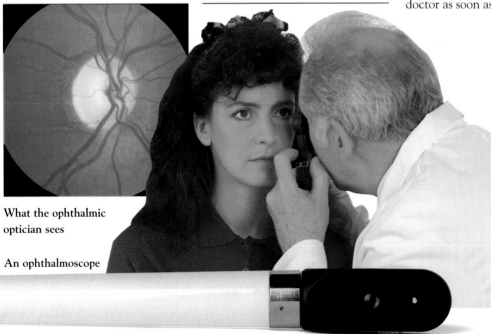

What the ophthalmic optician sees

An ophthalmoscope

Ophthalmoscopy
An ophthalmoscope is an instrument used to examine the inside of the eye. A light source and a series of lenses provide a highly detailed image of the back of the eye. It is used to diagnose disorders such as retinal detachment or degeneration, inflammation of the optic nerve, and damage to retinal blood vessels.

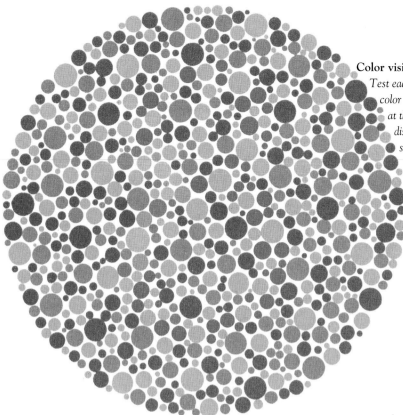

Color vision test
Test each of your eyes separately for red-green color vision by covering one eye and looking at this Ishihara's test plate. If you cannot distinguish between red and green, you will see the number 3, instead of the number 8. Color blindness is much more common in men than in women.

THE EFFECT OF AGING

The lenses of the eyes become less elastic with age. Therefore the nearest point on which the eye can focus progressively moves further away. Even if your vision has always been normal, you may start to need reading glasses at about 45 years of age.

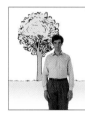

Normal vision
Young people's eyes can focus on the man in the foreground, and on the tree.

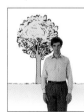

Aging vision
Older people may find that if distant objects are clear they cannot focus on the foreground.

Do you need glasses?
Hold this book 16 in (40 cm) away from your eyes and try to read the different sizes of print. If you cannot read normal-sized print you may need to wear glasses. If you usually wear glasses, try the test while wearing them. If you still cannot read the print you need some new lenses.

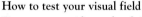

VISUAL FIELD TESTS

Both of these tests check your field of vision. You can carry out the first simple test for yourself.

How to test your visual field
Cover one eye with your hand. Stretch your other arm out to the side at shoulder height, with your thumb pointing up. Then, while looking straight ahead at a fixed object, see if you can detect your thumb moving when you wiggle it. If you cannot, you may have a restricted field of vision. Repeat with the other eye.

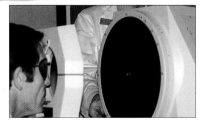

The professional approach
A more accurate assessment of visual field defects, used by ophthalmic opticians, involves the use of a screen on which points of light appear at different positions.

HEARING TESTS

Hearing tests assess how well you hear sounds of varying pitch and loudness.

IF YOU THINK that you are not hearing as well as you should be, ask your doctor to test your ears. Do not delay in consulting your doctor; most forms of hearing loss are easy to treat.

There are many different ways that your hearing can be checked. Some of these tests are complex and involve producing detailed graphs of the pattern of your hearing loss. Other methods are very simple and use only a tuning fork.

How sound travels

There are two ways that sound waves can reach your inner ear. They can either travel down the ear canal, (known as air conduc-tion) or they can pass directly through the skull into the inner ear (bone conduction).

Testing with tuning forks

If a tuning fork is tapped against a solid object it vibrates and emits a sound. By holding the fork near the opening of the outer ear canal your doctor can test the transmission of sound waves through the outer and middle ear. The fork is pressed against the skull behind your ear to test your bone conduction. In a healthy ear, air conduction is better than bone conduction, so the sound of the fork will seem louder when held near the ear.

Poor bone conduction is a sign that the inner ear, the hearing centers in the brain, or the connecting nerves are damaged.

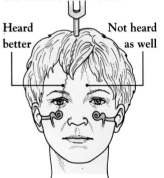
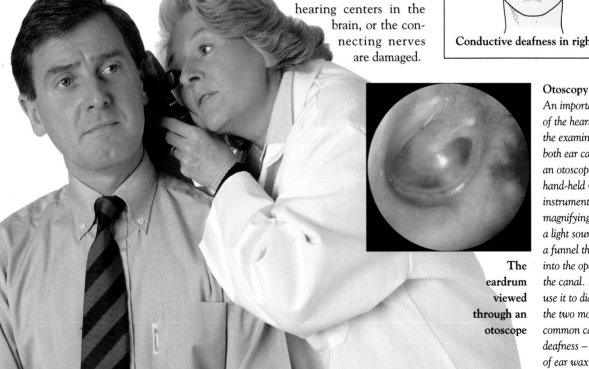

The eardrum viewed through an otoscope

Otoscopy
An important part of the hearing test is the examination of both ear canals with an otoscope. This hand-held viewing instrument has a magnifying lens, a light source, and a funnel that slides into the opening of the canal. Doctors use it to diagnose the two most common causes of deafness – build-up of ear wax and infection behind the eardrum.

AUDIOMETRY

An audiometer is a machine which transmits sounds at different frequencies and intensities. The person being tested sits in a soundproof room to cut out any background noise. At each frequency level the volume is decreased until the person being tested can no longer hear it. When these hearing thresholds are plotted on a graph, the pattern of any hearing deficit across the range of frequencies heard by the human ear is shown.

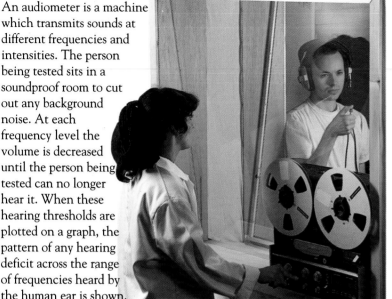

HEARING AND OLD AGE

For many people ageing is associated with a reduced sensitivity to higher-frequency sounds, making conversations difficult to follow. But this decline is often treatable. Removing wax from the ears may restore hearing.

Hearing aids
that selectively amplify high tones can improve many elderly people's hearing.

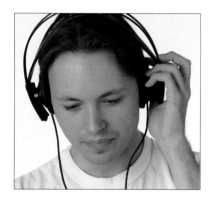

Out of range
Air conduction is measured by playing different sounds through headphones to one ear at a time. An oscillator is held behind the ear to record bone conduction.

WHO NEEDS A HEARING TEST?

- All children as part of their developmental assessment.
- A child who is slow in learning to talk – he or she may be suffering from a loss of hearing.
- Anyone who finds it difficult to follow conversations or who has persistent ringing or buzzing in their ears.
- An elderly person who has become confused – this may simply be due to poor hearing.
- People who are regularly exposed to loud noises.

IMPEDANCE AUDIOMETRY

To vibrate freely and transmit sound waves to the middle and inner ear, the eardrum must have equal pressure on each side. Impedance audiometry checks whether the eardrum is restricted in its movements. A probe, fitted inside the ear canal, transmits sound waves at the eardrum while air is pumped through at varying pressures. The different patterns of sounds reflected back from the eardrum are detected by a microphone in the probe and will reveal any middle ear disorders.

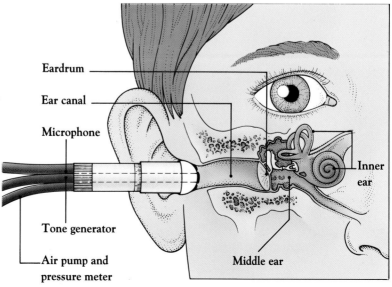

Eardrum

Ear canal

Microphone

Tone generator

Air pump and pressure meter

Inner ear

Middle ear

BLOOD TESTS

Analyzing your blood can provide clues to the diagnosis of a wide range of diseases.

BECAUSE BLOOD is made up of hundreds of different con-stituents whose concentration or appearance alters when an illness is present, blood tests are valuable diagnostic tools. They can reveal the presence of a disorder in a major body organ, a hormonal imbalance, an infectious disease, or a defect in the immune system.

Blood tests may be carried out on whole blood; on plasma which is the fluid in which platelets and red and white blood cells are suspended; or on serum, the fluid left behind after blood has clotted.

Analyzing the blood

To help assess the structure and function of blood cells, their shape, size, and appearance may be examined under a microscope. Blood groups can also be analyzed.

The chemicals present in the blood include: nutrients, amino acids, cholesterol, hormones, gases, enzymes which stimulate chemical reactions, ions, waste products, and any drugs or alcohol.

Some infectious diseases can be diagnosed if microorganisms, such as bacteria or fungi, are found in the blood. These microorganisms can be seen either under a microscope or by using a special "broth" to encourage them to grow.

The body's white blood cells release antibodies which are designed to kill invading microorganisms, so testing for a significant increase in the level of specific antibodies will show that an infection is present.

HAVING BLOOD TAKEN

Some blood tests require only a drop or two of blood, in which case a drop is drawn from the fingertip. When more blood is needed, it is taken from a vein at the front of the elbow using a sterile needle.

Since the circulation normally contains at least eight pints of blood, losing a little will not harm you. The procedure should not cause much discomfort. Providing sterile equipment is used, there is no risk of a blood-borne infection, such as AIDS or hepatitis B.

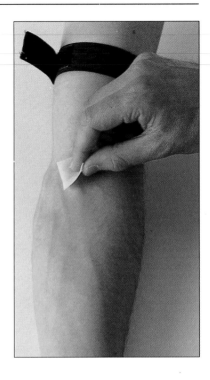

1 To make the vein more prominent, a soft tube or band is wrapped around the upper arm to act as a tourniquet. Skin over the vein is then cleaned with alcohol, prior to inserting the sterile needle.

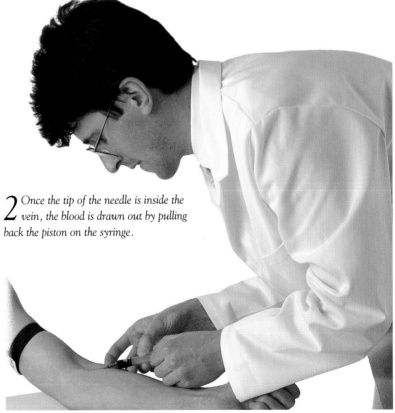

2 Once the tip of the needle is inside the vein, the blood is drawn out by pulling back the piston on the syringe.

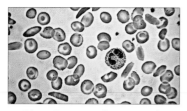

Sickle cell anemia *shows up under the microscope as deformed red blood cells with an elongated, sickle shape.*

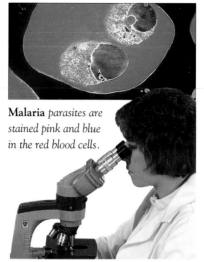

Malaria *parasites are stained pink and blue in the red blood cells.*

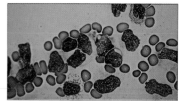

Acute lymphatic leukemia *shows up as abnormal-looking white blood cells with many more immature cells.*

MICROSCOPIC ANALYSIS

Examining a blood smear may reveal abnormal-looking blood cells which signify a particular blood disorder, or the presence of bacteria or parasites. Only red blood cells, white blood cells, and platelets are visible under the microscope. Other substances in blood are too small to be seen – they show up in a chemical analysis.

BLOOD PROTEIN ANALYSIS

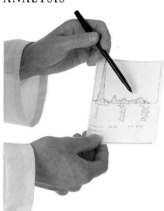

Measuring the level of different blood proteins, such as albumen, enzymes, hormones, and antibodies, can help diagnose disorders of the liver, kidneys, endocrine, and immune systems. Using a technique known as electrophoresis, which uses an electric field to separate out different blood proteins, a breakdown of the concentration of each protein in a sample of blood can be produced.

BLOOD SUGAR CONTROL

Many diabetics monitor how well their condition is being controlled by measuring their blood sugar (glucose) level regularly. If the blood sugar readings are running too high, the diabetic may need to increase the dosage of insulin or re-evaluate the foods in his or her diet.

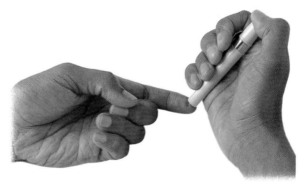

1 A drop of blood is obtained by pricking a fingertip. Some people use an automated device to make it easier to obtain a blood sample.

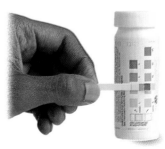

2 Holding the testing strip horizontally, a drop of blood, large enough to cover the chemically treated area, is applied.

3 By comparing the color change on the strip with the printed color scale on the container, the level of glucose in the blood sample can be determined.

URINE TESTS

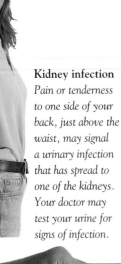

TESTING FOR GLUCOSE, PROTEIN, OR BLOOD

Kidney infection
Pain or tenderness to one side of your back, just above the waist, may signal a urinary infection that has spread to one of the kidneys. Your doctor may test your urine for signs of infection.

Some urine tests need to be done in the laboratory, but others can be performed in a doctor's surgery. A doctor can detect the presence and amount of glucose, protein, and blood in your urine. A test strip that has been impregnated with a range of chemicals is simply dipped into a urine sample. If any of these substances are present, the strip will change color.

1 Dipping the test strip
The strip is dipped in the sample and any excess tapped off against the side. Some strips have several separate colored squares, each of which tests a particular constituent in the urine.

A urine test is a simple way of gaining a wealth of information about the state of your health.

A URINE TEST CAN help confirm the existence of an infection, establish the presence of kidney disease, test for pregnancy, or monitor the control of diabetes.

If a bladder or kidney infection is suspected, you may be asked to follow certain procedures when giving your specimen, such as not taking the sample as soon as you start urinating – a midstream specimen is better because any microorganisms around the opening of the urethra will have been flushed away. Washing yourself thoroughly before giving a sample also helps prevent contamination by microorganisms in the genital area.

An early-morning specimen gives a better chance of finding the bugs, as they will have had all night to multiply their numbers. The more bugs, the easier they will be to see under the microscope.

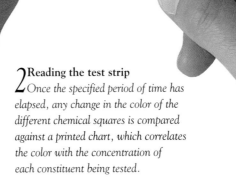

2 Reading the test strip
Once the specified period of time has elapsed, any change in the color of the different chemical squares is compared against a printed chart, which correlates the color with the concentration of each constituent being tested.

CHANGES IN YOUR URINE

The color of your urine may change from time to time. Some of these changes are normal; others may indicate a medical problem.

APPEARANCE	POSSIBLE CAUSES
Pale yellow or colorless	Urine may be diluted after drinking a large volume of fluids.
Darker yellow	Urine may be concentrated due to dehydration caused by sweating or a bout of diarrhea or vomiting.
Orange or red	Certain drugs may change the color of your urine – check with your doctor.
Brown	Broken-down red blood cells not being processed normally due to a liver or gall bladder disorder.
Pink, red, or smoky brown	Blackberries, beetroot, food dyes, and some drugs. If the color persists, the urine will be checked for blood.
Frothy	Protein leaking from a damaged or diseased kidney.

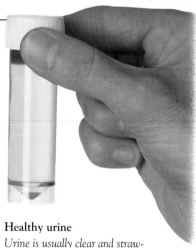

Healthy urine
Urine is usually clear and straw-colored, with only a faint odor.

WHAT IS ABNORMAL?

Blood, glucose, and large amounts of protein in the urine are all abnormal and may signal diabetes, infection, tumors, kidney disease, or prostate trouble in men.

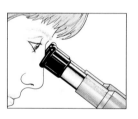

URINE UNDER THE MICROSCOPE

In addition to looking for signs of bacteria, which would confirm the presence of a urinary tract infection, urine may also be examined under the microscope to detect features of other disorders.

Cystourethrography

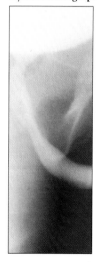

A substance that is opaque to x-rays is introduced into the bladder through the urethra, showing a detailed outline on x-rays taken during urination. This test is often used for children who have had urinary tract infections, to see if the cause is urine flowing back up one of the ureters as the bladder empties.

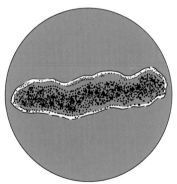

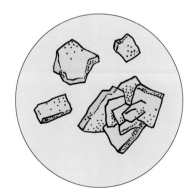

Casts *are a protein-like material that sometimes contain blood cells. Casts in the urine confirm the presence of kidney disease and are normally associated with a high protein loss.*

Crystals *are sometimes normal, but a large number of a particular crystal may indicate a specific metabolic disorder. For example, uric acid crystals are linked with gout and kidney stones.*

WARNING

If your urine starts to smell foul, changes color, becomes blood-stained, or starts to froth excessively, see your doctor as soon as possible for a urine test.

DENTAL HEALTH

DENTAL-CARE EQUIPMENT

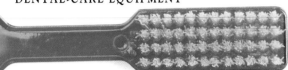

Toothbrush
*Choose a brush
that has soft,
rounded bristles
– harder bristles
may damage tooth
enamel and
puncture the gums.
You may also need
another brush with
a smaller head to
clean areas of the
mouth that are
difficult to reach.*

Daily brushing and flossing help to prevent tooth decay and gum disease.

THE TYPICAL WESTERN diet has so much sugar in it that it is almost impossible to prevent tooth decay completely. However, good dental care, eating fewer sugary foods, and having more regular check-ups by a dentist, can limit the damage.

By brushing your teeth every morning and evening, and after each meal, you will remove food particles, prevent the accumulation of plaque (a sticky coating of saliva, bacteria, and food deposits), stop bad breath, and keep your teeth and gums healthy.

Toothpaste
*Fluoride hardens
tooth enamel.
Therefore regular
brushing with any
toothpaste that
contains fluoride
will help to prevent
tooth decay.*

HOW TO KEEP TEETH AND GUMS HEALTHY

- Visit your dentist every six months.
- Brush your teeth every morning and evening with a fluoride toothpaste and ask your dentist whether your children need to take a fluoride supplement.
- Cut down on sugary foods. Finishing a meal with cheese will help neutralize the acids left around your teeth.
- Floss every day, but be careful not to pull the floss up too hard into your gums.
- Use toothpicks carefully: they can damage your gums.

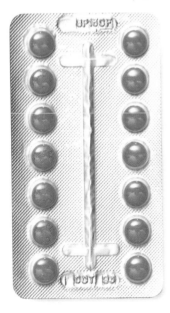

Disclosing tablets
*Chewing a disclosing
tablet releases a dye which
stains plaque red. You
need to improve your
brushing technique in any
red areas to stop decay.*

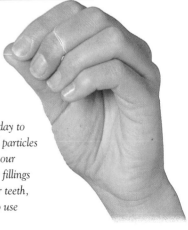

Dental floss
*Use dental floss once a day to
remove plaque and food particles
from the gaps between your
teeth. If you have many fillings
or uneven edges on your teeth,
you may find it easier to use
waxed floss.*

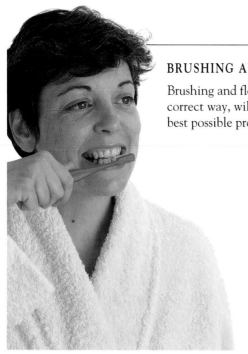

BRUSHING AND FLOSSING

Brushing and flossing your teeth every day, in the correct way, will keep them clean and provide the best possible protection from decay and gum disease.

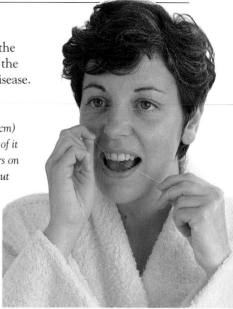

Flossing technique
Take about 12 in (30 cm) of floss and wind most of it round the middle fingers on each hand, leaving about 4 in (10 cm) to draw between your teeth. Slide the floss towards the gum line and then, with a sawing action, remove debris by flossing up and down each tooth in turn.

Brushing technique
The most efficient technique for cleaning teeth is to brush from side to side, and up and down, using small circular strokes. Children's teeth should be brushed in the same way as soon as the first teeth appear.

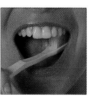

• First brush the inside, then the chewing, and finally the outer surfaces of the teeth. Clean the upper teeth first.

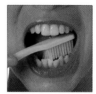

• Plaque builds up where the gums and teeth join, so brush away from the gum as you clean each tooth.

DENTAL CHECKUP

Regular checkups at the dentist, at least once or twice a year, are essential to maintain healthy teeth and gums. Early treatment of tooth decay and gum disease can prevent more serious damage. Wisdom teeth can be removed if they are impacted or if there is overcrowding.

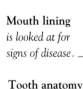

Mouth lining
is looked at for signs of disease.

Tooth anatomy
is inspected. Signs of overcrowding, irregular wear, and any missing teeth are noted.

Gums *are checked for signs of disease, such as bleeding, inflammation, and swelling.*

Dental x-rays *reveal disorders of the teeth and gums that cannot be seen just by looking inside the mouth.*

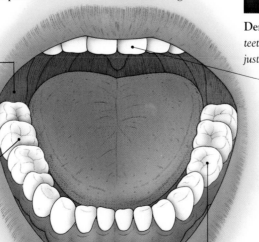

Dentures *are checked for correct fit and function.*

Biting surfaces *are examined for decay, excessive grinding, chipping, staining, and an abnormal bite.*

HEART WATCH

Early detection and treatment of heart and circulatory disorders, such as angina and high blood pressure, reduces the risk of heart disease.

DISORDERS OF THE heart and the circulatory system cause many different symptoms. These same warning signs can, however, relate to other more trivial problems.

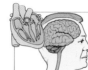

Dizziness and fainting
Most attacks of dizziness are not serious, but if they happen often, a heart or circulatory problem may be the cause, particularly if the feeling of light-headedness always occurs during exercise.

Fainting is usually harmless. It may be brought on by standing for a long time in a hot or stuffy atmosphere. Severe pain or a shock can cause fainting by overstimulating the vagus nerve which slows down the heart beat. If fainting is due to a serious heart disorder then it may occur during vigorous exercise. This, however, is rare.

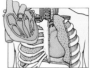

Chest pain
Most chest pain is not related to the heart at all. It is commonly caused by some form of muscle strain, heartburn, or a trapped nerve. Cramping central chest pain may, however, be due to coronary heart disease and should not be ignored. Contact your doctor immediately if it occurs.

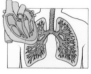

Breathlessness
It is quite normal to become a little out of breath during strenuous exertion, but severe breathlessness, or breathing difficulty when resting or doing only a gentle exercise, may be a symptom of heart failure.

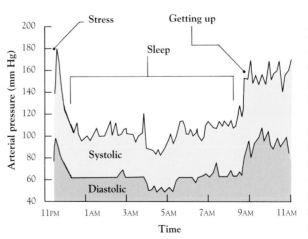

A fit heart
Regular exercise keeps you fit and reduces your risk of suffering from a heart disorder.

HIGH BLOOD PRESSURE

One in eight people in the US has high blood pressure, which means that their blood pressure remains high even when resting. Untreated, it increases the risk of having a heart attack, stroke, or other circulatory disease. Since it does not always cause symptoms, all adults should have their blood pressure routinely checked at least every three years. Low blood pressure is not a problem, unless associated with a recent accident or trauma.

Stress · Getting up · Sleep · Systolic · Diastolic

Arterial pressure (mm Hg): 200, 180, 160, 140, 120, 100, 80, 60, 40

Time: 11PM, 1AM, 3AM, 5AM, 7AM, 9AM, 11AM

Daily changes
Systolic and diastolic blood pressure readings fluctuate according to changes in activity. Blood pressure is at its highest during stress, pain, or physical exertion, and at its lowest during sleep.

Swollen ankles

Fluid retention in the tissues around the ankles is occasionally due to heart failure. More commonly, it is the result of a vein disorder aggravated by immobility.

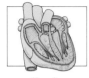

Palpitations

A fluttering or thumping sensation in the chest is usually due to a person becoming more aware of their heart beating, or of harmless extra beats.

HOW TO HELP SOMEONE HAVING A HEART ATTACK

Prompt first aid can save a life. If someone collapses or has symptoms of a heart attack, you should:

• Call for medical help immediately; most deaths occur at an early stage, and often could have been avoided.
• Loosen tight clothing around the neck and chest.
• Keep the victim as calm as possible.
• If breathing stops, start mouth-to-mouth resuscitation (see p299).
• If you cannot feel a pulse, begin external heart massage – if you have been trained to perform it correctly.

AM I HAVING A HEART ATTACK?

A heart attack occurs when an area of heart muscle is severely deprived of oxygen, due to a blockage in one of the coronary arteries. Pain that comes on during exertion and fades away quickly when you rest may be due to angina, in which the blood flow to the heart muscle is reduced. If the pain is not relieved by rest and lasts for 20 minutes or longer, you may be having a heart attack.

Chest pain
Most heart attack victims suffer chest pain – usually a dull, crushing pain like a weight on the chest lasting over 20 minutes.

Fever
There is almost always a slight fever that starts within 12 hours and lasts up to one week.

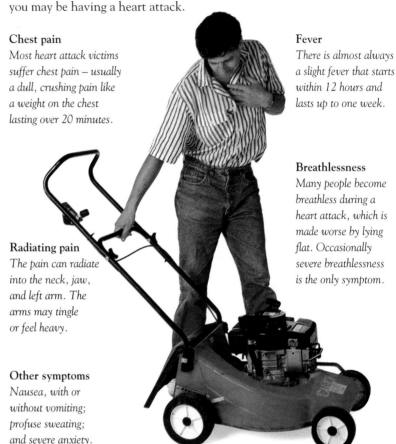

Breathlessness
Many people become breathless during a heart attack, which is made worse by lying flat. Occasionally severe breathlessness is the only symptom.

Radiating pain
The pain can radiate into the neck, jaw, and left arm. The arms may tingle or feel heavy.

Other symptoms
Nausea, with or without vomiting; profuse sweating; and severe anxiety.

IS YOUR HEART AT RISK?

The risk of heart disease increases with age and is more common in men than women. You are also at greater risk if anyone in your family has had a heart attack before the age of 60.

You cannot change heredity factors, but you can control your lifestyle. Eat a low-fat, high-fiber diet and take regular exercise to help reduce your cholesterol level. Stop smoking – cigarette smoking greatly increases the risk of heart disease. Drink alcohol in moderation – drinking to excess puts your heart at risk. Keep your weight under control, too. Obesity increases your chances of having high blood pressure and a high blood cholesterol level, which in turn increase the risk to your heart.

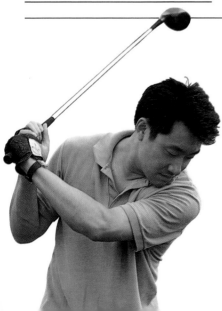

Chest pain while playing sport
is usually the result of a muscle strain, trapped nerve, or inflamed rib joint. But if the pain is severe or persists, or if there are other symptoms, consult a doctor.

TESTING FOR HEART DISEASE

To DIAGNOSE HEART disease, doctors listen to the heart with a stethoscope; study its electrical activity on an electrocardiogram (ECG); and image its shape, size, pumping action, valve function, and blood flow, using ultrasound and other specialized equipment.

The simplest test of the heart is to listen to it beating. The familiar "lubb-dupp" sounds made by the

Monitoring the heart's activities may reveal the presence of heart disease.

heart as it beats are caused by the heart valves slamming shut to prevent a back-flow of blood.

To your doctor, the sounds your heart makes may reveal a damaged valve, a congenital defect, or a damaged or diseased heart muscle

wall. However, not all unusual sounds are abnormal.

Listening to the heart cannot, however, reveal coronary heart disease. Specific tests such as an ECG, an exercise stress test, or cardiac blood pool imaging may be needed.

Recording an ECG
Electrodes are connected to the wrist, ankles, and six positions on the chest. Two electrodes are activated at a time to complete a circuit with the ECG machine.

ECG Machine

The heart's electrical activity is then recorded as a wave pattern.

Normal ECG

Abnormal ECG

An abnormal heartbeat
Damage to the heart muscle usually changes the wave pattern produced on an ECG. In this tracing, which shows six beats, the heart is beating fast and erratically. This is often due to coronary heart disease, although it can be caused by an overactive thyroid.

ELECTROCARDIOGRAPHY (ECG)

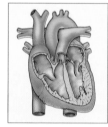

An electrocardiogram monitors the electrical activity of the heart. This activity is recorded, allowing the doctor to diagnose a wide range of heart disorders. In a healthy person, the passage of electrical impulses through the heart muscle follows a regular wave pattern with a characteristic shape. The unhealthy heart is equally predictable, with different heart disorders producing their own specific abnormal pattern of electrical activity. The ECG is not just one recording, but a series of recordings produced by attaching electrodes to different parts of the body. Each recording looks at the electrical activity at a slightly different axis through the heart. Analysis of the many different wave patterns allows not only the nature of the disorder to be established, but also the precise location of any heart muscle damage.

Having an ECG
In order to produce a clear tracing you must lie still, relax, and breathe normally. Your heart's activity is then recorded on a machine that will either print out the wave pattern on a moving sheet of paper or show it on a monitor.

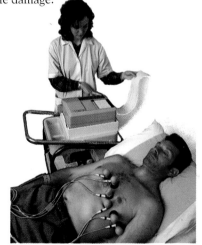

LISTENING TO THE HEART

To hear the noises made by each heart valve more clearly, the end of a stethoscope is placed at the four different sites that correspond to the positions of the four different valves. To make the sounds clearer, you may be asked to hold your breath, to lean forwards, or to lie on your left side.

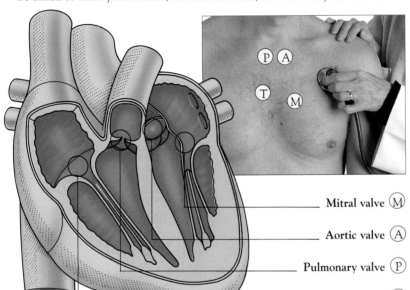

Mitral valve (M)

Aortic valve (A)

Pulmonary valve (P)

Tricuspid valve (T)

CARDIAC BLOOD POOL IMAGING

To see how well the heart pumps, a radioactive substance is injected into the bloodstream. When it reaches the heart the change in radioactivity shows the difference in blood volume between when the chambers contract and relax, reflecting the heart's pumping ability.

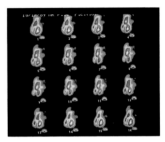

Scans *taken during the imaging show one complete heart cycle.*

EXERCISE STRESS TEST

To assess the heart's response to physical activity, the electrical impulses of the heart muscle are recorded during exercise. Testing is stopped if there are any signs of distress.

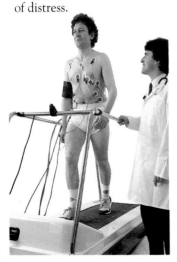

LIVING WITH A HEART CONDITION

People with many types of heart condition are now encouraged to live life to the full and not to regard themselves as being disabled.

Cigarettes
If you smoke, stop. This will prevent your heart from deteriorating.

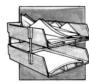
Relaxation
Leisure activities can avoid a potentially dangerous build-up of stress and tension.

Exercise
Improving your physical fitness can improve the overall function of both your heart and your circulation.

Sex
If you are fit enough to cope with the exertion of climbing stairs, sex is good for both your heart and your happiness.

Obesity
Losing excess weight through a calorie-controlled diet and a gentle exercise program will reduce unnecessary strain on the heart.

Alcohol
One or two drinks a day may be good for your circulation, but try to avoid drinking more because of its damaging effect on the heart muscle.

CANCER FACTS

More than one million people develop cancer each year in the US.

AFTER HEART DISEASE, cancer is the second most common cause of death in the US. New treatments and better screening have reduced the incidence of some types of cancer. The overall death rate, however, is still increasing because the average age of the population is rising. Cancer is mainly a disease of middle and old age. The more old people there are, the higher the number of cancer cases.

The main killer is lung cancer. Death rates from this cancer are still rising, especially for women. However, lung cancer can often be prevented as it is closely, though not always, related to smoking.

What is cancer?

The term cancer actually refers to at least 200 different conditions, involving almost every tissue or organ in the body. Cancer is a disease that causes cells to grow when they should not and to spread to tissues where they should not be.

What causes cancer?

Within the DNA (genetic material) of each cell there are thought to be certain genes which are concerned solely with the promotion of cell growth and replication.

Exposure to a cancer-causing factor, or carcinogen, can change genetic material and transform a normal cell into one that grows abnormally to produce a malignant tumor. Carcinogenic substances include tobacco (see p104), some foods (see p76), and radiation.

(see p104), (see p76)

CANCER TERMINOLOGY

- **Carcinoma** – any cancer arising from cells in the surface lining of a body structure.
- **Leukemia** – cancer of the white blood cells in the bone marrow.
- **Lymphoma** – cancer of a tissue in the lymphatic system.
- **Myeloma** – cancer of the plasma cells in the bone marrow.
- **Sarcoma** – any cancer arising from the body's supporting and connective tissues, such as the muscles, tendons, and bones.

WHICH CANCERS ARE MOST COMMON IN THE US?

The 10 cancers that occur most commonly in both sexes are shown in the table below. Rarer cancers make up the remainder of new cases each year.

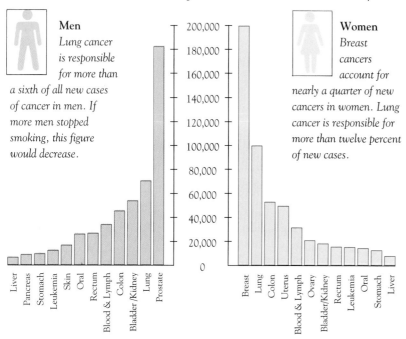

Men
Lung cancer is responsible for more than a sixth of all new cases of cancer in men. If more men stopped smoking, this figure would decrease.

Women
Breast cancers account for nearly a quarter of new cancers in women. Lung cancer is responsible for more than twelve percent of new cases.

Men chart (cancers left to right): Liver, Pancreas, Stomach, Leukemia, Skin, Oral, Rectum, Blood & Lymph, Colon, Bladder/Kidney, Lung, Prostate

Women chart (cancers left to right): Breast, Lung, Colon, Uterus, Blood & Lymph, Ovary, Bladder/Kidney, Rectum, Leukemia, Oral, Stomach, Liver

Scale: 0, 20,000, 40,000, 60,000, 80,000, 100,000, 120,000, 140,000, 160,000, 180,000, 200,000

Total numbers of new cancer cases in the US each year

HOW FAST DOES A CANCER GROW?

The smallest mass that can be detected by x-rays or scans is about 0.1 in (2 mm) in diameter. A tumor, such as the one shown below, may take a year to reach this size. Some, however, take only a few weeks.

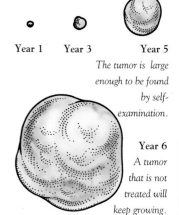

Year 1   Year 3   Year 5

The tumor is large enough to be found by self-examination.

Year 6
A tumor that is not treated will keep growing.

Q *Is cancer on the increase?*

A Cancer is not a new disease – there is evidence that it existed in ancient man. The apparent increase in the incidence of cancer is partly due to the fact that people now talk more freely about it and partly because people are living longer. Seventy percent of all new cancers occur in people over the age of 60.

Q *Is there an inherited tendency towards developing certain cancers?*

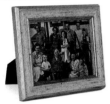

A The exact contribution of hereditary factors to the risk of developing cancer is not fully understood. Only a few rare cancers can be attributed solely to inheritance. Breast cancer, for instance, does run in families but will not affect everyone in the family. This suggests that other factors, such as diet, play a part.

Q *How is cancer treated today?*

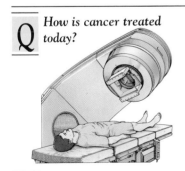

A Almost all cancers are still treated by surgery, often followed by radiotherapy and anti-cancer drugs to suppress or arrest the growth and replication of any cancer cells that remain.

Q *Do all cancers behave in the same way?*

A No two cancers are the same. They vary in the speed with which they spread, in their readiness to form a second cancer in another part of the body (known as metastasis), and in their response to treatment.

Q *Does the body have any natural defences against cancer?*

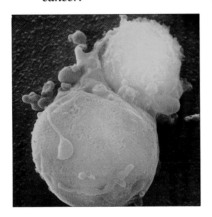

A Yes, the body's immune system fights cancer cells. This system recognizes the abnormal cancer cells as foreign bodies and then sends out T-lymphocytes to destroy them by binding onto them and interfering with their growth and replication. Anything that damages the immune system increases the risk of developing cancer.

Q *How is cancer diagnosed?*

A A pathologist is usually able to tell the difference between healthy cells and cancerous cells by examining a sample of suspect tissue or body fluid under a microscope. It may also be possible to predict whether a cancer is going to be fast- or slow-growing.

Q *Is cancer an inevitable part of aging?*

A Aging leads to the immune system becoming less efficient at detecting and killing cancer cells. This is why over one-third of all people who live beyond 70 will eventually be found to have some form of cancer.

Q *Why does cancer cause weight loss?*

A People who have cancer may suffer a marked reduction in weight in the later stages of their disease or just after surgery. This can simply be due to loss of appetite. The main reason, however, is that tumors use a lot of calories and nutrients to support their energy and growth needs.

Q *How successful are cancer treatments?*

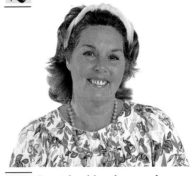

A Considerable advances have been made over the last few years. Cancers that had a poor outlook in the past, such as testicular, ovarian, and uterine cancer, Hodgkin's lymphoma, and some leukemias, can now be treated successfully. New drugs that can relieve symptoms help patients to continue leading active lives too.

267

CANCER WATCH

TO DETECT CANCER in its early stages, learn to recognize the various warning symptoms, examine yourself regularly, and have professional cancer screening.

Detecting cancer early means that there is a better chance of curing it.

The risk of developing cancer

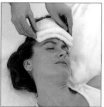

Statistics have revealed that cancer will develop at some time in about a third of the population. Treatment is most successful if it is started before too much damage has occurred, so learn to recognize the early warning signs of cancer.

Cancer may cause a variety of minor symptoms, such as feeling unwell or feverish, but unless these symptoms continue for several days,

there is no need to see your doctor. There are, however, other, more specific symptoms and signs of cancer that should always be taken seriously. These symptoms do not mean you have cancer, but you should see your doctor so that the possibility can be ruled out.

Coughing up blood-stained phlegm might be due to lung cancer, especially if you smoke now or once smoked, so see your doctor immediately. Hoarseness is usually due to laryngitis; however if it lasts longer than one week, or is recurrent, it could indicate a serious underlying disorder, including several types of cancer.

Unexplained lumps

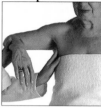

The presence of an unexplained lump or bump on any part of the body is one of the most significant signs of cancer, even though most of these swellings are not cancerous. Because of the slight risk, however, anyone who finds a persistent lump or swelling under the skin should see a doctor for a checkup. Women should examine their breasts for lumps once a month. Breast cancer is more easily treatable in the early stages.

SELF-EXAMINATION

Be thorough
You must examine every area of your body. For instance, men with facial hair should remember to feel for lumps beneath this hair.

Because you are the person most familiar with the look, shape, and feel of your body, you are in the best position to notice any significant changes that may indicate cancer or another health problem. Women should carry out regular self-examination of their breasts (see p274). Men should also get into the habit of examining their testicles for lumps, irregularities, or changes in firmness (see p227). Examining your skin is a vital check for skin cancer (see p270).

LOOKING OUT FOR CANCER

If you notice any of the following symptoms, contact your doctor as soon as possible:

• A scab, sore, or ulcer that fails to heal within three weeks, either on your skin or in your mouth or nose.
• A breast lump, change in breast shape, or discolored or blood-stained discharge from the nipple.
• Change in shape or size of a testicle.

• A wart or mole that enlarges, bleeds, or itches.
• Unexplained bruising.
• Rectal bleeding, particularly if the blood is mixed in with the stool.
• Bleeding from the vagina between periods, after sexual intercourse, or after the menopause.
• Coughing up any blood or blood-stained phlegm.
• Blood in the urine.

Swollen neck glands caused by an infection may cause difficulty swallowing. If this symptom persists or worsens, see your doctor who can check that it is not due to a cancer of the esophagus (gullet).

The abdomen and bowel

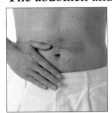

Persistent or recurrent abdominal pain is not usually due to cancer. Conditions like irritable bowel syndrome, gallstones, or a peptic ulcer are more likely causes.

A sudden alteration in your bowel habits, that is not the result of a change in diet or minor illness, must always be investigated by a doctor. It is normally caused by an intestinal disorder other than cancer, but the possibility of a malignant growth needs to be excluded.

See your doctor if you have any rectal bleeding. The most common causes are hemorrhoids or a small tear in the skin around the anus, when the blood will usually be bright red and seen on the toilet paper. If blood is actually mixed in with the feces, cancer of the bowel wall is a possible diagnosis.

DO NOT DELAY

If you develop a warning symptom of cancer, do not ignore it. In reality, a disorder other than cancer is far more likely. However, any delay in seeing your doctor will not only prolong your fears; it might also reduce your chances of successful treatment, if the diagnosis does turn out to be cancer.

Other symptoms

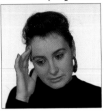

Losing weight for no apparent reason may be due to cancer, but other conditions, such as depression, may also be the cause.

Vaginal bleeding between your periods, after sex, or after the menopause, may be a symptom of cancer of the cervix or uterus, so see your doctor. There are, however, many other possible reasons.

Persistent or recurrent headaches may, very rarely, be due to a brain tumor. If so, the pain becomes more severe with time, is worse on waking, and is invariably accompanied by neurological symptoms, for instance, muscle weakness or loss of coordination.

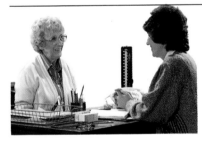

SCREENING TESTS

Screening can detect specific types of cancer early, before symptoms appear, so that any treatment needed can be started when it is most effective. Research is still in progress to evaluate how and when these tests should be done and at what ages. Some are recommended for people known to be at high risk; others are performed on wider target groups within the general population based on factors such as age or sex.

TEST	HOW OFTEN?	WHY IS IT DONE?	WHEN TO TEST MORE OFTEN
Cervical smear	Every one to three years for women aged 18 to 64 who have ever had sex.	Reveals abnormal cells that could develop into cancer of the cervix.	If you have ever had an abnormal smear or your doctor advises it.
Mammography (breast x-ray)	Every one to three years, starting at age 40 to 50.	Detects breast cancers in their early stages.	If you have had breast cancer or a family history of the disease.
Fecal occult blood	Once a year after age 45 to 50.	To detect any abnormalities of the lower bowel.	High-risk individuals (those with colitis or colon polyps).
Sigmoidoscopy/ colonoscopy	Everyone should be tested once at age 60.	To detect any abnormalities of the lower bowel.	Every three years if you have colitis or colon polyps.

SKIN WATCH

Everyone should examine their skin regularly for changes that may indicate health problems and to detect signs of cancer.

YOUR SKIN AND THE SUN

People who are exposed to strong sunlight over many years will develop wrinkles at a much younger age. This is caused by a breakdown in the elastic tissues under the skin's surface. Exposure to sunlight also increases the risk of suffering from all types of skin cancer.

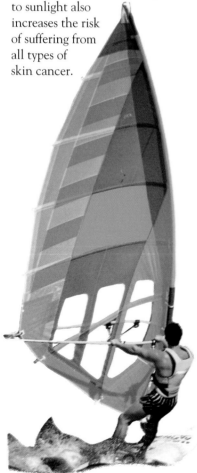

ALTHOUGH THE incidence of skin cancer has increased over the last 10 years, a great many cases could have been avoided easily by reducing the amount of exposure to sunlight. Because most skin cancers are curable if they are discovered and treated at an early enough stage, it is vital that you recognize any abnormal change in the appearance of your skin.

Everyone should examine their skin regularly, but some people are more at risk from skin cancer than others. Those who have a very fair complexion, who are over 30 years of age, and have sunbathed without adequate protection need to be particularly observant.

How to check your skin

Examine yourself in a well-lit room, preferably in front of a full-length mirror. Use a hand mirror to look at any inaccessible areas.

Get to know the appearance of your skin. To help you detect very subtle changes, draw outlines on a piece of paper of the front and back of your body. Mark on them your moles and any other significant blemishes. Each time you perform the examination, you can refer to these "skin maps".

Pay particular attention to those areas of your body that are often exposed to the sun, including your

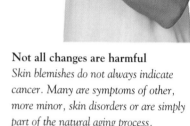

Not all changes are harmful
Skin blemishes do not always indicate cancer. Many are symptoms of other, more minor, skin disorders or are simply part of the natural aging process.

scalp. Men should remember to check under any facial hair. Skin cancer, however, can occur in any area of the body, even the soles of your feet, which rarely see sunlight.

What to look for

Changes that could signify the onset of cancer include a sudden change in skin color or texture (dark spots under a fingernail or toenail could be a warning sign of a malignant melanoma), a sore or an ulcer that fails to heal within three weeks, or a new mole or blemish that itches, bleeds, or changes shape, size, or color.

PREVENTING SKIN CANCER

• Sunbathe sensibly. If you are fair-skinned you should only sunbathe for 15 minutes when the sun is strong. Increase this time by around 30 minutes a day for the first week.
• Stay in the shade between 10AM and 2PM, when the sun is most intense and likely to burn your skin.

• Remember that a sun-hat and clothing are the best sunscreens.
• Use a sunscreen with a high protection factor if you are exposed to strong sunlight or if the sun is being reflected off water, sand, or snow.
• Sun lamps and sun beds may harm your skin, so do not overuse them.

HOW TO RECOGNIZE A MALIGNANT MELANOMA

A malignant melanoma is a type of skin cancer which can spread to other parts of the body. If it is not diagnosed at an early stage it can prove fatal. The tumor usually develops on an area of skin that is often exposed to the sun, and typically grows from an existing mole.

Healthy mole – *small, brown, circular, flat or evenly raised, and symmetrical.*

Unhealthy mole – *revealed by changes in shape, color, or size. Look for any new moles too.*

WHAT IS A SKIN BIOPSY?

If there is any abnormal change in your skin, your doctor may do a biopsy to assess its cause. Under local anesthetic, a small section of skin is removed and examined for signs of disease. The wound is then closed with sutures. If the doctor suspects cancer, a surrounding area of healthy looking skin may be removed as well to make the assessment more reliable.

COMMON SKIN DISORDERS

When you examine your skin for early signs of cancer you are more likely to find other skin disorders, which, although they can be distressing, are much less serious and respond readily to treatment. If you have a problem with persistent itching, an unsightly rash, or troublesome spots, see your doctor as soon as possible. Over-the-counter medication should not be used until a doctor has diagnosed your problem.

Ringworm
This fungal infection appears as rings of red, scaly skin, which are itchy. The same group of fungi also cause athlete's foot and rashes in folds of skin such as under the breasts. Antifungal drugs are used to kill off fungal cells.

Allergic dermatitis
Allergy reactions can cause redness, swelling, and itching. Steroid ointments and antihistamines help this condition.

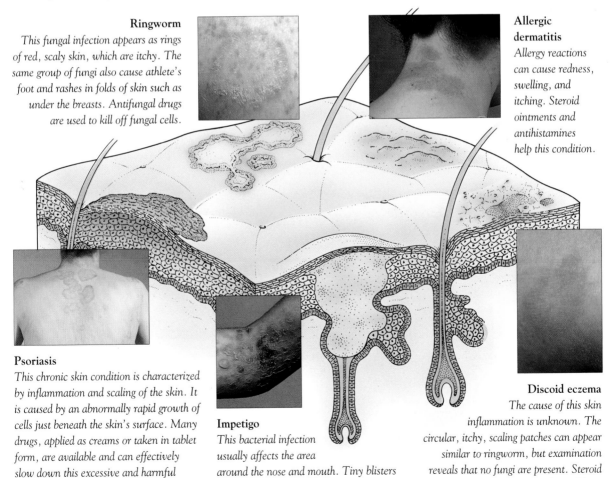

Psoriasis
This chronic skin condition is characterized by inflammation and scaling of the skin. It is caused by an abnormally rapid growth of cells just beneath the skin's surface. Many drugs, applied as creams or taken in tablet form, are available and can effectively slow down this excessive and harmful production of new skin cells.

Impetigo
This bacterial infection usually affects the area around the nose and mouth. Tiny blisters appear which then rupture and form a crust.

Discoid eczema
The cause of this skin inflammation is unknown. The circular, itchy, scaling patches can appear similar to ringworm, but examination reveals that no fungi are present. Steroid ointments alleviate the problem.

MOUTH AND BOWEL DISORDERS

Your mouth and bowel provide vital clues to your state of health.

THE TWO ENDS of the digestive tract, the mouth and the bowel, can easily be observed for signs of cancer or other illness. By checking inside your mouth and being aware of any changes in your normal pattern of bowel activity, you can help safeguard your health.

When to see your doctor

Bowel activity varies among the healthy population, from twice a day, to once a week. Changes in bowel activity can be due to a stomach upset, but they may also be caused by colitis, irritable bowel syndrome, or bowel cancer. Therefore, you should see a doctor if you have a persistent change in the frequency of your bowel movements.

Some stool types can indicate a disorder. See your doctor if your stools become pale, bulky, greasy, foul-smelling, and tend to float; tarry and black; or contain blood.

Over 90 percent of cancers in the colon or rectum occur in those over 50 and begin as polyps on the bowel lining. Some doctors therefore recommend annual tests, such as fecal occult blood testing, for everyone over 50.

EXAMINING YOUR MOUTH

Examine your lips, gums, tongue, teeth, and mouth lining regularly in front of a mirror in a good light. If you find any of the warning signs described below you should visit your doctor or dentist for a check-up.

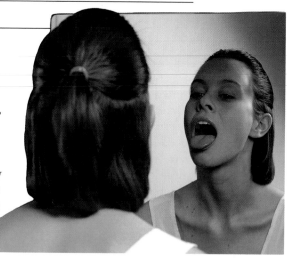

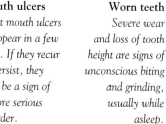

Mouth infection
Sore white patches on the tongue and mouth lining may be caused by a fungal infection (thrush).

Sore tongue
A sore, bright red, and unnaturally smooth tongue may be caused either by anaemia or a vitamin deficiency.

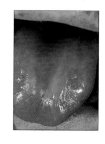

Bleeding gums
Red, swollen, and bleeding gums are early signs of gum disease and can be reduced by better mouth care such as regular flossing.

Lips
Painful blistering on the lip or inside the mouth may be due to a herpes infection.

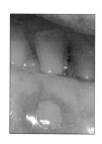

Mouth ulcers
Most mouth ulcers disappear in a few days. If they recur or persist, they may be a sign of a more serious disorder.

Worn teeth
Severe wear and loss of tooth height are signs of unconscious biting and grinding, usually while asleep.

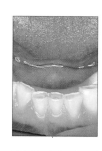

SIGNS OF MOUTH CANCER

See your doctor if you have:
• A bleeding ulcer or sore area in or around the mouth that does not heal within three weeks.

• A white patch, lump, or swelling.
• Recurrent mouth bleeding or numbness or pain in the mouth or throat with no apparent cause.

FIBER AND BOWEL CANCER

A high-fiber diet reduces the incidence of cancer of the colon and of the rectum. Evidence suggests that cancers in the large bowel are more common in those people with a sluggish bowel action. By speeding the passage of fecal material through the digestive tract, fiber reduces the time that cancer-causing substances in the feces are in contact with the bowel lining.

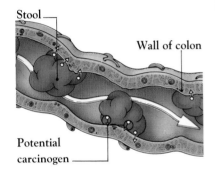

Stool

Wall of colon

Potential carcinogen

Hard, dry stools
A diet that is low in fiber will cause the stools to become hard and dry. Because these stools are less fluid, they cannot pass through the bowel quickly and potential cancer-causers are in contact with the bowel lining for a longer period of time.

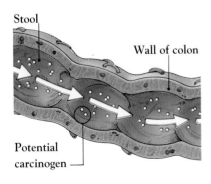

Stool

Wall of colon

Potential carcinogen

Soft, fluid stools
A diet that is rich in high-fiber foods, such as baked beans, bran, granary bread, and sweetcorn, increases the bulk of the stools. This speeds the stools' passage through the bowel and reduces the risk of cancer.

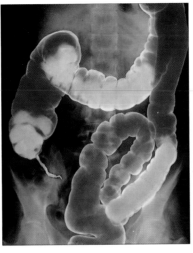

BARIUM X-RAYS

The bowel lining does not show up on x-rays so it must be coated with barium, which is opaque to x-rays, to show any abnormalities. Barium sulphate mixed with water is given as an enema or swallowed. It takes up to five hours before barium that has been swallowed reaches all the small bowel, while a barium enema is completed within 25 minutes.

Revealing the bowel
A barium x-ray enables a doctor to study the bowel in great detail.

FECAL OCCULT BLOOD

The presence of a minute amount of blood in the feces can be detected with a chemical indicator that reacts with blood. A thin film of the stool is smeared onto a chemically-coated piece of paper. If, when a drop of an oxidizing agent is added, the feces-covered paper turns blue, blood is present.

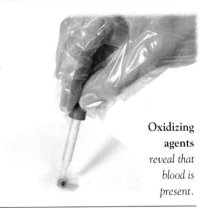

Oxidizing agents *reveal that blood is present.*

COLONOSCOPY AND SIGMOIDOSCOPY

A long, thin, flexible viewing tube called a colonoscope may be used to examine the lining of the colon (colonoscopy). The tube is lubricated and guided through the anus and rectum, into the colon. As the scope is withdrawn, the doctor examines each area of the colon wall that comes into view, removing any polyp or ulcer that could be malignant for analysis. The procedure for a sigmoidoscopy is similar, but only the lower part of the bowel is examined.

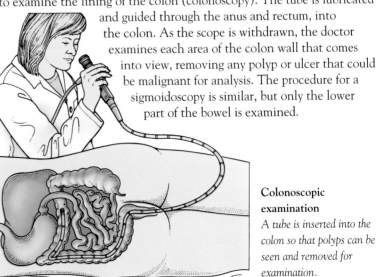

Colonoscopic examination
A tube is inserted into the colon so that polyps can be seen and removed for examination.

BREAST SCREENING

BREASTS DIFFER WIDELY in size, shape, and texture from one woman to another. By performing a monthly self-examination, you can become familiar with the normal characteristics of your breasts, and will therefore find it easier to notice any sudden changes.

If you find a lump
You should see a doctor at once if you find a lump or any change in your breasts. Worrying about your discovery will only waste time – keep in mind that some 90 percent of breast lumps are not cancerous.

All women over the age of 20 should examine their breasts every month for any changes.

An examination and a test such as mammography or ultrasound can rule out cancer and put your mind at ease. If a lump does turn out to be cancer, an early diagnosis is a great bonus, because it can be treated much more effectively in its early stages.

Further tests
Cancerous and benign lumps can feel the same, even to an experi- enced doctor, so further tests such as ultrasound, x-rays, or a biopsy may be required.

If a biopsy reveals that the lump is benign, then no more treatment will usually be needed. If it appears cancerous, or the diagnosis remains in doubt, surgery, such as removal of the lump, may be carried out. Radiotherapy or chemotherapy, and in some cases hormone thera- py, may also be offered.

BREAST SELF-EXAMINATION

Examine your breasts at the end of your period, when they are not swollen. It is important to do this every month so that you can detect any changes quickly. Some women's breasts are naturally lumpy, so getting used to what is normal for you is important. It is not just lumps that you have to look out for – coloured discharge from the nipple and an orange-peel appearance to the skin are other warning signs.

1 Sit or stand in front of a large mirror with your arms hanging loosely by your side. Be sure to sit up straight. Study the appearance, size, and contour of each breast. You should watch out for changes in the size of your breasts, one breast being lower than the other, a turned-in nipple, or puckering or dimpling of the skin. Gently lift your breasts so that you can see the undersides if they are not easily visible.

— Inverted nipple

Lump — Dimpling of the skin

Bloody or colored discharge

What to look for
An increase in size, or any dimpling or puckering of the breast, or changes in the nipple's size, shape, or color.

2 Raise each arm in turn and check for dimpling. Turn from side to side to observe the outline. Then raise both arms together and look at your nipples – they should both move upwards about the same distance.

MAMMOGRAPHY

Mammography is a type of x-ray that visualizes the internal structure of the breasts. One breast at a time is placed on an x-ray film and a plastic cover gently flattens the breast tissue. The procedure is usually painless, and the dose of radiation minimal. It shows a growth when it would still be too small to be felt by hand. If an abnormal area is found, further tests will need to be carried out.

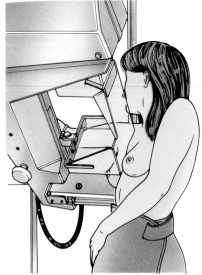

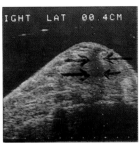

WARNING

Cancer of the breast is the most common cancer in women. The earlier a cancer is diagnosed and treated, the greater the chance of a successful recovery.

Breast ultrasound
This completely painless procedure involves passing sound waves through the breast tissue to identify any lumps.

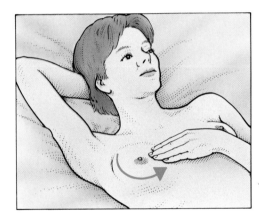

3 *To examine the right breast, lie in a relaxed position and put your right hand behind your head. Pressing gently but firmly with the middle three fingertips of your left hand, run your hand from beneath your armpit, first along the underside of your breast towards the center of your chest, then across the top half of the breast, and finally across the center of your breast over the nipple.*

MONITORING YOUR BREASTS
Changes that can be detected by self-examination

- A lump or lumpy area.
- An increase in the size of one breast only.
- Puckering or dimpling of the skin.
- A turned-in nipple (unless this is normal for you).
- Discharge from one nipple.
- A rash, or change in skin texture.
- Swelling of the upper arm or under the armpit.
- Enlarged or swollen lymph glands.
- Persistent pain in one breast area.

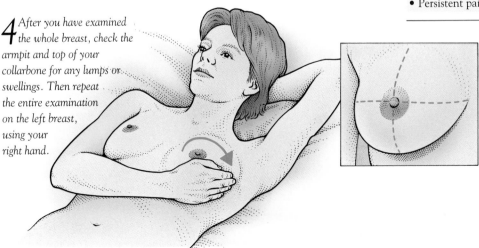

4 *After you have examined the whole breast, check the armpit and top of your collarbone for any lumps or swellings. Then repeat the entire examination on the left breast, using your right hand.*

5 *To help you remember to feel the whole breast, and to make it easier to describe any change you may find, divide each breast into imaginary quadrants with the nipple as the center. By examining your breasts regularly you will learn what is normal for your breasts.*

THE CERVICAL SMEAR

This test is thought to have saved thousands of lives since its introduction over 40 years ago.

CHANGES IN THE cervix can be detected by a cervical smear. Early "precancerous" changes, known as dysplasia, are easily detected and treated, thus preventing invasive cancer from developing.

An abnormal smear does not mean cancer. The most common abnormality is a mild dysplasia, where the abnormal cells will often disappear spontaneously within a few months. If this happens no treatment will be needed. If dysplasia persists, however, most doctors recommend that it is treated.

If the dysplasia is more severe, a colposcope is used to investigate. The colposcope is a high-powered microscope with its own light source which allows the surface of the cervix to be examined.

If cervical precancer remains undiscovered or untreated then it may progress to cervical cancer. Possibly one in three women with the severest grade of precancer will develop cancer. Since there is no way to predict who will develop cancer, all women with this condition should have treatment.

WHEN TO HAVE A SMEAR

Some doctors recommend that all sexually active women between the ages of 18 and 64 be tested every five years. However, as there is a risk that the smear may not be 100 per cent accurate and because the disease can spread rapidly, many gynaecologists advise more frequent screening. Have your initial smear within six months of first having sex. A second smear should be taken one year later. Then, have a smear at least every three years, if each test is normal.

HAVING A CERVICAL SMEAR

Although the availability and high success rate of this test have been well publicized, there are many women who still do not visit their doctors for a regular cervical smear test. The test itself is a simple, painless procedure that can detect abnormal changes in the cells on the surface of the cervix before any cancer appears. If the disease is caught at this point in its development then simple treatment will totally cure it. However, you will need to continue having regular cervical smear tests.

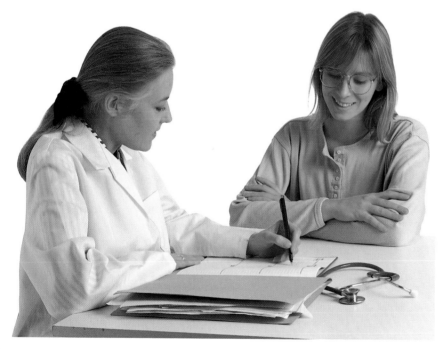

SCREENING SAVES LIVES

Screening for cervical cancer saves lives by allowing changes in the cervix to be monitored and any cancers to be discovered early when they are most treatable. Many women who have an invasive cervical cancer will not survive for more than five years, but 100 per cent of women whose precancers are detected by screening and treated will live out a normal life span.

1 *The doctor or nurse will probably ask you many background details, such as when your last period was, how many children you have had, what contraceptive methods you are using, and what the result of your last smear was.*

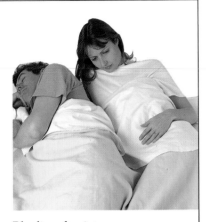

Bleeding after intercourse
Always have a smear if you experience this type of bleeding. It can be a sign of cervical erosion, a benign condition, or cervical cancer.

ASSESSING THE RISK

If you answer YES to one or more of the questions below, you may be more likely to contract cervical cancer and should have cervical smears more frequently.

- Were you very young when you began having sexual intercourse?
- Have either you or your partner had a lot of sexual partners?
- Have you been exposed to the genital wart virus? (Some types can put you at risk.)
- Do you smoke?
- Have you ever had a positive cervical smear?

WHAT A SMEAR LOOKS LIKE

Under the microscope, the cells are examined for abnormalities. If the smear shows any abnormal changes, further tests, such as colposcopy, will be performed to discover exactly what these changes mean.

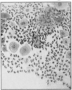 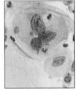

Normal smear   Abnormal smear

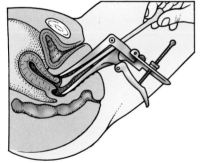

2 A speculum is gently inserted into the vagina to hold it open, so that the cervix can be seen by the doctor or nurse. A lubricant may be used to make insertion easier. The cervix will then be examined for any obvious signs of abnormality and a spatula will be used to gently scrape some cells from its surface.

3 The cells are scraped from the spatula onto the slide.

WHAT HAPPENS NEXT?

If there are abnormal cells your doctor may refer you for an examination with a colposcope. This instrument illuminates and magnifies the cervix. If there are any signs of precancer the specialist will take a small specimen known as a biopsy which will be examined in the laboratory. You will then be told what treatment is best suited to you.

If there is any suspicion of true cervical cancer, then the specialist will arrange for you to go into hospital for further tests.

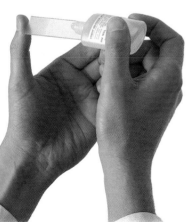

4 After the cells have been smeared onto the glass slide, it is then sprayed with fixative, before being sent to the laboratory for examination.

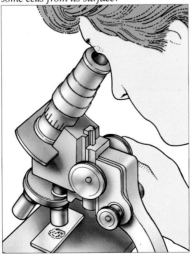

5 Each slide is carefully examined under a microscope by a laboratory technician and any abnormalities are reported to your doctor or clinic.

CONTRACEPTIVES

THERE ARE TWO MAIN types of contraceptive: barrier methods that physically prevent the sperm from reaching the egg, as with the condom, or chemically, as with a spermicide; and hormonal methods like the oral contraceptive pill that prevent ovulation and so conception. Vasectomy and sterilization are permanent methods available to those who do not want to have any more children.

Contraceptives allow men and women to plan when they will have children and to enjoy intercourse without fear of pregnancy.

Intrauterine contraceptive devices
(IUDs) are inserted into the uterus and work as a contraceptive by causing an inflammatory reaction in the lining of the uterus that stops the implantation of a fertilized egg.

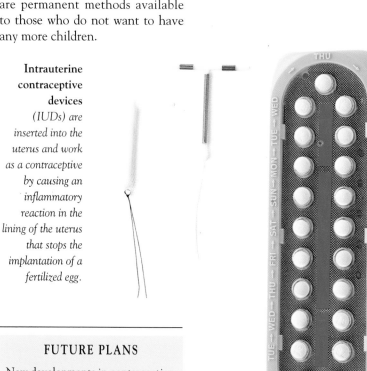

Spermicides *are made as creams, pessaries, foams, or gels. They destroy sperm chemically and most kill the AIDS virus. On their own, they are not very effective; but with a condom or diaphragm they work well. Some spermicides can damage the rubber in condoms or diaphragms.*

FUTURE PLANS

New developments in contraception that are being evaluated at present include a vaginal ring that releases synthetic progesterone for three months, the female condom, hormone implants, and skin patches.

The combined oral contraceptive pill *contains synthetic forms of two female sex hormones and prevents ovulation. The pill is the most successful contraceptive but it can have side effects. It should not be taken if you smoke and are over 35 years of age, if you are diabetic, if you have raised blood pressure, or if a close relative has developed heart disease or thrombosis at an early age. The progesterone-only minipill has to be taken with absolute regularity as it is less effective.*

The condom *can be bought over the counter and consists of a sheath of thin latex rubber, which is usually lubricated, and normally has a teat at the end to hold ejaculated semen. The condom should be rolled onto the erect penis before any genital-to-genital contact, because sperm can leak out prior to ejaculation. Condoms also protect against sexually transmitted diseases such as gonorrhoea and AIDS.*

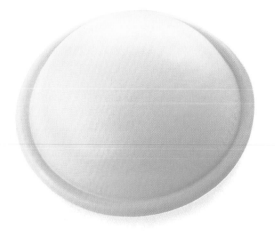

The vaginal sponge *is a disposable circular polyurethane foam sponge, impregnated with spermicide, which is moistened and pushed high into the vagina prior to sexual intercourse. Like the diaphragm, the sponge must be left in place for six hours afterwards. It has a loop attached making it easier to remove.*

The vaginal diaphragm *is a dome of thin rubber, with a coiled metal spring in its rim. It fits diagonally from behind the cervix across the front wall of the vagina to the ledge above the bone at the front of the pelvis. It needs to be used with a spermicide and to be fitted properly by a doctor or nurse, who will then teach you how to insert and remove it.*

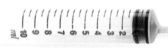

SUCCESS OF CONTRACEPTIVE METHODS

The efficiency of each method of contraception is measured by the number of pregnancies that will occur, on average, if 100 healthy young women use that method for a year. The benefits of using an effective method have to be weighed against its side-effects.

METHOD	USED PERFECTLY	USED LESS THAN PERFECTLY
Combined pill	Less than 1	1–2
Pill	Less than 1	1–4
Condom and spermicide	2	2–15
Diaphragm and spermicide	2	2–15
Spermicide alone (including sponge)	5–15	15–30
Hormone injection	Less than 1	N/A
IUD	1–3	N/A
Natural methods	2	2–20
Withdrawal	5	20
No contraception	90	N/A

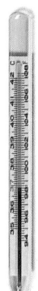

Injectable contraceptives *contain a synthetic progesterone hormone and are reliable for three months. Side effects such as irregular, heavy periods, and weight gain do occur.*

Natural methods *involve recording body temperature each morning. Ovulation causes a rise in temperature. Changes in mucus are also noted. These changes must be recorded for several months to accurately determine the pattern of ovulation. Around the time of ovulation women are at their most fertile and intercourse must be avoided.*

EMERGENCY CONTRACEPTION

If you make a mistake with your contraception some clinics offer a "morning-after" pill. High doses of estrogen and progesterone, taken within 72 hours, stop a fertilized egg implanting in the lining of the uterus.

GENETIC SCREENING

CYSTIC FIBROSIS FAMILY TREE

The gene for cystic fibrosis is inherited. If both parents are carriers of the defective gene, on average one in four of their children will be normal, 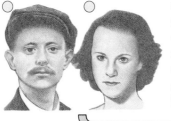 two in four will be carriers, and one in four will have the disease. To determine who is at risk, a family tree going back three generations is drawn up. It shows those with and without cystic fibrosis and highlights any blood relationship between partners.

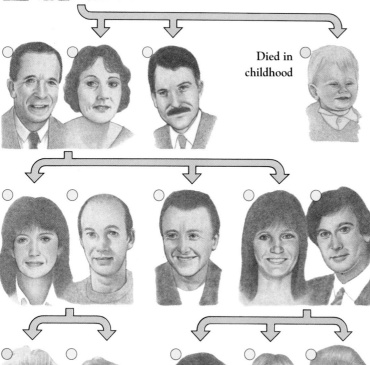

Died in childhood

GENETIC DISORDERS

Everyone carries between six and 10 faulty genes, which could harm their children if their partner has the same bad gene. Ask for a test if you have a family history of a genetic disorder.

KEY

○ Cystic fibrosis sufferer.

○ Carrier of the cystic fibrosis gene.

○ No cystic fibrosis gene.

Genetic disorders, such as cystic fibrosis and Down's syndrome, occur in about one in 50 pregnancies.

GENETIC COUNSELING provides couples with advice about the probability of bearing a child with a particular inherited disorder. This risk assessment is based on the type of condition being discussed, the way that condition is inherited, and which members of the family suffer from the condition or have the potential to pass it on.

Who needs counseling?

Having a child with an inherited disorder is one reason for requesting counseling. Others include: having a family member with an inherited condition; coming from an ethnic group which has a greater risk of a particular genetic disorder; marrying a blood relative; or having had previous miscarriages or stillbirths for no known reason.

The specialist will want to know about both families. If a couple already have one child with a disability, questions will be asked to determine if factors such as exposure to radiation, infection, or drugs during pregnancy may have caused the disability. If so, it is unlikely to affect any future children.

Making a decision

Once they know the risks, some couples may decide not to have children and are advised about contraception and sterilization. Others go on to have children. If tests during pregnancy reveal an abnormality, they can decide if they wish to have a termination.

CHROMOSOME ANALYSIS

Tests may be carried out on an unborn child to see whether it has a chromosomal abnormality such as Down's syndrome.

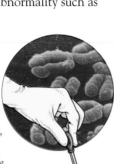

1 Cells from the fetus, obtained by amniocentesis or chorionic villus sampling, are allowed to grow and divide in a culture.

2 These cells are spread over a glass slide, before being examined through a high-powered microscope.

3 After matching the chromosomes into 22 pairs and one pair of sex chromosomes (X Y is male and X X female), they are inspected for any abnormalities. The most common fault is an additional chromosome on pair number 21, causing Down's syndrome.

SCREENING FOR ABNORMALITIES

POSSIBLE DISORDERS	WHAT ARE THEY?	PREGNANCIES AT RISK	SCREENING PROCEDURE	WHAT CAN BE DONE?
	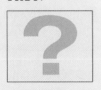			
Developmental abnormalities	Disorders occurring after fertilization. Many different parts of the body may be affected. Spina bifida is one such disorder.	Small risk in all pregnancies. Cause may be unknown or due to exposure to a toxic substance or infection during pregnancy.	An ultrasound scan, amniocentesis, or a blood test may detect some types.	Some of these defects can be prevented by good nutrition and vaccination before you get pregnant.
Chromosome abnormalities 	Damage occurs to the chromosome during the development of the egg or sperm; Down's syndrome is one example.	Increased risk if the mother is over 35 or if the father is elderly. May occur spontaneously even when both parents are under 35.	Chromosome analysis on foetal cells obtained by amniocentesis, chorionic villus sampling, or fetal blood sampling.	No specific treatment as yet. The parents' chromosomes should be checked before any future pregnancy.
Gene defects 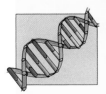	Disorders like hemophilia are caused by individual gene defects. The damaged gene is passed on to the next generation.	Almost no risk if there is no family history of these disorders. Certain conditions are more common in specific ethnic groups.	During early pregnancy, amniocentesis or chorionic villus sampling can reveal a few of these disorders.	For a few of these disorders, tests are now available that determine whether or not prospective parents carry the faulty genes.

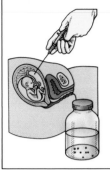

CONTROLLING YOUR ENVIRONMENT

The environment influences your health and your quality of life – so improving your environment will improve your health and wellbeing.

HUMANS ARE highly adaptable and able to live in many different types of climate. However, some regions are better for your health than others. You cannot alter the overall climate but, if you are aware of the potential risks in your own environment, you can control existing health problems and reduce the risks to your health.

The air you breathe
Avoid living at high altitude if you suffer from a respiratory disorder such as emphysema. The lower oxygen content in the air will make your condition worse.

Air pollution from car exhaust fumes and industrial pollution, at any altitude, is not good for your health, especially if you suffer from bronchitis or asthma. People with breathing difficulties should also try to avoid situations where they will be exposed to tobacco smoke.

The water you drink
Some studies show that people who live in soft water areas have a slightly higher incidence of heart disease, and a higher death rate, than people in hard water areas. The differences are too small to warrant moving from a soft to a hard water area but artificially softening water is not recommended.

If you are concerned about the purity of your drinking water you can switch to bottled mineral water or start to filter your tap water. Both these methods can, however, cause health problems if they are used incorrectly: bottled water that has been opened should be stored in the refrigerator to reduce the risk of bacterial contamination and the tap-water filter must be changed regularly.

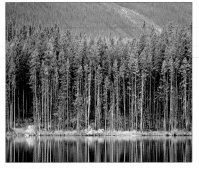

A healthy environment
An unpolluted environment promotes clean air, pure water, and therefore good health for you and your family.

Positive steps that will improve your water include replacing old lead-lined water tanks and pipes in your house and using fresh mains water whenever you boil the kettle.

The food you eat
Fertilizers, pesticides, additives, and preservatives, that are used in the production of our food, are claimed by some people to cause cancer, allergies, and, occasionally, hyperactivity in children.

The risk from chemicals in food are, however, far less important than those of an unhealthy diet containing too much fat, and those of alcohol and tobacco. People who buy only organic foods should check them carefully to be sure that they are in good condition since they have not been treated with preservatives. Because spoiled food is a serious health risk, preservatives are added to foods to stop them from becoming moldy.

Too much sunlight

Although many people worry about the harmful effects of radiation from nuclear power stations, the risks for most of the population are extremely small. In actual fact, there is a far greater threat to your health from the large doses of ultraviolet radiation that you absorb through lying in the sun for long periods of time. Therefore, if you sunbathe less, and avoid all unnecessary medical x-rays, you will help to keep your exposure to radiation within safe limits.

A little sunlight is needed every day to promote the production of vitamin D in the skin. However, too much exposure to the sun or to the ultraviolet rays of a sun lamp will prematurely age your skin. If you are very fair-skinned, it will also increase your chance of developing skin cancer. Children who suffer from recurrent sunburn are also more likely to develop skin cancer later in life.

Background radiation

People who work directly with sources of radiation have to take the most stringent safeguards to protect themselves. But there is probably nothing you can do to reduce the very small risk of developing cancer due to the low level of natural ionizing radiation that is present in the environment.

This background radiation comes from two main sources: cosmic rays from outer space and radon gas emanating mainly from uranium ores in the Earth's crust.

The level of natural radiation usually falls well within defined safety limits. However, in some cases, particularly where there is mainly granite rock beneath the soil, a higher-than-average amount of radon gas may be detected. If you live in a high-risk area, you can have the level of radon measured in your house. If there is a build-up of the gas, all you need to do to make your home environment safe again is to improve the ventilation.

Controlling your home environment
Many injuries occur in the home or at work. By instituting a few basic safety precautions, you can reduce this threat to you and your family's heath.

Environmental allergies

Hay fever and also some asthmas and eczemas are caused by allergic reactions to substances in your environment. If you are sensitive to pollen you should monitor the pollen count and try to avoid going outdoors on high-count days. Fitting indoor air filters and keeping your windows and doors shut will also help. A dust allergy can be eased by frequent vacuum cleaning and by using a spray every few months to eradicate house-dust mites from your bedding and soft furnishings.

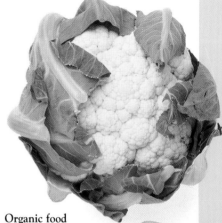

Organic food
You can ensure that you are not exposed to pesticides or food additives by choosing organic produce – but be sure it is really fresh before buying it.

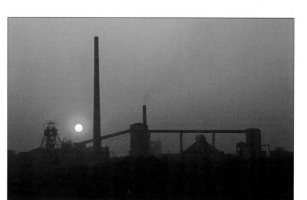

A hazardous environment
Exhaust fumes and uncontrolled industrial activity cause air pollution. This polluted air is thought to have caused the increase in the number of asthma cases in the industrialized West.

Safety in the Home

There are many simple steps that can be taken to reduce the risk of accidents occurring in the home.

IN THE GARDEN

- Put up fences to stop children running out into the road.
- Put play equipment on soft ground.
- Cover or fence off ponds.
- Remove any poisonous plants.
- Never leave children alone near a swimming pool.

IN THE BATHROOM

- Fix a secure hand grip on the side of the bath and next to the toilet.
- Install safety glass in the shower screen or replace it with a curtain.
- Fit a nonslip mat both in and alongside the bath.
- Mount electric heaters on the ceiling or high on the wall.

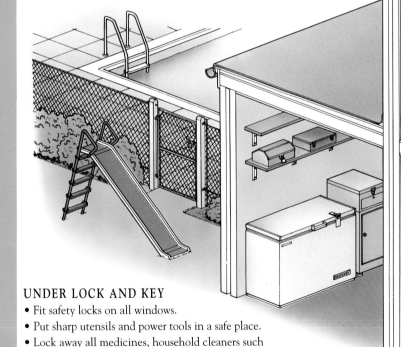

UNDER LOCK AND KEY

- Fit safety locks on all windows.
- Put sharp utensils and power tools in a safe place.
- Lock away all medicines, household cleaners such as bleach, and other chemicals.
- Attach a child-resistant lock to the deep freeze.

HIGH-RISK GROUPS

The young and the old are most at risk of suffering from an accident in the home. Toddlers and young children are naturally inquisitive and do not realize what is dangerous. Physical infirmities, such as less acute sight and slower reflexes, make it harder for elderly people to detect potential hazards and avoid accidents.

IN THE KITCHEN

- Fit a pan-guard to the stove.
- Place pan handles facing inward.
- Keep all plastic bags and small objects that could be swallowed by a child up high and out of reach of children.
- Store all chemicals in their original containers. Keep them tightly sealed.
- Always use potholders.

IN THE BEDROOM
• Do not smoke in bed.
• Fit dummy plugs to seal off unused wall sockets in a child's bedroom.
• Make sure your baby's crib conforms to all safety guidelines.

IN THE STAIRWAYS
• Ensure that stair carpets are secure.
• Make certain that your banister is strong and secure.
• Do not leave objects on the stairs.
• Keep the stairway brightly lit.
• Put gates at the top and bottom of the stairs if you have young children.

FIRE SAFETY
• Install smoke detectors.
• Keep safety guards around fires at all times.
• Have all gas, oil, and electrical heating systems serviced regularly.
• Make sure that all armchairs, sofas, bedding, curtains, nightclothes, and soft toys are made from flame-resistant materials.
• Keep a fire extinguisher in the house.
• Unplug electrical equipment at night.

IN THE LIVING AREA
• Use mats rather than a table cloth.
• Keep hot drinks out of reach of children.
• Remove glass doors, glass-topped tables, and furniture that has sharp edges if you have young children.

ACCIDENTS WILL HAPPEN
More people are injured in accidents at home than on the road. Yet many potential household hazards can be avoided by simply applying a little common sense. The majority of falls, for instance, happen at floor level, rather than at a height, and are due to tripping on loose or worn rugs, slippery surfaces, trailing wires, or general clutter.

SAFETY AT WORK

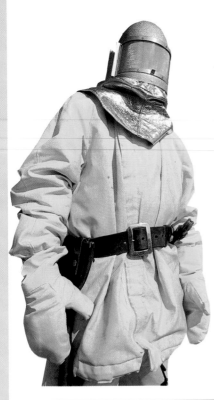

Whether you work in the open air, a factory, or an office, your workplace may be full of health hazards.

Dressed for safety

If you are likely to be exposed to any potentially toxic or cancer-causing substances, you must always wear the protective clothing and safety equipment provided by your employer.

THERE ARE MANY positive steps you can take to improve health and safety standards in your place of work. For instance, you should always use the safety equipment provided by your employer and follow all safety guidelines.

In addition, several industries offer regular screening programmes to detect early signs of any work-related disease. Ask your employer if any of these tests apply to your type of work.

Occupational hazards

Many occupations are prone to particular diseases and disorders. For example, welders are at increased risk of suffering from eye injuries.

IS YOUR JOB AFFECTING YOUR HEALTH?

No job is totally safe – even working behind a desk all day may lead to an increased risk of coronary heart disease. Many jobs have much more obvious health risks. If you are constantly exposed to loud noise, high temperatures, or excessive vibration you may be putting your long-term health under threat.

Noise – regular exposure to loud noise can cause deafness or tinnitus. Although wearing earplugs will avoid this problem, it is still one of the most common work-related disorders.

Dust – prolonged inhalation of mineral dust may reduce the elasticity of the lungs by causing fibrosis. Inhalation of organic dust can cause farmer's lung (a type of pneumonia).

Industrial solvents – contact with the skin or inhalation of industrial solvents through the lungs may cause allergic reactions. These powerful solvents may also damage the liver and kidneys.

Radiation – men exposed to radiation in nuclear plants can suffer sperm-cell damage. This may lead to a slightly higher risk of their children developing leukemia or congenital birth defects.

Stress – any problem at work that creates tension, for example, overcrowding or harassment, may lead to the development of a stress-related disorder such as a peptic ulcer or colitis.

Heat – workers who are exposed to high temperatures, for example in the steel industry, have an increased risk of suffering from muscle cramps, heat exhaustion, and even heat stroke.

Vibration – hand-held machinery which vibrates may damage the circulation to the finger-tips, resulting in painful and cold fingers. In extreme cases ulcers or gangrene may develop.

Pesticides – exposure to large amounts of pesticide may damage many parts of the body. Organs that are particularly at risk include the liver, kidneys, nervous system, ovaries, and testes.

HOW TO REDUCE HAZARDS IN THE OFFICE

Although the incidence of job-related illness is relatively low for the office worker, there are still a number of potential problems that can cause a variety of unpleasant and sometimes disabling symptoms. Preventive measures can reduce the risk to your health.

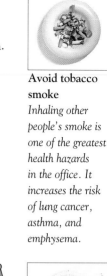

Avoid tobacco smoke
Inhaling other people's smoke is one of the greatest health hazards in the office. It increases the risk of lung cancer, asthma, and emphysema.

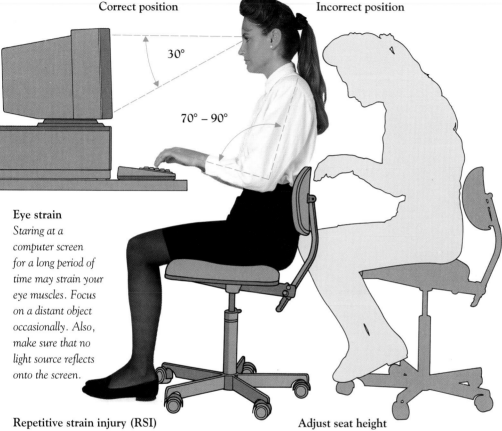

Correct position   Incorrect position

30°

70° – 90°

Eye strain
Staring at a computer screen for a long period of time may strain your eye muscles. Focus on a distant object occasionally. Also, make sure that no light source reflects onto the screen.

Regulate temperature
If you feel uncomfortably hot or cold, adjust the heating or air conditioning. Plants in the office can help humidify the atmosphere.

Repetitive strain injury (RSI)
RSI is caused by incorrect posture, such as typing on a keyboard set at the wrong height. Symptoms include pains in your wrists and arms and tingling or numbness in your hands. Rest is the only cure.

Adjust seat height
To avoid bad posture, sit in a relaxed position, feet flat on the floor, with your back straight and well supported. Use a foot rest if you cannot lower the chair.

Your height	Optimal desk height
4'11" (150 cm)	23" (57.5 cm)
5'4" (162 cm)	24" (60 cm)
5'6" (167 cm)	25" (62.5 cm)
5'9" (173 cm)	26" (65 cm)
6'2" (185 cm)	28" (70 cm)

Correct desk height
A correctly sited desk should allow you to type with your lower arms at an angle of between 70° and 90° to your abdomen. Also, the screen should lie within a 30° viewing angle of your direct line of vision.

PREVENTING INJURIES AT WORK

Accidents and injuries at work remain a major cause of death and disability. To keep the risks to a minimum:

- Always follow recommended safety procedures.
- Wear appropriate protective clothing.
- Use ear plugs or muffs if you work with noisy machinery.
- Tell someone in authority if you are worried about safety.
- If you take medication that makes you feel drowsy or dizzy, do not operate machinery or work at a height.
- Never drink alcohol during working hours.

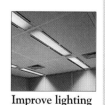

Improve lighting
Fluorescent lights should be filtered to cut out high-frequency flickering which causes headaches and eye fatigue. Use an adjustable desk lamp to improve office lighting.

287

HOLIDAY HEALTH

Illness and accidents can ruin a holiday – a few basic precautions will help you avoid endangering your health.

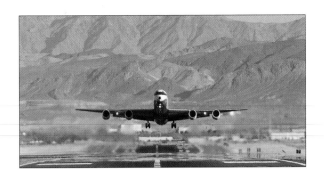

AT LEAST TWO MONTHS before you go on holiday check with your doctor or travel agent which vaccinations are recommended for each country you are going to visit. Some vaccinations take time to become effective or cannot be given at the same time as others. If you need malaria tablets you will have to start taking them a week before you travel and continue taking them for a month after you return.

Food hygiene
Many countries have low standards of hygiene. Fish and meat should always be well cooked, and, if the country you are visiting has very poor hygiene, you should avoid raw vegetables and salads and only eat fruit that can be peeled.

If the water quality is poor you should only drink, brush your teeth, and mix baby foods using bottled water or water that has been purified with sterilizing tablets or boiled

for more than five minutes. Remember not to eat ice cream or have ice in your drinks.

Enjoy yourself, but be sensible
Stay in the shade when the sun is at its brightest. Put sunscreen on any areas of exposed skin and drink plenty of fluids – but keep alcohol intake down. To protect yourself from insect and tick bites you should use an insect repellent. In tropical countries you need to sleep under a screen or mosquito net.

Leave your worries behind
Whether your trip abroad is for business or pleasure, ask your travel agent or insurance broker if you will need additional medical insurance.

Preventive measures
In many countries it is advisable to take sterile needles, syringes, and a suture kit (available at most pharmacies). This will reduce the risk of contracting hepatitis or AIDS through poorly sterilized needles.

CHOOSING SUNGLASSES

Ultraviolet light can harm your eyes, so sunglasses should be worn in strong sunlight or when it is reflected off water or snow, making the light more intense. Ask an optician which type of sunglasses to buy.

If you wear spectacles, you can have them fitted with photochromatic lenses which automatically darken in strong light. Alternatively, you can use clip-on filters or have your lens prescription made up into sunglasses.

Too much of a good thing
To avoid sunburn and heatstroke, increase the length of time you spend in the sun gradually, starting at 15 minutes a day.

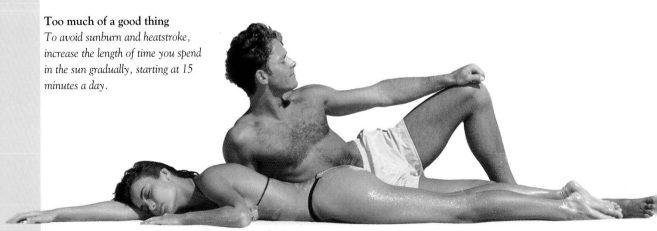

PRESCRIPTION DRUGS

If you need to take a drug that is subject to customs or prescribing restrictions in any country you are visiting, or if you are carrying needles and syringes because you are diabetic, a letter from your doctor explaining the situation will help. Make sure you have enough of your medication with you for the whole of your trip. If you have a medical disorder it is always advisable to check with your doctor that it is safe to travel.

BEWARE OF ANIMALS

Rabies is prevalent all over the world, including many parts of Europe, so stay away from stray or wild animals when you are abroad. Wash any scratch or bite with soap or detergent, rinse it thoroughly in clean water, and, if possible, swab it with alcohol. If the animal is a pet, try to find out the owner's name, address, and telephone number – even if it has a rabies certificate, it is still worth checking the animal is alive and well two weeks later.

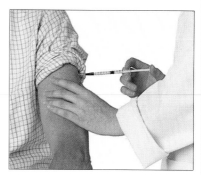

Immediate treatment is essential
If you are bitten, go to a hospital at once. If there is any doubt about the animal, you may need a course of rabies injections.

HOLIDAY FIRST-AID KIT

When you are planning your holiday, the possibility of falling ill or being hurt in an accident is probably the last thing on your mind. However, if you take your own basic first-aid supplies with you, you may save yourself a great deal of worry and expense.

You can buy a first-aid kit from your local pharmacy or make up your own, using a secure plastic box. Always keep it out of the reach of children. The objects shown below are some of the most useful first-aid items that you can take with you.

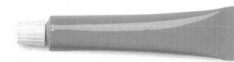
Sting relief

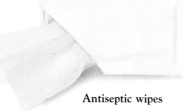
Antiseptic wipes

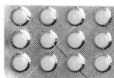
Travel-sickness tablets

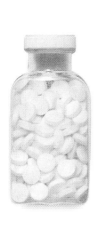
Painkillers – aspirin or acetaminophen

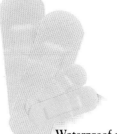
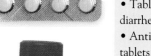
Waterproof plasters

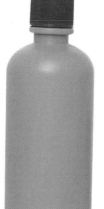
Calamine lotion

OTHER USEFUL ITEMS

• Tablets for diarrhea
• Antihistamine tablets
• Antiseptic cream
• Insect repellent
• Laxatives
• Liquid painkiller suitable for children
• Oral rehydration powders
• Safety pins
• Bandages
• Gauze dressings
• Scissors
• Thermometer
• Tweezers

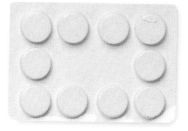
Indigestion tablets

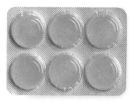
Lozenges for a sore throat

A SICK ENVIRONMENT

Chemicals in food

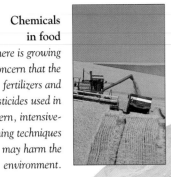

There is growing concern that the fertilizers and pesticides used in modern, intensive-farming techniques may harm the environment.

SOURCES OF POLLUTION

There is no consensus as to which of the many sources of environmental pollution pose the greatest threat to public health. Efforts to reduce the pollution of our air, water, and food are both costly and complex, requiring drastic changes in the lifestyle of the whole population.

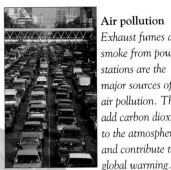

Air pollution

Exhaust fumes and smoke from power stations are the major sources of air pollution. They add carbon dioxide to the atmosphere and contribute to global warming.

Electric fields

A few scientists claim that long-term exposure to electromagnetic radiation from the cables between pylons can cause health problems.

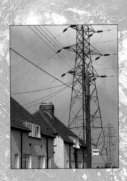

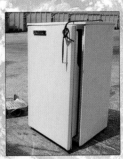

Chlorofluoro-carbons (CFCs)

CFCs are thought to be responsible for damaging the ozone layer that protects the Earth from harmful ultraviolet rays.

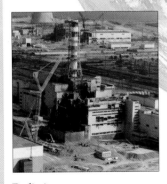

Radiation

The only people at high risk of cancer from exposure to radiation are those who have been within the vicinity of a nuclear accident or explosion.

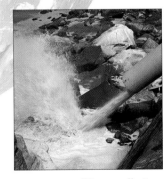

Water pollution

Lakes, rivers, and oceans are often polluted by man's destructive lifestyle, and even domestic water supplies do not always reach EC safety standards.

Environmental pollution is not new; in fact, in the West, the risk of dying of a pollution-based disease has decreased in the last century.

AIR, DRINKING WATER, and food are less polluted now than in Victorian times. Improvements in housing and sanitation have also reduced the risks to health from other environmental factors.

New environmental threats

Technological advances, such as the internal combustion engine, however, have created new threats to the environment and health.

The gases that make up exhaust fumes cause many health problems. Smog, produced by the action of sunlight on these fumes, can cause breathing difficulties for people with bronchitis, asthma, or heart disease; carbon dioxide adds to global warming; and lead is thought to interfere with children's intelligence and behavior. Switching to lead-free gas and fitting catalytic converters to cars will cut down on the emission of these gases and reduce environmental pollution.

Chlorofluorocarbons (CFCs) are another new and potentially lethal threat to human health. Used in spray cans, air conditioning units, refrigerators, and in the manufacture of insulation materials, they damage the ozone layer that surrounds the Earth and blocks out most of the sun's harmful ultraviolet radiation. The depletion of the ozone layer is likely to increase the incidence of skin cancer.

Towards a healthier future

Only a strong public commitment to achieving a healthier way of life will bring about the necessary changes in industry, farming, and transport that will remove all these environmental and health hazards.

HOW TO IMPROVE YOUR ENVIRONMENT

Everybody can make a contribution towards a safer and healthier environment by reducing pollution and conserving resources.

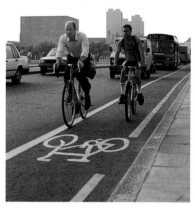

Transport
For short trips, leave your car at home and walk or cycle instead. This will cut down on air pollution.

Waste disposal
Recycle bottles, newspapers, and cans from your weekly refuse and dispose of articles like refrigerators carefully. These steps will help to save the Earth's precious resources.

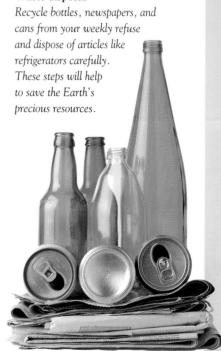

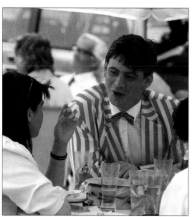

Passive smoking
Cigarette smoke pollutes the air. Inhaling other people's smoke in places such as restaurants, offices, and trains increases your risk of suffering from lung cancer.

SICK BUILDING SYNDROME

Occasionally people living in a particular block of flats or working in the same office develop a variety of minor symptoms at the same time. This condition, popularly referred to as sick building syndrome, usually involves buildings served by a closed ventilation system. The exact cause in most instances is never identified. Symptoms include extreme tiredness, headaches, blocked or runny nose, eye irritation, skin rashes, and nausea. To cure the condition, the building rather than the affected individuals must be treated.

ALLERGY

Allergic disorders, such as hay fever, are extremely common. Symptoms of these conditions, for example a runny nose, itchy eyes, dry cough, or inflamed, itchy skin, develop as a result of an exaggerated response by the body's immune system to substances that in other people would not cause any harm.

Allergic symptoms may be brought on by contact between the skin and the offending agent, by inhalation, by swallowing, or by exposure through the outer surface of the eye. Once an initial contact has caused sensitization of cells in the immune system, subsequent exposure rapidly produces symptoms.

Allergy-based diseases tend to run in families. For example 70 per cent of people with allergic eczema have a close relative with an allergic disorder. Therefore it is likely that a genetic factor is involved.

Allergies are an inappropriate reaction of the body's immune system to harmless substances.

SUBSTANCES THAT TRIGGER ALLERGIC DISORDERS

Pollen
Many people suffer from hay fever and asthma in the summer because they are sensitive to a particular type of tree or grass pollen.

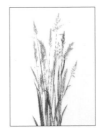

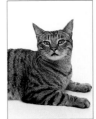

Animals
Allergies to animals occur because many people are sensitive to the tiny flakes of dead skin that are shed from animals' coats.

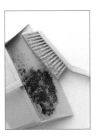

House-dust mites
However clean a house may appear, faeces from invisible dust mites in bedding and soft furnishings can cause allergies.

Feathers
Allergy to feathers is common but easy to deal with. Simply replace feather pillows and quilts for those with a synthetic stuffing.

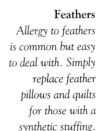

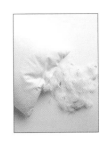

FOOD ALLERGIES

True food allergies, that involve the immune system, are extremely rare. Most reactions to food are caused by either food poisoning or an intolerance to a certain food due to a lack of a particular digestive enzyme.

Adverse reactions may sometimes start within just a few minutes of eating the "trigger" food. Symptoms include tingling in the mouth, swelling of the lips, abdominal distension, vomiting, abnormally loud bowel sounds, and diarrhea.

If you suffer from this kind of allergy the only effective treatment is to cut out the offending foods from your diet. To be safe, you should consult your doctor before starting yourself on an exclusion diet for a self-diagnosed food allergy.

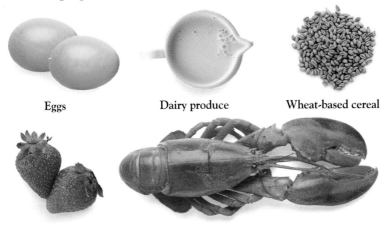

Eggs

Dairy produce

Wheat-based cereal

Strawberries

Fish and shellfish

Top five food allergies
These are the foods that most often cause allergic reactions. The symptoms they produce vary from one person to another.

ADDITIVES AT FAULT?

Allergy to a food additive is often cited as being a major cause of behavioural problems in children. However, scientific research has shown that this association is rare.

WHAT CAUSES AN ALLERGIC REACTION?

In a susceptible person, the surfaces of millions of cells, known as mast cells, are covered in immunoglobulin E molecules – a type of protein. Each of these molecules has a receptor that can interlock and rapidly bond with molecules of an allergen, such as pollen.

Once the allergen has locked on to the receptor, granules inside the mast cell are stimulated to release powerful inflammatory substances, such as histamine and prostaglandins. It is these chemicals which provoke the symptoms of an allergic reaction.

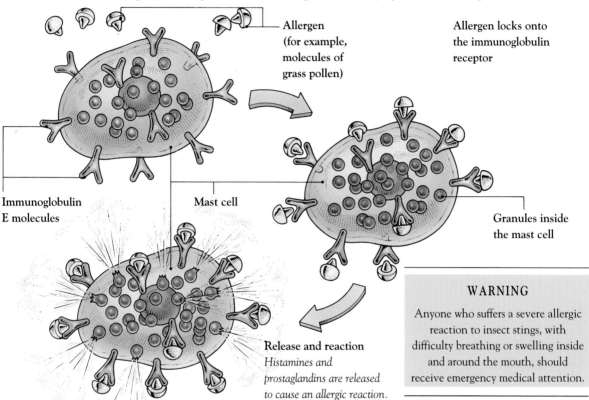

Allergen (for example, molecules of grass pollen)

Allergen locks onto the immunoglobulin receptor

Immunoglobulin E molecules

Mast cell

Granules inside the mast cell

Release and reaction
Histamines and prostaglandins are released to cause an allergic reaction.

WARNING

Anyone who suffers a severe allergic reaction to insect stings, with difficulty breathing or swelling inside and around the mouth, should receive emergency medical attention.

HOW ALLERGIES ARE DIAGNOSED

Doctors usually diagnose allergies simply by noting your symptoms and asking you when they occur. However, blood tests, which measure your level of immunoglobulin antibodies, provide a more accurate diagnosis and skin tests can identify the source of your reaction, as shown below:

1 Patches are soaked with each potential allergen and then taped to the skin (usually the back). Allergens may also be injected just below the surface of the skin.

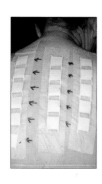

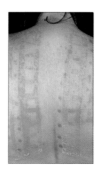

2 The patches are removed and allergy-producing substances leave an inflamed, red area. The test is not infallible – red areas do occur with substances to which you are not allergic.

TREATMENTS

Many allergy treatments are available. Sodium cromoglycate prevents histamine release from mast cells, antihistamine drugs can block the action of histamine, and corticosteroid treatment stops inflammation. Alternatively, you may be given doses of the allergen at fault, to promote tolerance to it. However, this desensitization treatment is becoming less common.

YOUR HOME MEDICINE CABINET

Medicines and first-aid supplies should be stored in a safe place.

MINOR ILLNESSES AND accidents can often be successfully treated without the aid of a doctor. To carry out this self-treatment, you should keep a small store of over-the-counter remedies and basic first-aid supplies in your home.

Medicines can be dangerous

All medicine and first-aid supplies should be kept in a cabinet that is not used to store anything except items for medical use. This cabinet should always be fitted with a childproof catch.

All drugs that are prescribed by your doctor should also be put into this cabinet. Tablets, especially, must not be left lying around the house – children can easily mistake them for sweets and eat them.

Planning ahead

If the accident or illness you are treating proves to be more serious than you first thought, you may need to seek help. Therefore, it is a good idea to put a list of emergency information, including the telephone numbers of your local doctor, hospital, and pharmacist, in the cabinet. A first-aid book that shows you how to perform basic emergency techniques may also prove useful and should be kept in or near the cabinet.

EACH TO THEIR OWN

Even if you have the same symptoms as another person, never use drugs that have been prescribed for them.

STORAGE AND SAFETY

Shown below are a selection of items that are always useful to have in your home medicine cabinet. Other medicines and items of first-aid equipment may be added according to your individual needs.

• Aspirin or acetaminophen.
• Cough mixture.
• Throat pastels.
• Sting relief.
• Antiseptic cream and liquid.
• Indigestion mixture.
• Calamine lotion.
• Adhesives.
• Bandages.
• Scissors.
• Tweezers.
• Sterile dressings.
• Safety pins.
• Eye drops.
• First-aid book.

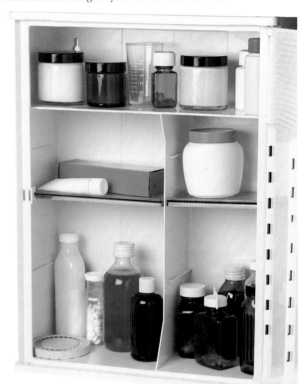

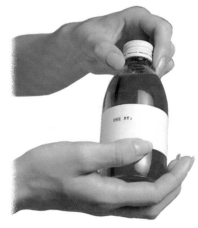

Correct containers
Never mix different drugs together in the same bottle. Medicines should be kept in their own containers so that you can follow the directions on the label.

Check the label
Many drugs cannot be taken by certain groups of people. For example, aspirin should not be given to children under 12 years of age. Read the label carefully for restrictions and expiration date.

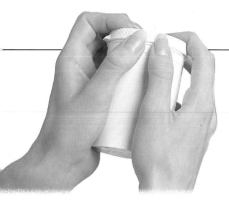

Close lids properly
The lid of any type of container should always be tightly closed. This will keep the medicine fresh and stop any accidental spillage. In addition, childproof caps are required by law to be used for many types of medicines that are taken by mouth.

Out of harm's way
A wall-cabinet, which is out of the reach of children, is the best place to store medicines. If your child swallows some pills, call a doctor at once. More detailed advice is given in the first-aid section (see p303).

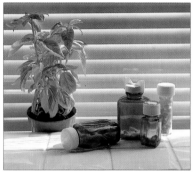

The harmful effects of the sun
Sunlight can cause a drug to deteriorate and lose its effectiveness. Therefore, all types of drugs, even those kept in an opaque container, should be kept out of direct sunlight.

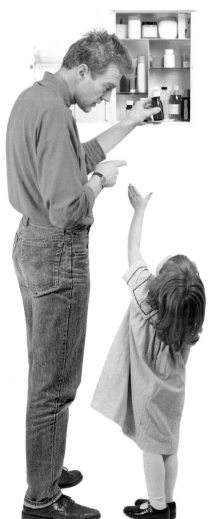

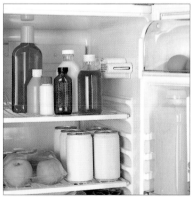

Special storage requirements
Some medications need to be stored in a particular way to stop them deteriorating or becoming toxic. Always follow the storage instruction that you are given by your pharmacist or doctor. For instance, if you are told to put a medicine in the refrigerator, you should do this – but make sure that it does not freeze.

WHEN TO DISPOSE OF YOUR MEDICATIONS

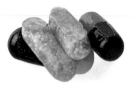

Medicines do not last for ever. With age, they can lose their effectiveness or become toxic. As soon as you notice any of the following warning signs you should dispose of the drug:

- The expiration date printed on the container has passed.
- Tablets that are over two years old or are cracked, powdery, or discolored.
- Ointments or creams that have hardened, discolored, or begun to separate.
- Tubes that are starting to crack or leak.
- Capsules that are soft, cracked, or stuck together.
- A medicine that has changed its smell.
- Bottles of eye drops that are over 28 days old.
- Liquids that are thickened or discolored.

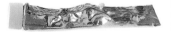

NEEDLES
If you inject yourself with a drug, such as insulin, ask your doctor or pharmacist how to dispose safely of your needles. If in doubt, return them to your pharmacist.

DEALING WITH A MAJOR EMERGENCY

Knowing how to give first-aid treatment can save an accident victim's life.

MAJOR EMERGENCIES include all life-threatening situations. The victim may not be breathing or may have no heartbeat. They could be suffering from severe burns, be bleeding profusely, or be unconscious. If treatment is not given promptly they may die.

The aim of first-aid treatment in a major emergency is to improve the victim's condition, or at least prevent it from worsening, and to get help quickly without further endangering either yourself or the victim. Knowing the order in which to give help is vital too – consult the chart shown below.

It is better to learn first aid in advance, rather than from a book in the midst of an emergency. Training is given by the Red Cross and the American Heart Association.

EMERGENCY CHECK-LIST

- **Is the victim breathing?** If not, try artificial respiration (see p299)
- **Is the victim's heart beating?** If there is no pulse, and if you know the technique, start CPR (see p299).
- **Is the victim unconscious?** Place them in the recovery position if they are still breathing (see p298).
- **Is there severe bleeding?** Control the bleeding (see p300).
- **Is the victim in shock?** If so, treat the shock (see p297).

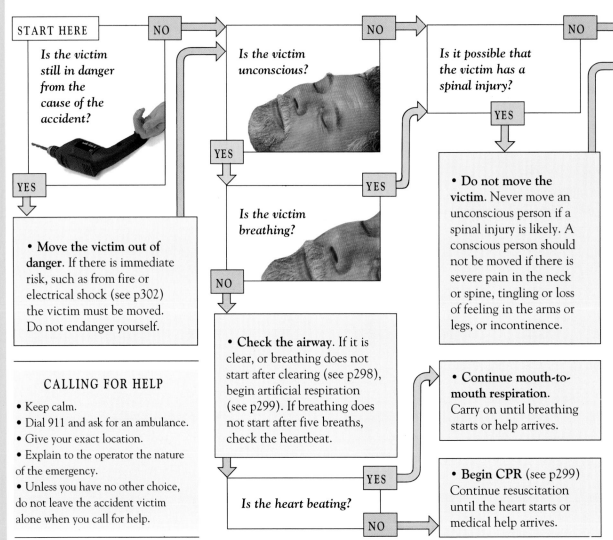

START HERE — NO

Is the victim still in danger from the cause of the accident?

Is the victim unconscious? — NO

Is it possible that the victim has a spinal injury? — NO

YES

Is the victim breathing? — YES

YES

- **Move the victim out of danger.** If there is immediate risk, such as from fire or electrical shock (see p302) the victim must be moved. Do not endanger yourself.

NO

- **Do not move the victim.** Never move an unconscious person if a spinal injury is likely. A conscious person should not be moved if there is severe pain in the neck or spine, tingling or loss of feeling in the arms or legs, or incontinence.

- **Check the airway.** If it is clear, or breathing does not start after clearing (see p298), begin artificial respiration (see p299). If breathing does not start after five breaths, check the heartbeat.

- **Continue mouth-to-mouth respiration.** Carry on until breathing starts or help arrives.

Is the heart beating? — YES / NO

- **Begin CPR** (see p299) Continue resuscitation until the heart starts or medical help arrives.

CALLING FOR HELP

- Keep calm.
- Dial 911 and ask for an ambulance.
- Give your exact location.
- Explain to the operator the nature of the emergency.
- Unless you have no other choice, do not leave the accident victim alone when you call for help.

- **Put the victim in the recovery position** (see p298). Now check for any signs of further injury. For instance, is there any bleeding? Is the victim suffering from burns, or in shock?

- **Try to stop the bleeding** (see p300). Apply pressure above and below the wound with your hand.

TREATMENT FOR SHOCK

1 Lay the victim down and raise both of his or her legs.

2 Loosen all tight clothing and wrap the victim in a coat or blanket to prevent heat loss. Do not use heat sources such as hot water bottles.

Shock may be caused by blood loss or severe burns. It needs urgent treatment as it can lead to unconsciousness. Symptoms are: pallor, rapid pulse, faintness, weakness, or cold skin. Fainting may be confused with shock. In a faint, however, the person becomes dizzy and then loses consciousness, but will regain consciousness in a minute or so.

3 Reassure the victim, but do not offer them food or drink.

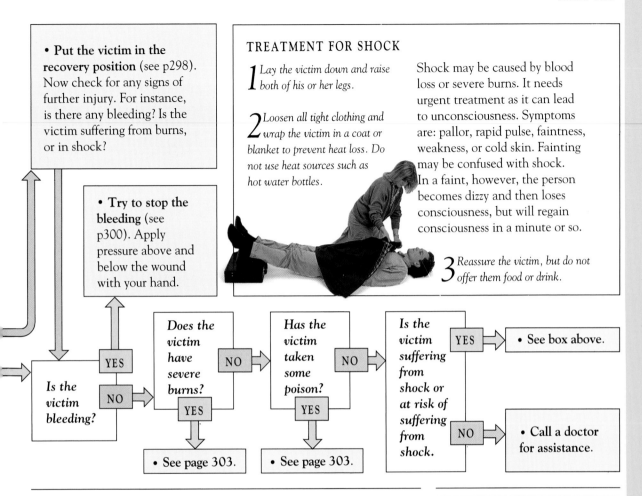

Is the victim bleeding?

NO → **Does the victim have severe burns?**

YES ↑

NO → **Has the victim taken some poison?**

YES → • See page 303.

NO → **Is the victim suffering from shock or at risk of suffering from shock.**

YES → • See box above.

NO → • Call a doctor for assistance.

YES (from bleeding) ↑

YES (burns) → • See page 303.

HOW TO DEAL WITH SEIZURES

Seizures usually stop in a few minutes and do not cause permanent harm. But you should call a doctor unless you know the victim is an epileptic. If this is the case, call for help if the fit continues for more than five minutes.

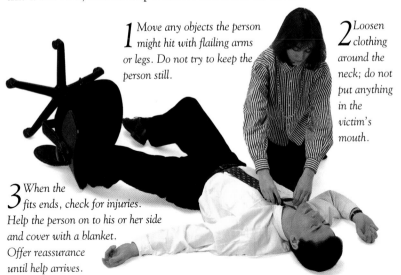

1 Move any objects the person might hit with flailing arms or legs. Do not try to keep the person still.

2 Loosen clothing around the neck; do not put anything in the victim's mouth.

3 When the fits ends, check for injuries. Help the person on to his or her side and cover with a blanket. Offer reassurance until help arrives.

WHEN TO CALL FOR AN AMBULANCE OR A DOCTOR

- **Unexplained drowsiness or loss of consciousness.** Help is needed at once, possible causes include a drug overdose, uncontrolled diabetes, or a brain disorder.
- **Severe bleeding.** Spurting blood or bleeding that does not stop within five minutes can be life-threatening.
- **Unexplained fits of any sort.**
- **Difficulty breathing.** If the person is at rest or asthmatic, help is needed.
- **Severe abdominal pain.** Seek help if vomiting does not relieve the pain, if it is on one side of the body only, if it continues for over three hours, or if there is sweating or faintness as well.
- **Sudden blurring of vision or seeing coloured haloes around lights.**

CHOKING – THE HEIMLICH MANEUVER

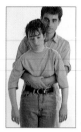

To dislodge an object, grasp the choking victim from behind. Place one fist, thumb-side facing in, under the breastbone. Clasp this fist with your other hand. Pull inwards and upwards with a thrusting movement. For children, use only one hand and less force. Turn babies upside down and press gently on the chest.

EMERGENCY TECHNIQUES

Breathing and blood circulation are necessary for life itself; if they stop, prompt action is vital.

WHEN TREATING AN unconscious victim, first check the airway, breathing, and circulation, using the initials of the words (ABC) to help you to remember the order.

How to keep the victim alive

Keeping the airway open is very important. If you place the victim in the recovery position this will stop him or her from choking on, or inhaling, vomit.

If breathing has ceased, you must use artificial respiration to force air into the lungs and keep the blood supplied with oxygen. This helps to prevent brain damage and death. If the heart has stopped beating, cardiopulmonary resuscitation (CPR) needs to be performed.

The Heimlich maneuver can be used to force a choking victim to expel any foreign object that is lodged in the throat.

THE RECOVERY POSITION

If an accident victim is unconscious, but is still breathing and there is no spinal injury, place them in the recovery position (lying on one side, head facing forward and downward). This position helps prevent choking or inhalation of vomit when the victim starts to regain consciousness.

PROTECT THE SPINE

If there is a spinal injury, the recovery position can cause further damage. In these cases, only use this position if the victim is vomiting.

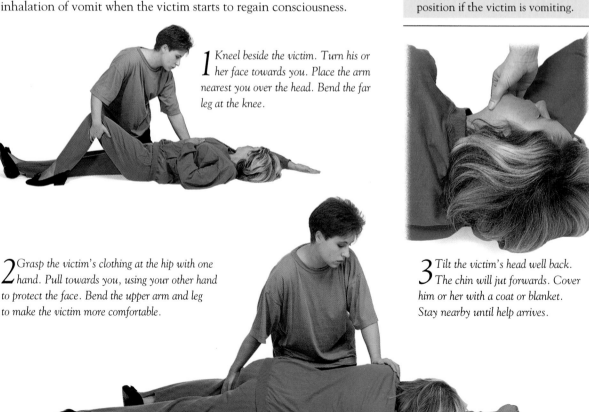

1 Kneel beside the victim. Turn his or her face towards you. Place the arm nearest you over the head. Bend the far leg at the knee.

2 Grasp the victim's clothing at the hip with one hand. Pull towards you, using your other hand to protect the face. Bend the upper arm and leg to make the victim more comfortable.

3 Tilt the victim's head well back. The chin will jut forwards. Cover him or her with a coat or blanket. Stay nearby until help arrives.

ARTIFICIAL RESPIRATION

If breathing has stopped, the victim's chest will not be moving and you will not be able to hear or feel the breath on your cheek. Carrying out artificial respiration may restore breathing. This procedure must be carried out quickly; brain damage can occur after only a few minutes without oxygen.

MOUTH-TO-NOSE

In poisoning or facial injury cases, mouth-to-nose respiration has to be used. Close the victim's mouth by pushing your hand against the chin, then breathe into the nose.

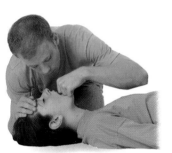
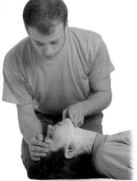
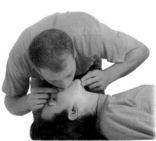
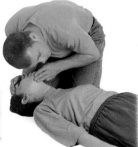

1 Send for medical help, if possible. Lay the victim on a firm surface. Clear the mouth of foreign objects such as dentures, dirt, or blood clots with your fingers.

2 Gently tilt the victim's head back. Place one hand beneath the neck and lift it up. To tilt the chin up, press down on the forehead with the heel of your other hand.

3 Take your hand from the forehead and pinch the victim's nostrils shut. Take a deep breath. Cover the victim's mouth with your mouth. Blow in to inflate the lungs.

4 Lift your head and listen for air leaving the lungs. Watch the chest fall. Now give four quick breaths. Proceed at 12 deep breaths a minute until the victim can breathe alone.

CARDIOPULMONARY RESUSCITATION (CPR)

If the person is not breathing, you may find that the heart is also not beating. If the heart has stopped, the victim will be unresponsive, the skin will be cold and discolored, and there will be no pulse. If the person is breathing, then his or her heart will be beating even if you cannot feel a pulse. CPR should only be carried out if the heart has stopped, since it can interfere with the heart's rhythm or stop it altogether.

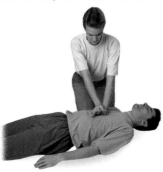

1 Place the heel of one hand 1 in (2 cm) above the point where the ribs meet the breastbone. Put your other hand on top. Lock your elbows. Push down about 5 cm (2 in), then release. Do not lift your hands.

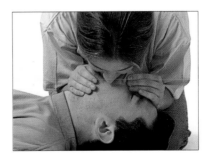

2 Repeat step one to compress the heart rhythmically 80 times per minute. Stop every 15 compressions to give two breaths by mouth-to-mouth respiration.

GET PROPER TRAINING

Do not attempt cardiopulmonary resuscitation unless you have detailed written instructions or have attended a first-aid class and learned the correct procedure. The steps listed here only outline the basic technique.

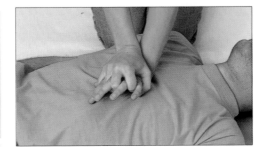

3 Feel for a pulse after every four full cycles of 15 compressions and two breaths, but do not stop CPR for more than a few seconds. Stop the heart compressions as soon as you feel a pulse. Continue mouth-to-mouth until the victim's breathing starts again.

WOUNDS, BRUISING, AND BLEEDING

Emergency treatment for bleeding and bruising aims to control the bleeding and stop swelling.

INJURIES TO THE BODY can cause bleeding either externally or internally. If there is a puncture, cut, abrasion, or scratch, the wound will bleed externally.

If the wound is very deep or cuts an artery, the bleeding must be stopped quickly to prevent shock, unconsciousness, and death.

Puncture wounds are narrow and deep, so there may not be much bleeding. However, they are still serious – there may be damage to internal organs. Always see a doctor if you receive a puncture wound. Abrasions or scratches can be very painful and carry a high risk of infection if they are not cleaned thoroughly.

Bruising is due to blood vessels beneath the skin's surface being broken and, as a result, bleeding.

Injuries to the brain or internal organs can cause life-threatening bleeding. Seek emergency medical help if the victim is bleeding from the ears or nose, coughing up blood, or has a swollen abdomen.

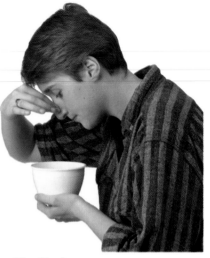

Nosebleeds
Lean forward, pinch your nostrils, and breath through your mouth. Seek medical help if the nose bleeds for over 20 minutes.

HOW TO CONTROL SEVERE BLEEDING

It is vital to know how to stop severe bleeding. Unless it is stopped it may cause the victim to go into shock, lose consciousness, and die.

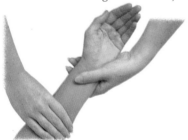

1 Raise the injured part above the level of the heart to reduce blood flow. Put pressure on the wound with your hand.

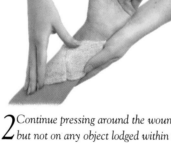

2 Continue pressing around the wound, but not on any object lodged within it. Pull the edges of a gaping wound together.

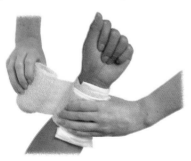

3 Cover with a clean bandage, tissue, or handkerchief, and maintain pressure. If blood seeps through, add more bandages over the existing ones.

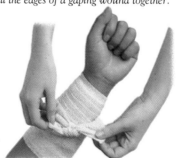

4 When the bleeding eventually stops, tie a clean bandage over the bandages that are already in place, knotting it directly over the wound.

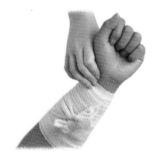

5 Finally, check that the arterial blood supply has not been cut off by the bandage. Feel for a pulse both above and below the wound.

WHEN TO SEEK HELP

You should seek medical help if:

• The wound is more than ½ in (1 cm) deep, gaping, or on the face.
• The bleeding does not stop.
• There is an object, such as grit or glass, stuck firmly in the wound.
• A dirty object caused the injury.
• The victim has not been immunized against tetanus.
• There are signs of infection such as fever, swelling, redness, or pain.

300

MINOR WOUNDS, CUTS, AND SCRAPES

Bleeding from minor wounds usually stops within a few minutes. If it does not, pressure can be applied to stop the bleeding. These injuries should be cleaned thoroughly to prevent infection or discoloration of the skin caused by grit or dirt remaining in the wound. If a cut is gaping it may need to be stitched.

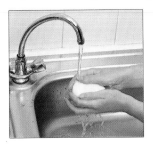

1 To reduce the risk of infection, wash your hands with soap and water before you treat or examine any wound.

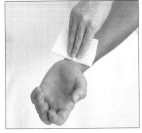

2 Using a clean, non-fluffy cloth, apply pressure directly over the wound until bleeding stops.

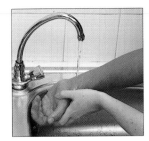

3 Wash the area with soap (or antiseptic solution) and running water. Remove any grit or dirt. Dry the wound.

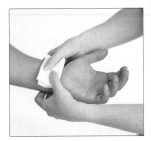

4 Cover the area with a sterile dressing or a clean bandage. Be sure to keep it free of dirt.

SPRAINS AND STRAINS

These injuries are caused by tearing or overstretching ligaments (sprains) or muscles (strains). Severe sprains are very painful and hard to distinguish from fractures. If in doubt about whether it is a sprain or a fracture, seek medical help. Both sprains and strains cause bruising.

Treating a sprain or strain
A combination of rest, ice, compression, and elevation (see p166) is usually the best treatment for soft tissue injuries, such as sprains, strains, or bruising.

BITES AND STINGS

Contamination can occur through animal saliva or snake or insect venom. In many countries, rabies is a threat in all animal bites and medical help must be sought quickly. Some people are hypersensitive to insect stings, suffering a severe reaction; this should be treated as shock (see p297). Bites from spiders, scorpions, snakes, and marine animals, such as jellyfish, need special treatment as venom may have been injected.

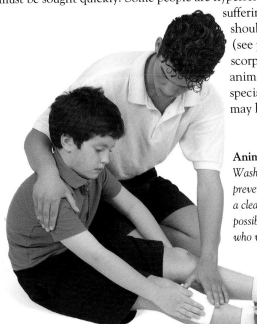

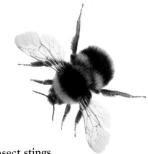

Insect stings
Scrape the sting away, but be sure not to squeeze the venom sac. Wash and apply an ice pack. Antihistamine or calamine lotion can reduce swelling.

Animal bites
Wash well with soap and water to prevent contamination. Cover with a clean bandage. If there is any possibility of rabies, see a doctor who will give antirabies vaccine.

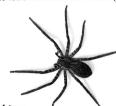

Spider bites
Keep the bitten area lower than the victim's heart and apply cold compresses. Get medical help immediately.

BURNS AND POISONING

Severe burns and all cases of poisoning require emergency medical attention.

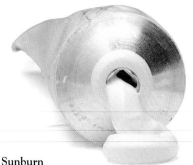

Sunburn

Treat mild sunburn as you would a minor burn, by cooling it with water. Calamine lotion may also be applied to soothe the skin. Stay out of the sun for a few days until the sunburn heals. Severe cases of sunburn should be seen by a doctor, who may prescribe a corticosteroid cream to relieve the symptoms.

B URNS CAN BE caused by dry heat, moist heat (scalds), electricity, friction, or corrosive chemicals.

The severity of a burn depends on its area and depth. The deepest burns leave a painless white or charred area. Burns that cover large areas of the body, particularly in a child, are always serious.

WARNING

- Do not put butter, oil, or grease on a burn.
- Do not use adhesive dressings.
- Do not use any fluffy material such as cotton wool.
- Do not prick blisters.

1 Do not touch the victim – you could receive a shock. Turn off the current or separate the victim from the power source with a dry, nonconducting object like a broom.

ELECTRIC SHOCK AND BURNS

Although an electric shock may have only caused a small burn, there may be serious internal damage. A severe shock can result in unconsciousness, stop the heart from beating, and cause breathing to cease.

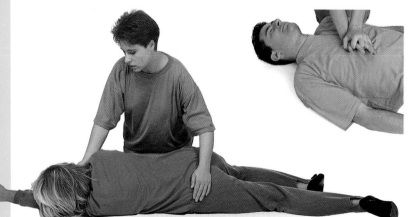

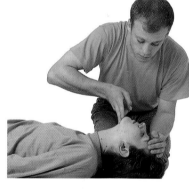

2 Check breathing and begin artificial respiration (see p299) if necessary.

3 Check the heartbeat after 5 breaths. Begin cardiopulmonary resuscitation (see p299) if there is no heartbeat.

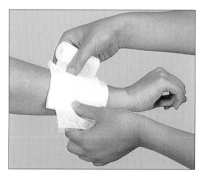

4 If the victim begins breathing place him or her in the recovery position.

5 Once the victim is breathing, treat any visible burns (see p303) and stay with the victim. Send for help.

TREATING BURNS

First-aid treatment for burns aims to remove the victim from danger, relieve pain, prevent infection, and prevent or treat shock. If the burn covers a large area or seems severe, get medical help immediately.

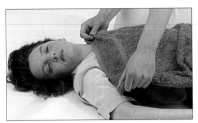

1 If the clothes are in flames, smother them with a blanket or roll the victim back and forth on the ground. Get help.

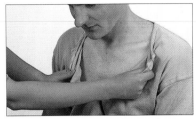

2 Remove wet clothing, but not dry, burned clothing that is stuck to the skin. Jewelry should be removed.

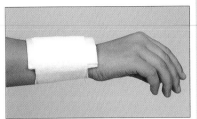

3 Apply a cold compress or immerse the area in cold running water. Cover the burn with a clean, wet, nonfluffy pad.

POISONING

Poisoning is always an emergency. Call your local poison control center. No matter how well the victim might feel, as there may be delayed complications. Never leave the victim alone. If he or she is conscious, try to find out what type of poison has been taken: it could save his or her life.

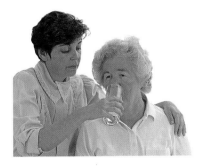

Noncorrosives
Conscious victims should drink eight ounces of water or milk. Stick your fingers down the throat to induce vomiting. Keep the victim face down.

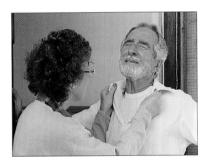

Poisonous gas
If poisonous gas has been inhaled, take the victim outside. Loosen any tight clothing around the neck to help the victim to breathe.

Poisonous plants
Certain plants such as toadstools, some berries and leaves, laburnum seeds, and foxgloves, are poisonous if eaten. Treat as for other types of poisoning. When abroad you may also encounter plants that cause an allergic reaction if they touch the skin. Wash well with soap and water, rub with alcohol, and apply calamine lotion.

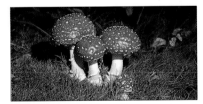

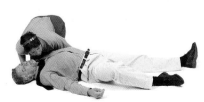

Unconscious victim
If the victim is drowsy or unconscious, do not induce vomiting or give liquids. Place him or her in the recovery position. If breathing or heartbeat stops, use artificial respiration (see p299) or CPR (see p299).

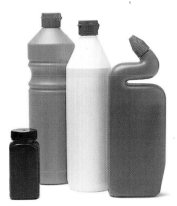

Corrosives
If a corrosive substance, such as bleach, has been swallowed, wash the mouth. Do not give drinks or induce vomiting. If artificial respiration is necessary use the mouth-to-nose method (see p299).

303

CARING FOR THE SICK

BASIC PATIENT CARE

- Establish a daily routine.
- Encourage the patient to do as much as possible for him or herself.
- Brush teeth and hair twice daily.
- Wash hair and cut nails regularly.
- Use a warm, moistened face cloth to gently wipe the corners of the eyes.
- Humidify the air by placing a bowl of water in the room.
- Use a back rest or triangular pillow to make sitting up more comfortable.
- Ask for a demonstration of the right techniques for lifting or giving a bedpan or bed bath from the nurse.
- Do not let visitors tire the patient.
- During vomiting, support the forehead with one hand and hold a bowl with the other. Sponge the face and give a mouth rinse afterwards.

Taking an adult's temperature
Holding the thermometer at the opposite end from the bulb, shake it until the mercury drops well below the normal mark. A normal reading is 98.6°F (37°C). Put the thermometer under the tongue. Leave for three minutes, then read it. Clean the bulb with antiseptic before putting the thermometer away.

The keys to a speedy recovery are relaxation, rest, and rehabilitation.

RELAXATION PREVENTS stress from hindering recovery. Rest helps the body's immune system to fight off invading cells, and its natural healing processes to repair damaged tissues. Rehabilitation gently introduces physical activities, sometimes using specific exercises to restore normal function, before the patient returns to everyday life.

Food and fluids
With a few exceptions, such as avoiding fried and fatty foods, most people who are ill should try to eat the same types of food as normal.

CHILDREN AND ILLNESS

If your child is feverish, try to bring the fever down with acetaminophen (see the label for the recommended dose). Bathe your child with tepid water and dress in thin cotton clothes. Cover with just a thin sheet. Wrapping a child in warm blankets will only raise his or her fever.

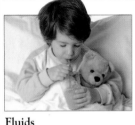

Fluids
Encourage a feverish child to drink plenty of liquid.

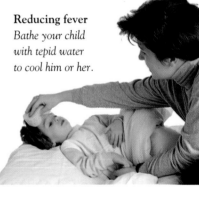

Reducing fever
Bathe your child with tepid water to cool him or her.

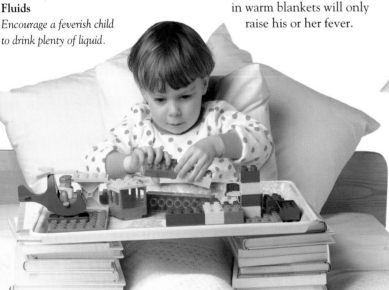

Play
During recovery, give your child jigsaw puzzles, crayons, or other toys to play with. Watching TV may also keep them amused.

A CHILD'S TEMPERATURE
A child can bite and break a glass thermometer so tuck it under the armpit or use a temperature strip on the forehead.

A balanced, varied diet promotes recovery from most illnesses. A special diet is only necessary if recommended by a doctor or in cases of diarrhea and vomiting.

During a bout of diarrhea and vomiting, water or fruit juice are the best drinks. Rehydration solutions, containing salt and sugar, are available from the druggist and may also be helpful. The first foods should be bland and low in protein. For fevers, drinking more fluids than usual replaces the water lost by increased sweating.

The bedridden patient

Being confined to bed tends to reduce appetite. For a few days this is not a problem, but during a long-term illness, a food supplement may be needed to preserve health.

For someone confined to bed, a bedside table stocked with drinks, tissues, reading materials, and a bell to call for assistance is useful. A bed tray is convenient both for serving meals and providing a firm surface for games, puzzles, or cards.

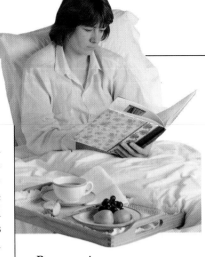

Room service
Most patients can feed themselves, if the meal is brought in on a tray. To coax a small appetite, be sure that the food looks and smells good.

Common sites of bedsores

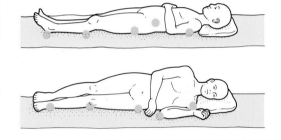

LONG-TERM ILLNESSES

Recovering from illness, injury, or surgery can cause boredom, discomfort, and embarrassment for the patient. Try to make the patient feel more comfortable and less vulnerable.

Since a high morale speeds recovery, try to create an atmosphere of calm and cheerfulness. The sickroom should be well lit, warm, quiet, uncluttered, well ventilated, and close to the bathroom. The bed should be comfortable and accessible from both sides.

Bed sores
occur when the body's weight cuts off the blood supply to areas of the skin in contact with the bed. Bedridden people must therefore be moved regularly.

THE ROAD TO RECOVERY

If you are caring for someone who has been ill, injured, or operated on, ask your doctor for clear guidelines on how best to monitor his or her progress. The following questions will help you give them the best possible care.

- How soon can the patient be allowed out of bed?
- Is there anything in particular that the patient must not do?
- When can the patient start walking again?
- Are there any symptoms or complications to look out for?
- When can the patient resume normal activities, such as driving and working?
- Is physiotherapy necessary?

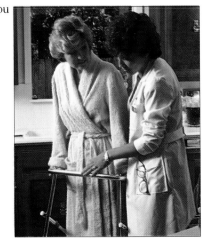

CARING FOR YOURSELF

When caring for someone else, do not neglect yourself.

- Take time off to relax and have fun; do not feel guilty about it.
- Ask for outside help, if needed.
- Make sure that you are receiving all the benefits you are entitled to.
- Look for a local self-help group if the person you are caring for has a specific medical disorder. The group can provide information and support.
- Get away. Your doctor may be able to refer you to facilities that can look after the person you are caring for, allowing you to take a break.

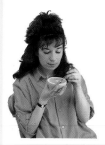

NUTRITION

Nutrition guidelines can help you check that you are eating the right foods in the right amounts.

WHAT YOU EAT influences how healthy you are. A balanced diet, rich in vitamins, minerals, and other nutrients can prevent deficiency diseases like scurvy as well as maintaining good health.

What is a balanced diet?

Scientists have identified a range of nutrients that must be present in the diet. The amounts that should be taken each day are called RDAs (Recommended Daily Amounts), RNIs (Reference Nutrient Intakes), and other terms.

These figures are only an average. If everyone took in the recommended amount of nutrients, most people would be well-nourished. Also, although these figures are given per day, you need not eat every nutrient, every day – you can achieve your intake of nutrients over a seven-day period.

But there are special circumstances, such as if you are ill or pregnant, which may increase the body's need for certain nutrients. A few people may not even need the recommended amount of nutrients.

So, when using these tables, you need not try to eat exactly what is recommended; eating roughly the right amount is good enough.

Are you eating too much fat and sugar?

In the West, most people eat too much refined sugar (added to tea, coffee, cakes, and biscuits) and fat (such as butter). This overconsumption causes tooth decay, heart disease, and other health problems. Nutritionists therefore recommend cutting down on sugar and fat.

Fiber
Most people in the US eat about 12 grams of fiber a day, half as much as is recommended. Fiber-rich foods include whole grain products, beans, and peas (see p41).

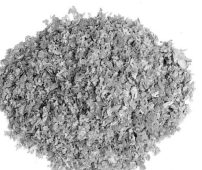

Sugar (simple carbohydrates)
Too much sugar can cause tooth decay, yet most people in the US get about 13 percent of their daily calories from sugar, instead of the recommended 10 percent. That is a difference of three teaspoons of sugar a day.

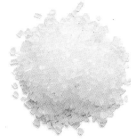

Starches (complex carbohydrates)
Starch should make up the major part of your diet (about 55 percent). Good sources of starch include potatoes, pasta, and bread, which provide energy and nutrients.

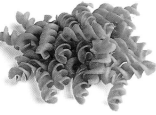

Salt
Nutritionists recommend that you eat about 4 grams of salt a day, yet most people in the US eat more than 8 grams a day. Studies suggest that salt may raise blood pressure, which in turn may increase your risk of developing coronary heart disease.

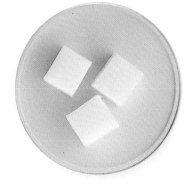

Fat
The western diet contains far too much fat for the good of your heart and health. Reduce the amount of saturated fat you eat and cut the total amount of fat you eat down to 30 percent of your daily calorie intake.

REFERENCE NUTRIENT INTAKE OF VITAMINS

(mg – milligram, µg – microgram, 1,000 µg = 1mg)

VITAMIN	INTAKE PER DAY (19 – 50 YEARS OF AGE)	EXAMPLES OF FOODS THAT CONTAIN THE VITAMIN
Vitamin A	700 µg (men) 600 µg (women)	Liver, fish-liver oils, egg yolk, and yellow-orange colored fruit and vegetables.
Vitamin B1 (Thiamine)	1.0 mg (men) 0.8 mg (women)	Whole grains (whole wheat bread and pasta), brown rice, liver, beans, peas, and eggs.
Vitamin B2 (Riboflavin)	1.3 mg (men) 1.1 mg (women)	Milk, liver, cheese, eggs, green vegetables, brewer's yeast, whole grains, and wheat germ.
Niacin	17 mg (men) 13 mg (women)	Liver, lean meats, poultry, fish, nuts, and dried beans.
Vitamin B6 (Pyridoxine)	1.4 mg (men) 1.2 mg (women)	Liver, poultry, pork, fish, bananas, potatoes, dried beans, and most other fruit and vegetables.
Vitamin B12	1.5 µg	Liver, pork, fish, yeast, eggs, and dairy products.
Folic acid	200 µg	Green leafy vegetables, nuts, and liver.
Vitamin C	40 mg	Citrus fruit, strawberries, and potatoes.
Vitamin D	No recommendation.	Oily fish (such as salmon), liver, eggs, cod-liver oil, and some cereals.
Vitamin E	No recommendation.	Margarine, whole grain cereals, and nuts.

REFERENCE NUTRIENT INTAKE OF MINERALS

MINERAL	INTAKE PER DAY (19 – 50 YEARS OF AGE)	EXAMPLES OF FOODS THAT CONTAIN THE MINERAL
Calcium	700 mg	Dairy products, green leafy vegetables, and beans.
Iodine	140 µg	Salt water fish and shellfish.
Iron	8.7 mg (men) 14.8 mg (women)	Meats, fish, liver, egg yolks, bread, some green leafy vegetables, cereals, nuts, and beans.
Magnesium	300 mg (men) 270 mg (women)	Nuts, soy beans, milk, fish, green vegetables, whole grain cereals, and hard water.
Potassium	3500 µg	Bread and whole grain cereals, beans, and bananas.
Selenium	75 µg (men) 60 µg (women)	Meat, fish, shellfish, whole grain cereals, and dairy products.
Zinc	9.5 mg (men) 7.0 mg (women)	Lean meats, fish, shellfish, beans, eggs, nuts, whole grain cereals, and whole wheat bread.
Sodium	1,600 mg	Processed foods, smoked meat, and table salt.
Fluoride	No recommendation.	Fish, soy beans, and drinking water in many areas.
Copper	1.2 mg	Liver, shellfish, peas, nuts, and dried beans.

IMMUNIZATION

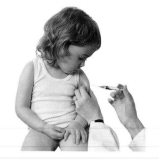

Immunization protects against infectious diseases.

TRAVEL IMMUNIZATION

Ask your doctor, pharmacist, or travel agent for a list of all the immunizations that are needed for the countries you plan to visit. Some vaccines must be given two months before you travel, so make sure you are immunized in plenty of time.

SINCE THE INTRODUCTION of an immunization program, the incidence of serious infectious illnesses has declined dramatically. Because smallpox has been eradicated, this vaccination is no longer needed. However, if immunization against the diseases listed in the table below was to stop, it is highly likely that epidemics would occur.

How does vaccination work?

Active immunization involves introducing a toxin or an infectious organism, which has been altered or killed, into the body. This stimulates the immune defenses in the same way as a genuine infection. By tricking the body into producing antibodies against this infection, the immune system is then ready to deal rapidly and efficiently with any subsequent exposure.

Passive immunization involves being injected with ready-made antibodies against the infection. This type of immunity provides immediate protection, but is only short-lived as the body kills antibodies it does not recognize as its own.

Are there any after-effects?

There are usually no side effects. To be safe, children are kept at the surgery or clinic for 10 minutes after the injection in case there is an immediate allergic reaction. This, however, is very rare.

Children may cry more than usual, become irritable, or refuse to eat after immunization. If they are not better within a few days they should be taken to the doctor. If children vomit within 30 minutes of swallowing the polio vaccine they need to be immunized again.

CHILDHOOD IMMUNIZATION SCHEDULE

To give your child the best possible protection early in life, he or she should be immunized against preventable infectious disease. The age at which your child will be given these vaccines will vary from clinic to clinic but will be approximately at the ages shown in the table below:

AGE	INJECTION	ORAL
2 months	Diphtheria, whooping cough, and tetanus.	Poliomyelitis
3 months	Diphtheria, whooping cough, and tetanus.	Poliomyelitis
4 months	Diphtheria, whooping cough, and tetanus.	Poliomyelitis
15 months	Measles, mumps, rubella (German measles)	
4 – 5 years	Diphtheria and tetanus booster.	Polio booster
5 – 6 years	Mantoux skin test (TB)	
10 – 14 years	Rubella (if missed earlier)	
15 – 19 years	Tetanus booster	Polio booster

REACTIONS TO VACCINES

Adverse reactions are extremely rare. There is a much greater risk of serious illness, handicap, or death from an infection such as measles, than from the vaccine. However, you should seek immediate medical help if your child starts to scream or cry continuously, becomes drowsy or restless, vomits several times, develops a swollen face or lips, suffers from a seizure, or has breathing difficulties after being vaccinated.

FAMILY HEALTH RECORD

Every illness you have, every immunization you are given, and every medication you take, form a part of your health record. By photocopying this page and filling it in for each member of your family, you can monitor when your child should be immunized and help your doctor diagnose your family's disorders.

Name _____ Date of birth _____

Name and telephone number of doctor(s) _____

Blood type _____ Allergies _____

IMMUNIZATIONS

Diphtheria, tetanus, and whooping cough		Poliomyelitis		Measles, mumps, and rubella		Other immunizations	
Age usually administered	Date of vaccine	Age usually administered	Date of vaccine	Age usually administered	Date of vaccine	Type	Date of vaccine
2 months		2 months		15 months			
3 months		3 months		10 – 14 years (rubella –if missed earlier)			
4 months		4 months					
4 – 5 years (diphtheria and tetanus booster)		4 – 5 years (booster)		Mantoux skin test (TB)			
				Age usually administered	Date of vaccine		
15 – 19 years (tetanus booster)		15 – 19 (booster)		5 – 6 years			

MAJOR ILLNESSES/SURGERY

	Date	Treatment/outcome

MEDICATIONS

	Date started	Date stopped

CHECKUPS/TESTS

	Date/result	Date/result	Date/result
Blood pressure			
Blood cholesterol			
Dental examination			
Cervical smear			
Mammogram			
Eye examination			

GLOSSARY

A

Abdomen
The area of the body between the hips and chest, below the ribs. It contains the stomach and other organs, such as the liver, kidneys, and intestines.

Abscess
A build-up of pus, for example at the root of a tooth, which results in pain as it swells.

Absorption
The process whereby nutrients pass from the digestive tract into the bloodstream.

Additive
A substance added to food to preserve, color, or flavor it.

Aerobic
The use of oxygen to generate energy and growth. The term is applied both to certain bacteria and to human muscles during sustained exercise.

Amino acids
Chemical units made up of nitrogen, carbon, and oxygen, that make proteins. There are 20 different amino acids in human proteins, but a single protein molecule may contain thousands of amino acid units.

Amniocentesis
Removal of a small amount of fluid from the womb of a pregnant woman so that tests may be carried out to detect abnormalities in the fetus.

Anerobic
Able to function without oxygen. Certain bacteria are anerobic, while some muscle cells in the body can work anerobically for a short time.

Antibiotic
A substance (such as penicillin) extracted from a mold, or other living structure, that kills bacteria.

Antibody
A protein made by the body to combat invading micro-organisms and other threats to health, such as cancer.

Artery
A blood vessel with muscular walls. The arteries carry oxygenated blood from the heart to the rest of the body.

Arthritis
Painful swelling and stiffness of the joints that may sometimes cause deformity.

B

Bacteria
Microorganisms which are found in air, soil, and water. Some can cause disease in humans and animals. Other bacteria, such as those that live in the intestine and help digest food, are useful.

Benzodiazepine
A group of tranquilizing drugs widely used to treat anxiety, stress, and insomnia.

Beta-blocker
A type of drug prescribed to slow down the heart rate. Used to treat heart conditions, raised blood pressure, and the symptoms of anxiety.

Bile
Greenish-brown liquid formed in the liver from broken down blood cells and other waste. It is stored in the gall bladder and helps the digestion of fats.

Biopsy
Test in which a few cells or small pieces of tissue are taken from the body and examined in order to diagnose cancer and other illnesses.

Blood pressure
The pressure of the blood as it is pumped through the body's main arteries. Blood pressure rises and falls depending on the body's activity level.

Bone
The hard, strong material containing calcium that forms the body's skeleton.

Bone marrow
The soft tissue that lies inside some areas of bone, where red blood cells are made.

Bowel
The name for the small and large intestine. It runs from the stomach to the anus and forms part of the digestive system.

C

Caffeine
A naturally occurring drug that acts as a stimulant. It is present in tea, coffee, and cola.

Calorie
A unit used to measure the energy content of foods.

Cancer
A condition in which some of the body's cells grow too fast and spread to other parts of the body, causing tumors in organs and leading, if unchecked, to serious illness and death. Cancer is caused both by genetic and environmental factors.

Capillary
A tiny tube with thin walls that carries blood between small arteries and veins, allowing oxygen and nutrients out to the tissues and collecting waste products.

Carbohydrate
A compound of carbon, oxygen, and hydrogen. Carbohydrate foods such as starch and sugar provide the body with energy.

Carbon dioxide
A gas formed from carbon and oxygen which is a by-product of metabolism in humans and animals.

Carcinogen
A substance or agent that causes cancer, such as radiation, tobacco smoke, or asbestos fibers.

Cardiopulmonary resuscitation (CPR)
A technique that attempts to restart breathing and heartbeat by using both mouth-to-mouth resuscitation (blowing into the mouth) and cardiac compression (rhythmically pressing on the chest).

Cardiovascular
Concerning the heart and its circuit of blood vessels.

Cartilage
Strong, elastic tissue that lines and protects the ends of bones inside joints.

Cell
The smallest unit of the human body, which is made up of billions of cells. Each cell has a nucleus and a surrounding membrane.

Central nervous system (CNS)
The brain and spinal cord make up the CNS.

Cervix
The lower end of the uterus, which has a small passage running through its center. During childbirth, the cervix opens gradually to allow the baby to be born.

Chemotherapy
A medical treatment in which drugs are used selectively to kill cancer cells in the body.

Chlorofluorocarbons (CFCs)
Chemicals used in aerosol sprays and a variety of electrical appliances, such as refrigerators, which are known to destroy the Earth's protective layer of ozone.

Cholesterol
A chemical found in certain foods, such as eggs, and produced in the liver from saturated fat. High levels of cholesterol in the blood increase the risk of heart disease, but some cholesterol is essential for life.

Chorionic villus sampling
A test performed early in pregnancy in which a sample of tissue is taken from the placenta to see whether the baby has any abnormalities.

Chromosome
A structure within the nucleus of a cell that carries genes, the instruction codes that determine inherited characteristics.

Cirrhosis
A liver disease in which cells are severely damaged and scarred; it is often caused by heavy alcohol consumption.

Colitis
An inflammation of the colon that causes severe bloody diarrhea and sometimes stomach pains and fever.

Collagen
A protein in the body that holds cells and tissues together and forms an important part of bones, cartilage, and skin.

Coronary
The two arteries that supply blood to the heart. The term is commonly used to describe a heart attack.

Corticosteroid
A group of hormones released by the adrenal gland. Synthetic versions are used to treat a wide variety of conditions including asthma and arthritis.

D

Dementia
A progressive deterioration of the brain, mostly affecting elderly people. Symptoms may include loss of memory, confusion, paranoia, depression, and delusions.

Diabetes mellitus
A condition in which the lack of the hormone insulin makes the body unable to use the energy from carbohydrates. The condition causes sugar to be lost in the urine.

Digestion
The extraction of nutrients from food so that they may be absorbed from the intestines into the body.

Diuretic
A type of drug used to increase the amount of water excreted from the body.

DNA
Molecules that carry genetic information on chromosomes.

E

Emphysema
A chronic lung disease in which loss of elastic tissue makes the lungs less efficient.

Enzyme
Any protein substance in the body that stimulates chemical activities, such as in digestion, without being changed itself.

Epidemic
An outbreak of a disease that spreads quickly.

Esophagus
A muscular tube that takes food from the mouth to the stomach.

Estrogen
One of several female hormones, produced mainly by the ovaries, which are responsible for the healthy functioning of the female reproductive system.

F

Fecal occult blood
A simple test that determines whether or not there is blood in the feces.

Fetus
The name given to the human embryo from the eighth week of pregnancy until birth.

Fiber
The indigestible part of fruit, vegetables, and cereals, also called roughage. It aids normal bowel function.

Fitness
Being in good physical health so that daily activities can be performed with ease.

Fluoride
A mineral that strengthens tooth enamel, helping to prevent dental decay.

G

Gastritis
Inflammation of the stomach lining.

Gene
A unit of DNA within a chromosome. The 100,000 human genes determine our inherited characteristics.

Glaucoma
A disease of the eye caused by raised pressure within the eyeball. Glaucoma can progress to blindness if not treated.

Glucose
Released from the digestion of starch and sucrose, this sugar is the body's main energy source.

H

Hamstring
One of a group of muscles at the back of the thigh that help bend the knee.

Heart attack
A sudden failure of the blood supply to the heart muscle.

Heart massage
A method of resuscitating the victim of a heart attack by pressing on the chest to restart the heart.

Hemoglobin
A protein that gives red blood cells their color and allows them to carry oxygen to tissues.

Hernia
The bulging of the intestine through a weak part of the abdominal wall.

Hormone
A chemical that circulates in the bloodstream and helps control functions such as growth and sexual development.

Hormone replacement therapy (HRT)
A treatment that may be used to replace hormones in women who have had their ovaries removed surgically or who are going through menopause.

Hyperactive
Abnormally active, usually refers to children with behavioral problems.

Hypoglycemia
An unusually low level of sugar in the blood, causing dizziness and sweating.

Hypothalamus
A gland at the base of the brain, which indirectly controls hunger, thirst, and many other functions.

Hypothermia
A dangerously low body temperature. The elderly and infants are more likely to suffer from this condition.

I

Immunity
The body's capacity to resist disease by producing antibodies that fight against it.

Inflammation
The reaction of the body's tissue to infection or injury, causing pain, swelling, redness, and increased heat in the area.

Insulin
A hormone produced by the pancreas depending on the level of sugar in the blood. Synthetic insulin is injected regularly by some diabetics.

J

Joint
The point where two or more bones meet, surrounded by a protective lining and connected by ligaments.

K

Kidneys
Two organs located in the abdomen on either side of the spine which filter waste products from the blood, excreting them as urine.

L

Lactic acid
A by-product of anerobic activity in the muscles, which causes pain and stiffness until it is carried off to the liver.

Laryngitis
Inflammation of the larynx, the part of the throat that holds the vocal cords.

Leukemia
A type of cancer in which white blood cells multiply and interfere with blood-forming processes in the bone marrow.

Life expectancy
Based on statistical evidence, this is the average age to which an individual may be expected to live.

Ligament
A band of strong, elastic tissue that connects and supports the joints within the body.

Liver
An organ in the abdomen that produces proteins for blood plasma, stores glucose, and regulates amino acid levels. Together with the kidneys, it clears the blood of waste.

Lymph
A body fluid containing white blood cells, proteins, and fats.

M

Malignant
Any disease or condition that develops rapidly and is potentially fatal.

Malnutrition
Ill-health due to lack of adequate food.

Mammogram
An x-ray of the breast, used to screen women for signs of breast cancer and to diagnose the disease.

Melanoma
A tumor on the skin, usually composed of darkly pigmented cells. It may be either malignant or benign (not harmful).

Membrane
A thin layer of tissue that covers, lines, or connects the body's organs or cells.

Metabolism
All the various chemical processes occurring in the body that result in growth, production of energy, and elimination of waste.

Molecule
The simplest chemical compound that can exist, in which two or more atoms are linked by a chemical bond.

Muscle
Bundles of specialized cells capable of contraction and relaxation to create movement. The three types of muscle are skeletal, smooth, and cardiac.

N

Nervous breakdown
Behavior that is thought to be part of a crisis of severe anxiety or tension. Often includes tearfulness, episodes of shouting and screaming, and social withdrawal.

Nutrient
The essential dietary factors – carbohydrates, fats, proteins, vitamins, and minerals.

O

Obesity
A condition of extreme overweight. An obese person is 20 percent or more over the maximum desirable weight for his or her height.

Organ
A collection of various tissues that work together to perform a specific function.

Osteoarthritis
Degeneration of a joint and its cartilage leading to pain, stiffness, and loss of function. The condition affects almost everyone over 60, women more severely than men.

Osteoporosis
A disorder in which loss of bone substance makes the bones brittle and more easily fractured.

Ozone
An atmospheric gas comprised of oxygen atoms. A layer of this gas surrounds and protects the Earth from the harmful effects of the sun's radiation.

P

Palpitations
The sensation of having a rapid and unusually forceful heartbeat, which may be felt after strenuous exercise, in tense situations, or after suffering from a severe fright or shock.

Peristalsis
A wave-like movement that results from rhythmic, involuntary contraction and relaxation of muscles in the walls of the digestive tract. These movements pass food and waste through the digestive system.

Physiotherapy
Physical treatments that are used to prevent or reduce joint stiffness and to restore muscle strength.

Plaque
A sticky coating on the teeth consisting of saliva, bacteria, and food debris. It is the chief cause of tooth decay. If allowed to accumulate, a hard deposit may be formed on the tooth.

Polyp
A growth that projects, usually on a stalk, from the lining of the nose, the cervix, the intestine, the larynx, or any other mucous membrane in the human body.

Processed food
Food which has been treated or converted by means of special processes, including the adding of substances for the purpose of preservation or to improve flavor or color.

Progesterone
One of several sex hormones produced in the ovaries. It is necessary for the healthy functioning of the female reproductive system.

Prostaglandin
One of a group of fatty acids that acts in a similar way to hormones. Synthetic prostaglandins are used as drugs.

Protein
A molecule consisting of hundreds or thousands of amino acids linked to form long chains. Proteins in the diet supply the body with amino acids.

Psychosomatic
A term describing physical disorders that have been caused or worsened by psychological factors.

Psychotherapy
The treatment of mental and emotional problems by psychological methods. The patient talks to a therapist and establishes a relationship that helps him or her deal with conflicts and difficulties.

Pulse
The rhythmic expansion and contraction of an artery as blood is forced through it, pumped by the heart.

R

Radiotherapy
Treatment of cancer and some other diseases by x-rays or other sources of radioactivity. The radiation passes through the diseased tissue, destroying or slowing down the development of abnormal cells.

Radon
A colorless, odorless, tasteless, radioactive gas produced by the radioactive decay of radium.

Refined foods
Foods that have been treated to remove "unwanted" ingredients, causing valuable substances like fiber to be lost.

Rehabilitation
Treatment aimed at enabling a person to live an independent life following injury, illness, alcohol or drug dependence.

Respiration
The movement of air in and out of the lungs. The term is also used to describe the use of oxygen by body cells to obtain energy.

Roughage
The indigestible parts of foods that contain cellulose and provide dietary fiber. This fiber adds bulk to the feces, helping the bowel to function better.

Rubella (German measles)
A viral infection that is minor in children but more serious for adults. When a woman in early pregnancy contracts rubella, serious birth defects may result.

S

Saccharide
A type of sugar.

Saturated fat
Fat containing fatty acids that have the maximum quantity of hydrogen atoms. Animal fats, found in meat and dairy products, are largely saturated and tend to increase the amount of unwanted types of cholesterol in the blood.

Secretion
The manufacture and release, by a cell, gland, or organ of chemical substances such as sweat or skin oils (sebum).

Seizure
A sudden episode of uncontrolled electrical activity in the brain, sometimes referred to as a fit. Epilepsy is a disorder in which there are recurrent seizures.

Shock
Physiological shock can cause a dangerous reduction of the flow of blood throughout body tissues. The condition may be caused by serious injury, loss of blood, or a heart attack, and can lead to collapse, coma, and death if not treated.

Side effect
A consequence of medication or therapy that is additional to the intended effect. It is usually undesirable.

Spasm
An involuntary and often powerful contraction that may affect one or more muscles.

Sphincter
A ring of muscle around a natural opening or passage that serves as a valve to regulate inflow or outflow.

Spleen
An organ in the upper left abdomen that helps to fight infection by producing antibodies. It also controls the quality of circulating red blood cells by removing those that are worn-out.

Sprain
Tearing of the ligaments that hold together a joint, due to a sudden pull or overstretching. It causes painful swelling.

Strain
The tearing or stretching of tendons or muscle fibers as a result of suddenly pulling them too far. Bleeding into the damaged area causes pain, swelling, spasm, and usually a bruise.

Stress
Mental or emotional tension leading to interference with a person's wellbeing. Long-term stress can damage health and produce symptoms such as depression, indigestion, insomnia, and muscular pains.

Stroke
Damage to part of the brain caused by an interruption to its blood supply or by blood leaking through the walls of its blood vessels. Strokes are a leading cause of death in the West. They are more common amongst older people, and affect men more than women.

Systole/diastole
Contractions of the heart (systoles) alternate with resting periods (diastoles). The blood pressure reaches its highest level at systole and then falls during the diastole. These points are measured when a blood pressure reading is taken.

T

Tendon
A strong, flexible, and fibrous cord that joins muscle to muscle or muscle to bone.

Testosterone
The most important of the male sex hormones, it is responsible for the healthy functioning of the male reproductive tract.

Therapy
The treatment of any disease or abnormal mental or physical condition.

Tinnitus
A whistling, ringing, or other noise in the ear. The condition is usually associated with some loss of hearing and can be caused by continuous exposure to loud noise.

Tissue
A collection of cells within an organism which are specialized to perform a particular function. Examples include muscle tissue and nerve tissue.

Toxic
Poisonous, harmful, or even deadly.

Tumor
An abnormal mass of tissue that forms when cells in a specific area reproduce at an increased rate. Tumors may be either benign (noninvading) or malignant (cancerous).

U

Ulcer
An open sore on the skin or on a mucous membrane that results from the destruction of surface tissue.

Ultrasound
Sound with a frequency greater than the human ear's upper limit of perception. Ultrasound waves passed through the skin and reflected back provide clear images of internal organs, or of a developing fetus, without the hazards of x-rays.

Ultraviolet radiation
Ultraviolet rays in sunlight cause tanning and produce vitamin D in skin – but harmful effects such as skin cancer may result from excess exposure.

Unsaturated fat
Fats that have the desirable effect of helping to decrease unwanted types of cholesterol in the blood. Most vegetable fats are unsaturated.

Uterus
The organ in which the fertilized egg normally becomes embedded and in which the baby develops before birth. It is also known as the womb.

V

Vaccine
A substance given to induce immunity against an infectious disease by sensitizing the body's immune system to a particular disease-causing bacterium, toxin, or virus.

Varicose veins
Visibly enlarged or twisted veins just beneath the skin.

Vein
A blood vessel that returns blood to the heart from the various organs and tissues of the body.

Virus
A submicroscopic infectious agent only one half to one hundredth the size of the smallest bacteria. Viruses cause disorders ranging from the common cold to rabies.

X

X-ray
Invisible electromagnetic energy that is produced when high-speed electrons strike a heavy metal. X-rays are used increasingly for medical diagnosis and treatment. The rays can produce images of bones, organs, and internal tissues, and can also be used to damage cancer cells.

INDEX

Index:
Susan Bosanko

Editorial assistance:
Nikki Carroll

Design assistance:
Desmond Plunkett

Illustrations:
Paul Bailey, Peter Ball,
Russel Barnet, Joanna Cameron,
Karen Cochrane, David Fathers,
Tony Graham, Andrew Green,
Kevin Marks, Coral Mula,
Gilly Newman, Lydia Umney,
John Woodcock

Photography:
Elizabeth Barrington
Steve Bartholomew
Steve Curd
Yaël Freudmann
Susanna Price
Tim Ridley
Clive Streeter

Airbrushing:
Roy Flooks, Imago,
Richard Manning, Janos Marffy

**The photograph on page 48 (bl)
was taken on the premises
of the Rock Garden Café,
Covent Garden, London**